ADVANCES IN

Surgery

Editor-in-Chief
John L. Cameron, MD

ELSEVIER

PHILADELPHIA LONDON TORONTO MONTREAL SYDNEY TOKYO

ADVANCES IN
Surgery

VOLUMES 1 THROUGH 56 (OUT OF PRINT)

VOLUME 57

12. Liver Transplantation for Colorectal Liver Metastases: Is It Appropriate?, *by Jenna N. Whitrock, Stephen J. Hartman, Ralph C. Quillin III, and Shimul A. Shah*

13. Transanal Total Mesorectal Excision for Rectal Cancer *by Sue J. Hahn, Ameer Farooq, and Patricia Sylla*

14. New Techniques for Intraoperative Parathyroid Localization , Colleen M. Kiernan and Carmen C. Solórzano

15. What Mesh Should be Used in Hernia Repair? *by Ansley Beth Ricker, Matthew N. Marturano, and Brent D. Matthews*

16. Prehospital Resuscitation: What Should It Be?, *by James E. Manning, Jonathan J. Morrison, and Paul E. Pepe*

17. What is the Role of Whole Blood Transfusions on Trauma Patients? *by John M. Porter and Joshua P. Hazelton*

18. Does Carotid Intervention Improve Cognitive Function?, *by Bahaa Succar and Wei Zhou*

19. Can Colorectal Surgery Be Performed as an Outpatient Surgery? *by Abier Abdelnaby and Analena Alcabes*

VOLUME 56

1. Failure to Rescue After the Whipple: What Do We Know? *by Elizabeth M. Gleeson and Henry A. Pitt*

2. Management of Necrotizing Pancreatitis *by Thomas K. Maatman and Nicholas J. Zyromski*

3. Should We Utilize Routine Cholangiography? *by L. Michael Brunt*

4. Reducing Firearm Injury and Death in the United States?, *by Joseph V. Sakran and Nicole Lunardi*

5. Reducing Complications After Surgery for Benign Anorectal Conditions?, *by Alton Sutter and Vitaliy Poylin*

6. Private Equity and Its Increasing Role in US Healthcare *by Kristen M. Beyer, Lyudmyla Demyan, and Matthew J. Weiss*

7. Facts and Fallacy of Benchmark Performance Indicators *by James P. Byrne and Elliott R. Haut*

8. Transcarotid Artery Revascularization: Is It Better than Carotid Endarterectomy?, *by Patric Liang and Marc L. Schermerhorn*

9. Endovascular Repair of Descending Thoracic Aortic Aneurysms *by Michol A. Cooper, Zain Shahid, and Gilbert R. Upchurch Jr.*

10. What Surgeons Need to Know About Gene Therapy for Cancer, *by Shanmugappiriya Sivarajah, Kevin Emerick, and Howard L. Kaufman*

11. Is There a Place for Hyperbaric Oxygen Therapy?, *by Kinjal N. Sethuraman, Ryan Smolin, and Sharon Henry*

12. Endoscopic Treatment of Gastroesophageal Reflux Disease, *by William S. Richardson, Jessica Koller Gorham, Nicole Neal, and Robert D. Fanelli*

13. Direct Peritoneal Resuscitation for Trauma *by Samuel J. Pera, Jessica Schucht, and Jason W. Smith*

14. What is the Best Inguinal Hernia Repair?, Jennwood Chen and Robert E. Glasgow

15. Do all Patients Get the Same Care Across Hospitals? *by Adrian Diaz and Timothy M. Pawlik*

16. What Is the Role of Neoadjuvant Endocrine Therapy for Breast Cancer?, *by Anna Weiss and Tari A. King*

17. What Is the Best Treatment for Acute Limb Ischemia? *by Elizabeth G. King and Alik Farber*

18. Endovascular Repair of Complex Aortic Aneurysms, *by Guilherme B.B. Lima, Marina Dias-Neto, Emanuel R. Tenorio, Aidin Baghbani-Oskouei, and Gustavo S. Oderich*

19. Is There a Role for Rib Plating in Thoracic Trauma? *by Chaitan K. Narsule and Anne C. Mosenthal*

Editor: John Vassallo (j.vassallo@elsevier.com)
Developmental Editor: Akshay Samson

Printed in the United States of America.

Editorial Office:
Elsevier
1600 John F. Kennedy Boulevard,
Suite 1800
Philadelphia, PA 19103-2899

International Standard Serial Number: 0065-3411
International Standard Book Number: 978-0-443-29308-5

ADVANCES IN
Surgery

CONTRIBUTORS

AHMED ABDELKARIM, MD, Research Scholar, Department of Surgery, Division of Vascular and Endovascular Surgery, UC San Diego, La Jolla, California, USA; Center for Learning and Excellence in Vascular & Endovascular Research (CLEVER), UC San Diego, San Diego, California, USA; Altman Center for Clinical and Translational Research, La Jolla, California, USA

CHARLOTTE ARIYAN, MD, PhD, Associate Attending, Department of Surgical Oncology, Memorial Sloan Kettering Cancer Center, New York, New York, USA

ANDREW BARNES, MD, Resident Physician, Department of General Surgery, Ochsner Medical Center, New Orleans, Louisiana, USA

MARYLISE BOUTROS, MD, FACS, FRCSC, Professor, Department of Surgery, McGill University, Montréal, Québec, Canada; Colorectal Surgeon and Research Director of the Digestive Diseases Institute, Department of Colorectal Surgery, Ellen Leifer Shulman and Steven Shulman Digestive Disease Institute, Cleveland Clinic Florida, Weston, Florida, USA

ERROL L. BUSH, MD, Surgical Director, Advanced Lung Disease and Lung Transplant Program, Division of Thoracic Surgery; Associate Professor, Department of Surgery, Johns Hopkins Medical Institutions, Baltimore, Maryland, USA

DYLAN CARROLL, MD, Fellow, Department of Surgery, University of Louisville, Louisville, Kentucky, USA

THOMAS W. CHENG, MD, Integrated Vascular Surgery Resident, PGY1, Division of Vascular and Endovascular Surgery, Dartmouth-Hitchcock Medical Center, Lebanon, New Hampshire, USA

SEAN CLEARY, MD, MSc, MPH, Professor of Surgery, Division of Hepatobiliary and Pancreas Surgery, University of Toronto, Toronto, Ontario, Canada

AMANDA M. DANN, MD, Assistant Professor, Division of Surgical Oncology, Department of Surgery, University of Texas Southwestern, Dallas, Texas, USA

ADRIAN DIAZ, MD, MPH, Resident, Division of Surgical Oncology, Department of Surgery, The Ohio State University Wexner Medical Center, James Comprehensive Cancer Center, Columbus, Ohio, USA

DEAN M. DONAHUE, MD, Director, Thoracic Outlet Syndrome Program, Division of Thoracic Surgery, Department of Surgery, Massachusetts General Hospital, Director, Thoracic Outlet Syndrome Program, Boston, Massachusetts, USA

PHILIP A. EFRON, MD, Professor, Department of Surgery, University of Florida College of Medicine, Gainesville, Florida, USA

ALIK FARBER, MD, MBA, FACS, DFSVS, Interim Chief, Department of Surgery, Associate Chief Medical Officer for Surgical Services, Chief, Division of Vascular and Endovascular Surgery, Boston Medical Center, Interim Chair, Department of Surgery, Professor of Surgery and Radiology, Boston University Chobanian and Avedisian School of Medicine, Boston, Massachusetts, USA

SHELDON FELDMAN, MD, Professor, Department of Surgery, Division of Breast Surgery, Montefiore Breast Cancer Center, Montefiore Medical Center, Bronx, New York, USA

CARLOS FERNÁNDEZ-DEL CASTILLO, MD, Professor of Surgery, Clinical Co-director, GI Cancer Center, Director, Pancreas and Biliary Surgery Program, Department of Surgery, Massachusetts General Hospital, Harvard Medical School, Boston, Massachusetts, USA

ANDREW M. FLEMING, MD, Resident Physician, Department of Surgery, The University of Tennessee Health Science Center, Memphis, Tennessee, USA

LEONARDO E. GARCIA, MD, Surgery Resident, General Surgery, Division of Colorectal Surgery, Department of Surgery, Johns Hopkins School of Medicine, Baltimore, Maryland, USA

RICHARD GARFINKLE, MD, MSc, PhD, Fellow, Division of Mayo Clinic Colon and Rectal Surgery, Rochester, Minnesota, USA; Division of Colon and Rectal Surgery, Jewish General Hospital, Montréal, Québec, Canada

SUSAN L. GEARHART, MD, MEd, Associate Professor, Division of Colorectal Surgery, Department of Surgery, Johns Hopkins School of Medicine, Baltimore, Maryland, USA

DAVID G. GREENHALGH, MD, FACS, Chief of Burns, Burn Department, Shriners Children's Northern California, Sacramento, California, USA; Professor, Emeritus, Department of Surgery, University of California, Davis, California, USA

JONATHAN B. GREER, MD, Assistant Professor of Surgery and Oncology, Division of Gastrointestinal Surgical Oncology; Director, Peritoneal Surface Malignancy Program, Johns Hopkins University School of Medicine, Baltimore, Maryland, USA

HALLBERA GUDMUNDSDOTTIR, MD, Fellow, Division of Hepatobiliary and Pancreas Surgery, Mayo Clinic, Rochester, Minnesota, USA

JOSEPH R. HABIB, MD, Surgery Resident, Department of Surgery, New York University Langone Health, New York, New York, USA

MOHAMMED HAMOUDA, MD, Research Scholar, Department of Surgery, Division of Vascular and Endovascular Surgery, UC San Diego, La Jolla, California, USA; Center for Learning and Excellence in Vascular & Endovascular Research (CLEVER), UC San Diego, San Diego, California, USA; Altman Center for Clinical and Translational Research, La Jolla, California, USA

JOHN W. HARMON, MD, FACS, Professor, Department of Surgery, Johns Hopkins University, Baltimore, Maryland, USA

LISA JACOBS, MD, MSPH, Associate Professor of Surgery, Johns Hopkins University, Baltimore, Maryland, USA

AMMAR A. JAVED, MD, Assistant Professor, Department of Surgery, New York University Langone Health, New York, New York, USA

SANDY KAVALUKAS, MS, MD, FACS, Assistant Professor, Colorectal Surgery, Department of Surgery, University of Louisville, Louisville, Kentucky, USA

JESSICA KOLLER GORHAM, MD, FASC, ABOM, Program Director, Department of General Surgery, Ochsner Medical Center, New Orleans, Louisiana, USA

LIZA LAQUIAN, MD, Assistant Professor, Department of Surgery, University of Florida College of Medicine, Gainesville, Florida, USA

MAHMOUD B. MALAS, MD, MHS, RPVI, FACS, Professor and Chief, Department of Surgery, Division of Vascular and Endovascular Surgery, UC San Diego, La Jolla, California, USA; Center for Learning and Excellence in Vascular & Endovascular Research (CLEVER), UC San Diego, San Diego, California, USA; Altman Center for Clinical and Translational Research, La Jolla, California, USA

MAUREEN P. McEVOY, MD, Assistant Professor, Department of Surgery, Division of Breast Surgery, Montefiore Medical Center, Montefiore Breast Care Center, Bronx, New York, USA

BARAAH M.A. MOHAMED, MD, General Surgery Resident, York WellSpan Health, York, Pennsylvania, USA

FARZAD MOKHTARI-ESBUIE, MD, Postdoctoral Research Fellow, Department of Surgery, Johns Hopkins University, Baltimore, Maryland, USA

HALA MUADDI, MD, MSc, PhD, Surgeon, Division of Hepatobiliary and Pancreas Surgery, Mayo Clinic, Rochester, Minnesota, USA

NIKHIL PANDA, MD, MPH, Resident, Division of Thoracic Surgery, Department of Surgery, Massachusetts General Hospital, Boston, Massachusetts, USA

TIMOTHY M. PAWLIK, MD, PhD, MPH, MTS, MBA, Professor and Chair, Division of Surgical Oncology, Department of Surgery, The Ohio State University Wexner Medical Center, James Comprehensive Cancer Center, Columbus, Ohio, USA

JESSICA M. RUCK, MD, PhD, General Surgery Resident, Division of Thoracic Surgery, Department of Surgery, Johns Hopkins University School of Medicine, Baltimore, Maryland, USA

NILOUFAR SHABABI, MD, Postdoctoral Research Fellow, Department of Surgery, Johns Hopkins University, Baltimore, Maryland, USA

REENA S. SURESH, MBChB, Colorectal Research Fellow, General Surgery, Division of Colorectal Surgery, Department of Surgery, Johns Hopkins School of Medicine, Baltimore, Maryland, USA

LI TING TIAN, MBBS, General Surgery Resident, Department of Surgery, The Johns Hopkins Hospital, Baltimore, Maryland, USA

JONAH D. THOMAS, MD, MS, General Surgery Resident, Department of Surgery, Massachusetts General Hospital, Harvard Medical School, Boston, Massachusetts, USA

BRIAN VISCOMI, MD, Resident, Department of General Surgery, Ochsner Medical Center, New Orleans, Louisiana, USA

NOLAN M. WINICKI, MS, Student, Department of Surgery, Johns Hopkins University School of Medicine, Baltimore, Maryland, USA

CHRISTOPHER L. WOLFGANG, MD, PhD, Professor, Chief of Hepatobiliary and Pancreatic Surgery, Department of Surgery, New York University Langone Health, New York, USA

ELIZABETH H. WOOD, MD, Assistant Professor, Department of Surgery, The University of Tennessee Health Science Center, Memphis, Tennessee, USA

ADVANCES IN
Surgery

CONTENTS

VOLUME 58 • 2024

these patients may further be complicated by the need for chronic immunosuppression. The underlying principles continue to include optimization of nutritional status, and preservation of bowel length when possible. However, there have been several recent advances in both the medical and surgical management of the disease. Understanding the contribution of the mesentery to inflammation, new surgical techniques such as the Kono-S anastomosis and extended mesenteric resection is decreasing the need for repeated resections.

Poverty and Its Impact on Surgical Care **35**

Adrian Diaz and Timothy M. Pawlik

In this article, the authors explore the intricate relationship between poverty and surgical care, underscoring its multifaceted nature and its profound impact on access and outcomes. Poverty extends beyond financial constraints to encompass barriers related to healthcare infrastructure, geographic isolation, education, mental health, and social determinants of health, resulting in persistent disparities in access to high-quality surgical care, especially for those in persistently impoverished areas and access-sensitive surgical conditions. Additionally, the authors delve into the complex intersection of poverty, race, and ethnicity, emphasizing the heightened risks faced by minority patients in surgical care.

Is Hyperthermic Intraperitoneal Chemotherapy Appropriate for Colon Cancer? **49**

Nolan M. Winicki and Jonathan B. Greer

Colorectal cancer (CRC) with peritoneal metastases is a complex disease and its management presents significant clinical challenges. In well-selected patients at experienced centers, CRS/hyperthermic intraperitoneal chemotherapy (HIPEC) can be performed with acceptable morbidity and is associated with prolonged survival. Based on the results of recent randomized controlled trials, HIPEC using oxaliplatin after CRS with shortened perfusion periods (30 minutes) is no longer recommended. There is a movement toward utilizing mitomycin C as a first-line intraperitoneal agent with extended perfusion times (90–120 minutes); however, there is currently little prospective evidence to support its widespread use.

Breast cancer related lymphedema (BCRL) affects many breast cancer survivors and drastically affects their quality of life. There are several surveillance methods for BCRL that are critical at early detection. Prevention of BCRL involves knowledge of alternatives to aggressive axillary surgery, avoidance of axillary surgery, and de-escalation of axillary surgery. There are also techniques to better delineate the anatomy in the axilla to avoid taking nodes that drain the upper extremity. A multidisciplinary approach with medical oncology and radiation oncology can also help avoid unnecessary surgery or radiation that can together strongly increase the risk of BCRL.

Pancreatoduodenectomy is a complex surgical procedure with a high rate of morbidity, of which surgical-site infections (SSIs) make a large portion. Reduction of SSI rates is critical to decrease hospital lengths of stay, readmissions, delays in adjuvant therapies, and financial health care burden. Current clinical guidelines recommend the administration of cefoxitin as surgical prophylaxis prior to pancreatoduodenectomy. In April 2023, a randomized controlled trial was published in *JAMA* which showed that piperacillin-tazobactam as perioperative surgical prophylaxis prior to pancreatoduodenectomy decreased 30 day SSI rates (primary outcome), clinically relevant postoperative pancreatic fistula, postoperative sepsis, and *Clostridium difficile* infection rates.

Current Management of Diverticulitis 87

Richard Garfinkle and Marylise Boutros

Over the last few decades, our understanding of the pathophysiology and natural history of sigmoid diverticulitis has greatly improved. This knowledge has challenged many of the traditional principles in the management for diverticulitis, such as routine antibiotic administration in all cases, number-based recommendations for elective surgery, and the necessity for an end colostomy in emergency surgery. This review will cover the breadth of management for sigmoid diverticulitis, covering both uncomplicated and complicated disease as well as elective and emergent disease presentations. New and emerging concepts in management will be highlighted with a particular focus on level-1 data, when available.

Repair of Parastomal Hernias 107

Andrew M. Fleming and Elizabeth H. Wood

Parastomal hernias are an inevitable consequence of ostomy formation and their repairs remain a challenge to many surgeons. With multiple systems of classification and a multitude of techniques for hernia repair ranging from suture to mesh repair, the literature remains sparse with regards to the optimal method of repair. The authors describe the most commonly adopted techniques, discuss preventative measures, and review

This is a comprehensive review of carotid artery revascularization techniques: Carotid Endarterectomy (CEA), Transfemoral Carotid Artery Stenting (TFCAS), and Transcarotid Artery Revascularization (TCAR). CEA is the gold standard and is particularly effective in elderly and high-risk patients. TFCAS, introduced as a less invasive alternative, poses increased periprocedural stroke risks. TCAR, which combines minimally invasive benefits with CEA's neuroprotection principles, emerges as a safer option for high-risk patients, showing comparable results to CEA and better outcomes than TFCAS. The decision-making process for carotid revascularization is complex and influenced by the patient's medical comorbidities and anatomic factors.

the surgeon decides source control is indicated, they must determine the optimal approach and timing. As soon as culture and sensitivity data are available, de-escalation to narrower spectrum agents is essential to decrease the risks of antibiotic toxicity and resistance. Importantly, surgeons should participate in antibiotic stewardship in their patients.

Historically, stage IV melanoma carried a dismal prognosis and surgical resection was the only potential treatment offering long-term survival or palliation of symptomatic disease. With modern systemic therapies that can provide durable disease control for many patients with metastatic disease, we are actively redefining the role of surgery in metastatic melanoma. Contemporary treatment strategies can employ surgical resection in the upfront setting followed by adjuvant therapy, or used in tailored approach following systemic therapy. The combination of surgical resection and modern therapies has been associated with good long-term survival.

The incidence of early-onset colorectal cancer has been rising over the last two decades. Tumors in young patients have distinct features compared to older patients. They predominantly arise in the distal colon and rectum and have poor histological features. Patients tend to present at a more advanced stage and be exposed to more aggressive management approaches; however, this has not translated into a significant survival benefit compared to their older counterparts. This chapter will share current evidence on risk factors and management options for early onset colorectal cancer with a focus on rectal cancer.

The Role of Surgery for Stage IV Breast Cancer **293**

Baraah M.A. Mohamed and Lisa Jacobs

Surgery for the management metastatic breast cancer has traditionally been considered a palliative procedure. However, some retrospective publications indicated that there may be a survival benefit to surgery in the presence of metastatic disease. Recent randomized trials will be reviewed for both management of the intact primary tumor in de novo breast cancer and systemic secondary metastases.

Current Status of Laparoscopic Liver Resection **311**

Hala Muaddi, Hallbera Gudmundsdottir, and Sean Cleary

The evolution of laparoscopic liver surgery, originating in the 1990s, has been marked by significant advancements and milestones, overcoming initial technical hurdles and gaining widespread acceptance within the surgical community as a precise and safe alternative to open procedures. Along this journey, numerous challenges emerged, leading to the accumulation of evidence and the development of guidelines aimed at assisting surgeons in determining the safety, suitability, and complexity of laparoscopic liver resection. This chapter provides a thorough examination of key aspects of laparoscopic liver resection, including difficulty scoring systems, criteria for patient selection, technical considerations, outcomes across different types of liver lesions, and the innovative solutions developed to address challenges, thus offering a comprehensive overview of laparoscopic liver resection, and highlighting its evolving significance in modern hepatobiliary surgery.

Advances in Surgery 58 (2024) 1–17

ADVANCES IN SURGERY

Current Thoughts on Burn Resuscitation

David G. Greenhalgh, MD[a,b,*]

[a]Burn Department, Shriners Children's Northern California, 2425 Stockton Boulevard, Sacramento, CA 95817, USA; [b]Emeritus, Department of Surgery, University of California, Davis, CA, USA

Keywords

• Burns • Resuscitation • Crystalloid • Colloid • Albumin • Glycocalyx • Endothelium

Key points

- There continue to be many unknowns in burn resuscitation.
- The endothelial glycocalyx is involved in regulating edema, but its role is being challenged.
- There are many mechanisms that are involved in edema: hydrostatic and osmotic pressures, intercellular and intracellular water transport, and lymphatic resorption.
- While the crystalloid versus colloid debate continues, it appears that using colloid reduces fluid requirements during burn shock.
- Albumin is the most common choice for use as a colloid, but plasma may protect the endothelial glycocalyx.

INTRODUCTION

Burn care has greatly improved so that survival of a patient with a massive burn is common [1]. Despite improvements in other aspects of care, the initial resuscitation of a patient with a burn greater than 25% total body surface area (TBSA) still remains problematic. Over-resuscitation, coined by Dr Pruitt and Saffle as "fluid creep" continues to be a problem [2,3]. It is felt that the classic formula, the Parkland Formula (4 mL/kg/% TBSA burn, give half during the first 8 hours), over-estimates fluid requirements [4,5] and leads to excessive volumes. To compensate for this "over-estimate," multiple different formulas have

*Burn Department, Shriners Children's Northern California, 2425 Stockton Boulevard, Sacramento, CA 95817. *E-mail address:* dggreenhalgh@ucdavis.edu

https://doi.org/10.1016/j.yasu.2024.04.001
0065-3411/24/

been developed to initiate lower starting volumes. The American Burn Association, in their Advanced Burn Life Support course, has suggested using a "Consensus Formula" which starts at 2 mL/kg/% TBSA burn in an attempt to reduce fluid requirements [6]. In addition, burn surgeons at the United States Army Institute for Surgical Research have developed a "Rule of 10s" (Fluids in mL/hour = 10 × % TBSA burn + 100 mL/kg/hour for every 10 kg body weight above 80 kg) in order to reduce the starting rate [7]. They and others suggest that a higher starting rate will lead to a higher fluid delivery, so initiating resuscitation at a lower rate reduces total fluid delivery [4,5].

There are many reasons why "fluid creep" has not been resolved. The first concern is that little attention is paid to excessive urine outputs during resuscitation. To compensate for "human errors," the "Burn Navigator" (Arcos Medical, Missouri City, Texas) was developed. It is a computer-decision algorithm that detects urine output and suggests adjustments in fluid rates [8,9]. There have also been attempts to use more modern devices to measure the adequacy of resuscitation than urine output, but these noninvasive monitors of cardiac function have failed to improve resuscitative volumes [10]. Other indicators, such as lactic acid and hematocrit, also lead to excessive volumes, but their changes lag behind those of urine output [11,12]. Finally, the choice of resuscitative fluid has also been debated for decades. The issue of whether to use crystalloids versus colloids for resuscitation continues to be debated. If a colloid is used, the best type of colloid is also unresolved.

The goal of this review is to summarize some of the latest concepts of the pathophysiology of burn shock, discuss the best methods of monitoring adequacy of fluid delivery and finally, evidence to support the optimal fluid to use during initial burn resuscitation.

GENERAL CONTENT

Pathophysiology of Initial Burn Shock

All forms of injury or inflammation lead to edema formation. For major burns, resuscitation of initial burn shock often requires dozens of liters of resuscitative fluids. The basic principles of edema formation after a burn were thoroughly reviewed by Demling in 2005 [13]. The capillary response is different for superficial versus full thickness burns. For partial thickness burns, edema peaks around 12 hours post-burn with 90% of the volume peaking at 4 hours. Fluid starts to be resorbed at 4 hours and edema is resolved around 4 days. With full thickness burns, there is loss of the dermal vascular plexus and lymphatic activity is impaired, so edema tends to peak around 18 hours. Since the major resorption of interstitial fluid is through the lymphatics [14], edema persists for longer periods. Increased compartment pressures and high ventilator pressures can inhibit lymphatic flow and lead to prolonged edema. In addition, destruction of extracellular matrix proteins below the skin increases interstitial compliance and osmotic pressures to promote tissue edema.

The classic theory on fluid shifts between the intravascular space and interstitial space is based on the *Starling principle* [15]:

$$J_v = K_f(P_c - P_i) + \sigma(\pi_p - \pi_i)$$

(J_v = fluid filtration rate, K_f = capillary filtration coefficient, P_c = capillary hydrostatic pressure, P_i = interstitial hydrostatic pressure, σ = reflection coefficient, π_p = plasma oncotic pressure, π_i = interstitial oncotic pressure).

Recently, the role of the intraluminal endothelial cell glycocalyx has been emphasized [16–21]. The glycocalyx is composed of proteoglycans, glycosaminoglycan chains, glycoproteins [22], and soluble plasma proteins. Many investigators have found that several glycoproteins, especially *syndecan*, are released in the plasma of patients suffering trauma and burns. In a study, the amount of glycocalyx shedding, measured by serum syndecan levels, was found to be proportional to burn severity [23]. The glycocalyx acts as an endothelial cell osmotic barrier, so it is felt to be more involved in regulating capillary leakage than isolated endothelial cells. Several publications have suggested that the Starling principle should be modified to include the role of the glycocalyx, called the *Modified Starling principle* where π_g (oncotic pressure of the subglycocalyx space) replaces π_i [16,18,24]:

$$J_v = K_f(P_c - P_i) + \sigma(\pi_p - \pi_g)$$

The transfer of fluid into the interstitial space is even more complex than either of the Starling principles [19,24–26]. First of all, the lateral sides of endothelial cells are bound by 3 complexes: *tight junctions, adherens junctions, and gap junctions.* The adherens junction is the main "gait" that opens to allow fluids to flow between cells. There are intraluminal endothelial cell receptors that bind either vascular endothelial growth factor (VEGF); or α-thrombin, histamine, platelet-activating factor, plus others, that open the adherens junction to allow transfer of water and small ions. The molecular mechanisms involved in edema formation, involving signaling through the Rho pathway to activate muscle-like f-actin and myosin to pull apart the adherens junction is reviewed by Komarova, and colleagues [26]. Typically, only water and small molecules pass between endothelial cells. The majority of large molecules (such as albumin) pass inside the cell (transcellular) through clathrin-coated pits, caveolae, or vesicular vacuole organelles. In addition, the extraluminal basement membrane of endothelial cells influences fluid flow, but this typically is only a problem of chronic diseases such as diabetes mellitus [16]. Finally, the pericytes surrounding the endothelial cells add another layer that restricts fluid loss. How each of these permeability regulators influences burn shock has not been completely elucidated.

Recently, there have been challenges to the participation of the glycocalyx in burn-induced edema [24,27,28]. These authors suggest that the glycocalyx may not cover the gaps between endothelial cells, and the bulk of fluid shift is through the larger intracellular pores that transfer large molecules. Therefore, they challenge that the "Modified Starling Principle" may not be applicable to trauma-induced edema. They also suggest that the turnover and replacement of the healthy endothelial glycocalyx is rapid, so its loss may not be prolonged. Clearly, more research needs to be performed to understand all the complexities of the fluid leak in burn patients.

Selecting the Type of Fluid for Burn Resuscitation

The optimal type of fluid to be used in burn resuscitation has been debated for decades. Using colloids for burn resuscitation was promoted in the very early publications, followed by strict crystalloid resuscitation formulas in the 1960s, and now the shift is back to colloid solutions. As a matter of fact, the crystalloid versus colloid debate has continued for decades. The question of which type of crystalloid or colloid has also been debated. Fortunately, recent clinical trials have suggested some answers to these questions.

Crystalloids

There are several advantages for using crystalloids for any intravenous resuscitation. Crystalloids are effective most of the time, especially with smaller burns. The risk of infection from a crystalloid is lower than for a colloid. Crystalloids are less expensive and easier to store than colloids. They have also been suggested for the first-line treatment for sepsis by the Surviving Sepsis Campaign [29], and are readily available since they have no special storage requirements. The disadvantage of crystalloid resuscitation is that it dilutes the intravascular proteins that maintain the osmotic force that keeps fluids inside the capillaries. No one has determined how low colloid levels need to go before the osmotic forces push fluid to the interstitial space. One prospective study randomized burn patients, after resuscitation, to receive albumin to maintain a normal level of 3.5 to 5 g/dL or allow levels to drop to 2 g/dL. They found no differences between the groups concluding that it is not necessary to replete albumin levels to normal levels of 2.5 to 5 g/dL [30]. It is not known, however, whether serum albumin levels less than 2 g/dL increase interstitial edema, but it would not be surprising. It is not uncommon for the massively burned patient to have albumin levels drop to as low as 0.7 g/dL, so the concept that adding colloids at such low levels is reasonable. The other rationale against the use of crystalloids for fluid resuscitation is that, in theory, one needs to give 3 to 4 times the lost volume. This concept is derived from the knowledge that water and electrolytes flow freely between the intravascular and interstitial spaces. Since the major problem is "fluid creep," one would worry that the use of crystalloid would increase the risk of over-resuscitation. Recent studies, however, question the belief that there is a need to replace fluid losses in a 3 to 4 times ratio with crystalloids [20].

When crystalloids are chosen, one must also choose which crystalloid to use. It is obvious that one must avoid a hypotonic fluid in order to prevent water from entering the cells and causing more edema. In the past, studies were performed with hypertonic saline (3%), with the idea of trying to prevent further intravascular water loss and potentially "pull" fluids back into the intravascular space [31,32]. It was also felt that hypertonic saline might have an immune enhancing effect, but a study by Bulger, and colleagues, demonstrated that early (pre-hospital) administration of 3% saline did not improve the outcomes of trauma patients [33]. Hypertonic saline is now rarely used in most burn centers and isotonic crystalloids are most commonly used for initial burn resuscitations. The use of 0.9% (normal) saline has also been abandoned because of the risk of hyperchloremic metabolic acidosis. Several studies have been performed in non-burn patients that compare the use of normal saline versus different isotonic crystalloids and have found that a "balanced" solution, one that contains electrolytes closer to those of plasma, leads to improved outcomes [34–37]. The most commonly used solution used for burn resuscitation is lactated Ringer's (LR) solution [38]. The question that remains is whether other commercially available "balanced" solutions are better than LR for the patient. While there are no studies in burns, several trials in other patients (sepsis, other diagnoses) have not led to convincing evidence to choose one balanced isotonic solution over LR.

Colloids

The most pressing question for burn resuscitation has been whether to add a colloid, either albumin or plasma, to the resuscitation. As stated earlier, the rationale for using colloids is based on the concept that when serum protein levels get so low, there is little intravascular osmotic force to prevent ongoing fluid loss associated with little drive to return fluids into the capillaries. The very early formulas did use colloid [39,40], but colloids were later abandoned because studies suggested that albumin rapidly left the intravascular space [41], and infection risks were not minimal. Two centers, one in Pittsburgh [42,43] and another in Israel [44], did use fresh frozen plasma (FFP) with good success. The use of albumin was almost completely stopped after a 1998 Cochrane study suggested that its use in sepsis increased mortality [45]. Subsequent large studies in sepsis patients suggested that albumin use might be beneficial [46–49], and a 2012 Cochrane review suggested that, at least, albumin use did not increase mortality [50]. There are 2 strategies for albumin use in burn resuscitation: (1) the immediate use of albumin; or (2) the use of albumin as a "rescue" when it appeared that crystalloid resuscitation rates were too high.

Immediate use of albumin. The classic method for measuring the final volume of fluid provided in 24 hours is to measure mL/kg/% TBSA burn. For example, the 24-h target for the Parkland formula is 4 mL/kg/% TBSA burn. For a 100 kg man with 80% TBSA burns, the expected volume would equal $4 \times 100 \times 80 = 32{,}000$ mL (32 L) in 24 hours. If the patient received 40 L, then he would have received 5 mL/kg/hour or 1 mL/kg/hour above the Parkland formula. Several early studies investigated the benefit of immediate use of albumin. In the first immediate use study, Recinos, and colleagues, (1975) compared the use of 2.5% albumin with LR and found that albumin reduced fluid requirements [51]. In children, albumin reduced the volume from 5.2

(LR) to 3.4 mL/kg/% TBSA burn, and in adults, from 2.9 to 2.0 mL/kg/% TBSA. Jelenko, and colleagues (1979), had 3 arms to his study: LR, hypertonic lactated saline, and hypertonic lactated saline with 1.25% albumin [52]. The 24-h outcome for LR was 5.7 mL/kg/% TBSA, hypertonic lactated saline was 3 mL/kg/% TBSA, and the combination 2 mL/kg/% TBSA. Goodwin, and colleagues (1983), compared LR with LR + 2.5% albumin and found similar reductions (3.81 vs 2.98 mL/kg/% TBSA) and improved cardiac function with albumin use [53]. Unfortunately, he also found that albumin treatment was associated with increased interstitial lung water that was not noticed in the LR group. After that study, immediate use of albumin was rarely used until more than 2 decades later, when Cooper, and colleagues (2006), found an insignificant reduction with the immediate use of albumin [54]. More recently, a group from Spain published their experience with using high-dose albumin at the start of resuscitation and gradually decreasing the concentration throughout the first 48 hours after burn injury. This "Biologic Engineering Technology–'BET'" formula led to a decreased 24-h volume of 2.58 mL/kg/% TBSA burn and improved lactate levels [55].

Albumin for "rescue". The concept of "fluid creep" was stressed during the early 2000s, so burn caregivers started using albumin to reduce fluid needs in those patients who seemed to be receiving excessive crystalloid volumes [2,3]. The focus was on using albumin as a "rescue" to reduce fluid requirements in those patients receiving excessive crystalloids. The first publication of the use of albumin as a "rescue" for excessive crystalloid volumes came from Salt Lake City, Utah. They developed a nurse-driven resuscitation protocol to limit excessive fluid administration [56]. After 12 hours, if burn patients were receiving crystalloids at greater than twice the Parkland Formula (>8 mL/kg/% TBSA burn), they were switched from LR alone to a 2/3 LR + 1/3 5% albumin solution. They then compared the outcomes of those patients receiving LR alone with the LR/albumin group. Despite the albumin group having more inhalation injury, longer time to resuscitation, higher volumes of resuscitation (9.4 vs 6.4 mL/kg/% TBSA burn), multivariate analysis found that albumin treatment led to a reduced mortality for the albumin group (odds ratio 0.27, 95% confidence interval 0.07–0.97) [57]. The next year, the US Army burn surgeons developed a fluid reduction program for burn-injured soldiers who were being transported from Europe to the United States. They dictated that patients receive 5% albumin if crystalloid resuscitation was greater than 6 mL/kg/% TBSA burn at 12 to 18 hours [58]. They also added vasopressin if there was hypotension. Compared to 2 years prior, the new protocol reduced the composite endpoint of abdominal compartment syndrome plus death from 36% to 18%. Similar reductions in extremity compartment syndromes and renal failure were reported by Dulhunty, and colleagues [59]. The Utah group subsequently published 2 respective reviews, one in adults [60] and another in children [61], that both showed that, when crystalloid resuscitation was too high, the addition of albumin markedly reduced the in/out (I/O) ratio. Park, and colleagues, from Michigan, developed a similar rescue protocol and compared outcomes before and after the new practice [62]. They found that albumin rescue improved mortality, ventilator days, P_a/O_2 ratios, pneumonia rate, abdominal compartment syndromes, and vasopressor use. They also found no significant reduction in total fluid volumes. A study by Dittrich, and colleagues, found that adding albumin between 8 and 12 hours reduced crystalloid volumes in children [63]. Around the same time, 2 meta-analyses also suggested that albumin treatment was beneficial or at least not harmful [64,65]. When a survey was sent to burn caregivers in 2009, the majority of the respondents (91%) stated that their preferred resuscitation fluid was LR, but 50% admitted to adding albumin within 24 hours. More recent studies continue to support the use of albumin for resuscitation "rescue." Comish, and colleagues, reported their use of 25% albumin when the crystalloid resuscitation was failing, and they found albumin reduced fluid requirements and improved urine output [66].

A proposal for a prospective, randomized, multi-center trial to compare LR to LR + albumin for burn resuscitation, summited to the United States Department of Defense, was turned down because the funding agency felt that a prior observational trial should be performed to assist with the design of the prospective trial. The Department of Defense subsequently funded the *A*cute *B*urn *R*es*U*scitation *P*rospective Multicenter Observational *T*rial (ABRUPT) (ClinicalTrials.gov - NCT03144427) [67]. This study involved 21 burn centers in the United States and Canada. Investigators had the choice to resuscitate with either isotonic crystalloid or crystalloid + albumin to a target urine output of 0.5 to 1 mL/kg/hour. Patients had to be ≥18 year old, have burns ≥20% TBSA burn, and have resuscitation data collected for 48 hours. If they received colloids other than albumin or had excision within 48 hours, they were excluded. A total of 400 patients were accrued with 21 being excluded for minor protocol violations. Of the remaining 379 patients, two-thirds received albumin and one-third received only crystalloid. Multiple logistic regression analysis revealed that those patients receiving albumin were older, had larger total and full-thickness burns, and higher Sequential Organ Failure Assessment scores. Those patients receiving albumin were provided much higher initial fluid volumes than those in the crystalloid group. The highest volumes were in the group that received albumin within 12 hours (Fig. 1). Closer evaluation revealed that caregivers gave albumin to those patients whose crystalloid requirements were higher than expected. If the early crystalloid rate was very high, albumin was started earlier. When one plots the volume of crystalloid given prior to and after the administration of albumin, one can observe rapidly increasing volumes that abruptly drop at the time of albumin administration (Fig. 2). This finding was identical to the studies in Utah revealing that albumin rapidly reduced fluid requirements [60,61].

Interestingly, the ABRUPT trial revealed that the total fluid provided in the first 24 hours to the entire cohort was 4.6 ± 2.2 mL/kg/% TBSA burn. The crystalloid group received 3.7 ± 1.7 and albumin group 5.2 ± 2.3 mL/kg/%

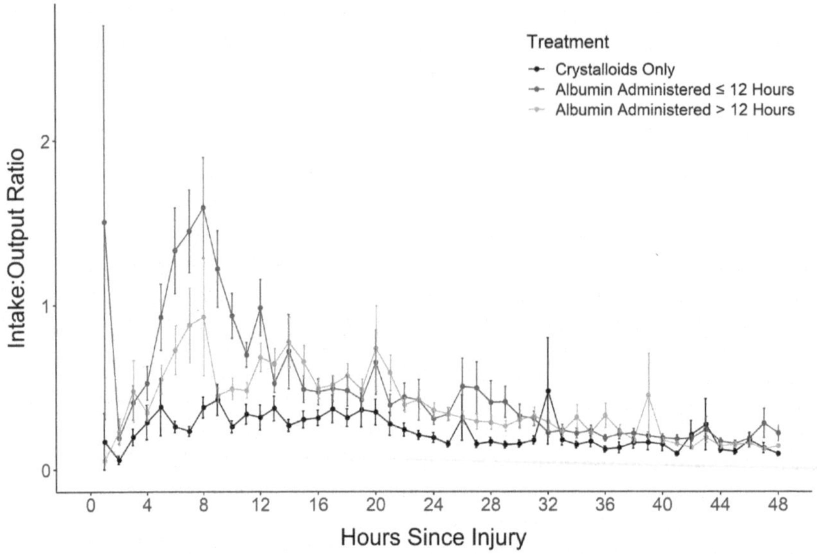

Fig. 1. The intake/output (I/O) ratios of 3 groups of patients from the *A*cute *B*urn *R*es*U*scitation *P*rospective Multicenter Observational Trial (ABRUPT). Those patients who received only crystalloid (lactated Ringer's [LR] solution) had a relatively low I/O ratio throughout the first 48 hours. Those patients who received LR + Albumin within 12 hours had the highest I/O ratios, while those who received LR + Albumin ≥12 hours had I/O ratios of intermediate values. Treatment with albumin rapidly reduced the I/O ratios. (*From* Greenhalgh DG, Cartotto R, Taylor SL, et al. Burn Resuscitation Practices in North America: Results of the Acute Burn ResUscitation Multicenter Prospective Trial (ABRUPT). Ann Surg. 2023;277(3):512 to 519 with permission.)

TBSA burn. Despite efforts to reduce fluids, in large burns, the Parkland formula appears to be fairly accurate. This study demonstrated that in North America, the use of albumin is dictated by the trajectory of fluid delivered. When too much crystalloid is required, most caregivers add albumin to the resuscitation fluid to rapidly lower fluid requirements.

Other questions were addressed in the ABRUPT trial. One issue was whether mechanical ventilation increases fluid requirements during burn shock. Mackie, and colleagues, suggested that increased intrathoracic pressures from positive ventilatory pressures lead to the need for increased venous pressure to return blood to the heart. The increased pressure leads to higher volumes for resuscitation [68,69]. The finding that the ABRUPT study found that ventilated patients required 1.32 mL/kg/% TBSA burn more fluids in 48 hours than patients not being ventilated supports this supposition. The other question was to address: when is burn resuscitation completed? While the actual timing of completion of resuscitation is unknown, the assumption was made that completion of resuscitation occurs when hourly fluid rates equals the sum of calculated daily fluid requirements (based on 1500 × body surface

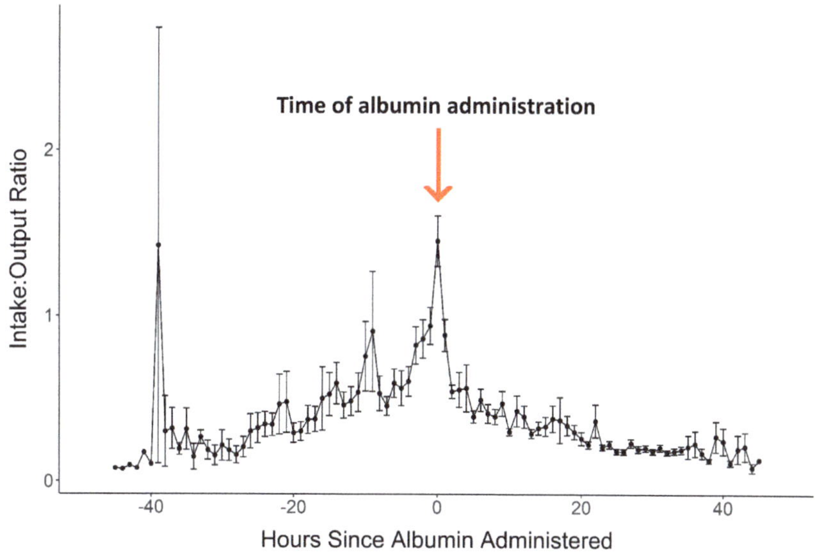

Fig. 2. The I/O ratios before and after albumin administration. The arrow demonstrates the time of albumin administration. The I/O ratio increased significantly prior albumin administration (values to the left of the *arrow*). At the time that albumin was given, there was a precipitous drop in the I/O ratio (values to the right of the *arrow*). This plot reveals that the addition of albumin to crystalloid resuscitation rapidly reduces fluid requirements during burn shock resuscitation. (*Modified from* Greenhalgh DG, Cartotto R, Taylor SL, et al. Burn Resuscitation Practices in North America: Results of the Acute Burn ResUscitation Multicenter Prospective Trial (ABRUPT). Ann Surg. 2023;277(3):512 to 519 with permission. The only modification was the addition of the arrow and label "Time of albumin administration".)

area [BSA], or on the 4 mL/kg for the first 10 kg, 2 mL/kg for the second 10 kg and 1 mL/kg for the remaining 10 kgs of the patient's weight) plus a calculation of the patient's evaporative loss ([25 + BSA] × % TBSA burn = mL/hour).

Post-resuscitation fluid rate = Daily fluid needs + evaporative losses (in mL/hour).

Post-resuscitation fluid rate = (1500 × BSA) + ([25 + BSA] × % TBSA burn) (in mL/hour).

Based on this assumption, it appeared that burn resuscitation was completed around 24 hours in the crystalloid group, but around 48 hours for the larger burn patients who received albumin (Fig. 3).

Lessons learned from the ABRUPT trial did lead to changes in the design of the subsequent prospective, randomized trial funded by the Department of Defense: *A*cute *B*urn *R*es*U*scitation *P*rospective Multicenter *T*rial 2 [ABRUPT2] (ClinicalTrials.gov–NCT04356859). The ABRUPT trial revealed that any fluid (crystalloid or colloid) is effective when resuscitating smaller, superficial burns, so the inclusion criteria was tightened to include total burns ≥25% and full thickness burn ≥20%. Patients are randomized to receive LR or 2/3

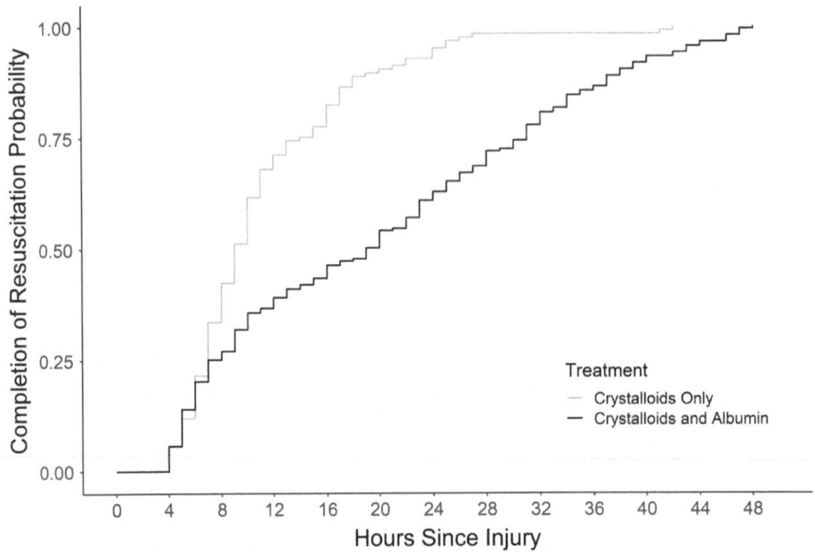

Fig. 3. The graph shows the difference between times to completion of resuscitation for either the crystalloid group and LR + Albumin. The plot was based on the assumption that resuscitation was complete when total fluid rates equaled daily fluid requirements plus calculated evaporative loss (see text). Resuscitation was completed around 24 hours for the crystalloid group, but delayed until 48 hours for the LR + Albumin group. (*Taken from* Greenhalgh DG, Cartotto R, Taylor SL, et al. Burn Resuscitation Practices in North America: Results of the Acute Burn ResUscitation Multicenter Prospective Trial (ABRUPT). Ann Surg. 2023;277(3):512 to 519 with permission).

LR + 1/3 5% albumin starting between 8 and 12 hours. The ABRUPT2 is ongoing, with 28 burn centers participating. As of mid-October 2023, 89 patients are enrolled with a goal of 400 patients accrued. Hopefully, the question of whether to provide albumin to major burns will be decided.

Choosing a Colloid

The next question is to decide which colloid to use. First of all, it is quite clear that the use of hydroxyethyl starch should not be used for any resuscitation since there have been large, multicenter sepsis trials that demonstrated increased risks for bleeding, renal failure, and death [70,71]. While hydroxyethyl starch has been used in burn patients [72–74], at least 1 study suggested that it increased mortality and renal failure [74]. In addition, gelatins and dextran solutions should also not be used [75]. The compelling question is whether to choose albumin versus plasma as the colloid of choice. As stated earlier, FFP has been successfully used by the burn centers in Pittsburgh [42,43] and Israel [44]. With the recent studies that suggest that preserving the endothelial glycocalyx may be important to reduce fluid leakage, the use of FFP makes sense. At least 1 study demonstrated that in rats, the use of

FFP ameliorated burn-related endothelial dysfunction, based on Evans Blue Dye extravasation in lungs, compared to treatment with LR [76]. The addition of albumin was also not protective. The protective effect of FFP was not as convincing since it did not alter the levels of syndecan-1 levels compared to LR treatment. Another retrospective study suggested that FFP reduced fluid requirements when compared to historic use of crystalloids by the Parkland formula [77]. The question of whether FFP is a better colloid than albumin for burn resuscitation is worthy of investigation. Is the albumin in FFP the primary effector of its benefit? Or do the other proteins provide additional benefit for burn resuscitation? The next prospective, randomized study should compare the effects of albumin versus FFP as the colloid choice.

Unanswered Questions

A major unanswered question is what the best endpoints are for determining the adequacy of burn resuscitation. Urine output is quite simplistic and has not solved the problem of fluid creep. One problem is that the responsiveness to increased urine outputs is often delayed so that fluid rates are not turned down. Some suggest that "permissive hypovolemia" or "permissive oliguria" should be practiced, but it is not clear how low of a urine output should be tolerated [78]. Urine output is not helpful when a patient develops intra-abdominal hypertension or syndrome. The use of lactate or base deficit levels are helpful but tend to have delayed changes that are not timely enough to prevent over-resuscitation [11,12,79–81]. Hemoglobin levels are often increased due to hemodilution, but the return to normal levels occurs hours after completion of resuscitation. The efficacy of more complex or invasive monitoring methods have not been effective and tend to over-resuscitate [10,82]. Better strategies supported by well-designed studies are needed to improve the monitoring of burn resuscitation.

Modifying the response to injury

A final question is whether the signals that increase capillary leak can be blocked to prevent the massive fluid shifts? For burns, the one major strategy used to decrease the response to injury and reduce fluid needs is with the use of high-dose vitamin C. The idea is that high levels of ascorbic acid have antioxidant activities that reduce capillary leakage and thus the needs for fluids. The major driver of this strategy came from investigators in Japan who showed that the use of intravenous vitamin C at 66 mg/kg/hour dramatically reduced burn resuscitative volumes [83]. Since their publication, many other centers have adopted the strategy [84–87], but some have suggested that there may be an increase in the risk of renal failure [86]. Discussions with many of the practicing centers reveal that they often have to provide fluid boluses toward the end of resuscitation, suggesting that there may be a diuretic effect in addition to the antioxidant activity [87]. It seems that the use of high-dose vitamin C has decreased as of late.

As of now, the only other method for slowing or nearly eliminating the initial burn shock is to excise the burn. Clinical experience indicates that early excision (during the first 24 hours) greatly reduces fluid requirements. Whether blocking agents can be developed to slow edema formation is a great goal, but, as of yet, no specific agent has been found. Just like for sepsis, attempts to find the "magic bullet" to block the inflammatory response have been unsuccessful. There are so many redundancies in the signals that initiate the inflammatory response that it is unlikely that any single or combination of blocking agents will inhibit the fluids shifts in response to any injury.

DISCUSSION

There has been a great amount of knowledge gained about the signals that turn on the inflammatory response and allow for the major fluid shifts that lead to the massive resuscitative needs after a large burn. We have learned a great deal about how pathogen-associated molecular patterns and damage-associated molecular patterns signal through pattern-recognition receptors to produce cytokines and other cellular signals. In addition, the signals that increase fluid shifts through the endothelial cell lining are also well-known. Despite this knowledge, there has been little that the clinician can do to control this response to injury. One problem is that no one can predict when a burn might occur, and once the process has started, we are unable to immediately turn it off. We are still treating capillary leak and the subsequent hypovolemic shock with resuscitative fluids. Our measures of adequacy of this resuscitation are also quite crude–still relying on urine output. Research needs to continue to develop methods to slow the process and reduce the well-known complications of excessive resuscitation. It seems that there has been a more recent trend to use colloids as a good option to reduce these fluid needs. It seems that we are getting closer to a new burn resuscitation formula that will reduce unnecessary fluid volumes. While there has been progress, there is still a long way to go.

SUMMARY

The complexities of burn edema continue to be learned. The molecular mechanisms that create the intravascular leak are fairly well understood, but there are different pathways for fluids to leak out of the capillaries. The intercellular bonds holding the adherens junctions open up after signals from the proteins (VEGF, histamine, etc.) open up to allow for water and electrolytes to pass to the interstitial space. But there are intracellular pathways that also transport large molecules such as albumin. In addition, the role of the endothelial glycocalyx is still being resolved. Outside the vessels, pericytes also contribute to the regulation of fluid loss, and finally, the lymphatic system is the primary method of fluid resorption.

While mechanisms of fluid shifts are better understood, fluid creep remains a problem. There are no accurate indicators of adequate resuscitation, so caregivers still rely on the crude measurement of urine output. The recent studies, however, suggest that using colloids, either albumin or FFP, reduce total fluids compared to crystalloids. Even if crystalloids are chosen first, if their infusion rate seems too high, the addition of colloids rapidly decreases fluid requirements.

Hopefully, the current multi-center, prospective, randomized trial comparing LR to LR + 5% albumin will confirm the benefit of using colloids for burn resuscitation.

CLINICS CARE POINTS

- Crystalloid resuscitation is adequate for smaller (<20% TBSA) burns.
- Larger and deeper burns (≥25% TBSA, ≥20% full thickness) benefit from the use of colloid.
- If the rate of crystalloid seems too high, the addition of albumin reduces fluid requirements.
- The question of whether FFP has advantages over albumin still needs to be investigated.
- Close monitoring of urine output improves outcomes.
- The use of more advanced resuscitation measures needs to be investigated.

Disclosure

The author is Principle Investigator of one current Department of Defense Grant (W81XWH-19-1-664.JW180038, Acute Burn ResUscitation Prospective Multicenter Trial 2 [ABRUPT2]) (ClinicalTrials.gov – NCT04356859) that compares the use of albumin to lactated Ringer's solution, and one completed Department of Defense grant (W81XWH-16-2-0048, *A*cute *B*urn *Res*U*scitation *P*rospective Multicenter *T*rial [ABRUPT]) (ClinicalTrials.gov – NCT03144427) that are described in the paper.

References

[1] Martens S, Romanowksi K, Palmieri T, et al. Massive pediatric burn injury: a 10-year review. J Burn Care Res 2023;44(3):670–4.
[2] Pruitt BA Jr. Protection from excessive resuscitation: "pushing the pendulum back". J Trauma 2000;49(3):567–8.
[3] Saffle JI. The phenomenon of "fluid creep" in acute burn resuscitation. J Burn Care Res 2007;28(3):382–95.
[4] Rizzo JA, Coates EC, Serio-Melvin ML, et al. Higher initial formula for resuscitation after severe burn injury means higher 24-hour volumes. J Burn Care Res 2023;44(5):1017–22.
[5] Chung KK, Wolf SE, Cancio LC, et al. Resuscitation of severely burned military casualties: fluid begets more fluid. J Trauma 2009;67(2):231–7 [discussion 237].
[6] Pham TN, Cancio LC, Gibran NS, et al. American Burn Association practice guidelines burn shock resuscitation. J Burn Care Res 2008;29(1):257–66.
[7] Chung KK, Salinas J, Renz EM, et al. Simple derivation of the initial fluid rate for the resuscitation of severely burned adult combat casualties: in silico validation of the rule of 10. J Trauma 2010;69(Suppl 1):S49–54.
[8] Salinas J, Chung KK, Mann EA, et al. Computerized decision support system improves fluid resuscitation following severe burns: an original study. Crit Care Med 2011;39(9):2031–8.

[9] Rizzo JA, Liu NT, Coates EC, et al. Initial Results of the American Burn Association Observational Multicenter Evaluation on the Effectiveness of the Burn Navigator. J Burn Care Res 2022;43(3):728–34.

[10] Paratz JD, Stockton K, Paratz ED, et al. Burn resuscitation–hourly urine output versus alternative endpoints: a systematic review. Shock 2014;42(4):295–306.

[11] Choi J, Cooper A, Gomez M, et al. The 2000 Moyer Award. The relevance of base deficits after burn injuries. J Burn Care Rehabil 2000;21(6):499–505.

[12] Cochran A, Edelman LS, Saffle JR, et al. The relationship of serum lactate and base deficit in burn patients to mortality. J Burn Care Res 2007;28(2):231–40.

[13] Demling RH. The burn edema process: current concepts. J Burn Care Rehabil 2005;26(3): 207–27.

[14] Petrova TV, Koh GY. Organ-specific lymphatic vasculature: From development to pathophysiology. J Exp Med 2018;215(1):35–49.

[15] Starling EH. On the absorption of fluids from the connective tissue spaces. J Physiol 1896;19(4):312–26.

[16] Kottke MA, Walters TJ. Where's the leak in vascular barriers? a review. Shock 2016;46(3 Suppl 1):20–36.

[17] Cardenas JC, Dong JF, Kozar RA. Injury-induced endotheliopathy: What you need to know. J Trauma Acute Care Surg 2023;95(4):454–63.

[18] Basas VA, Schutzman LM, Brown IE. Implications of the regulation of endothelial glycocalyx breakdown and reconstitution in severe burn injury. J Surg Res 2023;286:110–7.

[19] Chi Y, Liu X, Chai J. A narrative review of changes in microvascular permeability after burn. Ann Transl Med 2021;9(8):719.

[20] Myburgh JA, Mythen MG. Resuscitation fluids. N Engl J Med 2013;369(13):1243–51.

[21] Finfer S, Myburgh J, Bellomo R. Intravenous fluid therapy in critically ill adults. Nat Rev Nephrol 2018;14(9):541–57.

[22] Mouta-Bellum C, Kirov A, Miceli-Libby L, et al. Organ-specific lymphangiectasia, arrested lymphatic sprouting, and maturation defects resulting from gene-targeting of the PI3K regulatory isoforms p85alpha, p55alpha, and p50alpha. Dev Dynam 2009;238(10):2670–9.

[23] Luker JN, Vigiola Cruz M, Carney BC, et al. Shedding of the endothelial glycocalyx is quantitatively proportional to burn injury severity. Ann Burns Fire Disasters 2018;31(1):17–22.

[24] Levick JR, Michel CC. Microvascular fluid exchange and the revised Starling principle. Cardiovasc Res 2010;87(2):198–210.

[25] Cusack R, Leone M, Rodriguez AH, et al. Endothelial damage and the microcirculation in critical illness. Biomedicines 2022;10(12).

[26] Komarova YA, Kruse K, Mehta D, et al. Protein interactions at endothelial junctions and signaling mechanisms regulating endothelial permeability. Circ Res 2017;120(1): 179–206.

[27] Hahn RG, Dull RO, Zdolsek J. The extended starling principle needs clinical validation. Acta Anaesthesiol Scand 2020;64(7):884–7.

[28] Dull RO, Hahn RG. The glycocalyx as a permeability barrier: basic science and clinical evidence. Crit Care 2022;26(1):273.

[29] Evans L, Rhodes A, Alhazzani W, et al. Surviving sepsis campaign: international guidelines for management of sepsis and septic shock 2021. Intensive Care Med 2021;47(11): 1181–247.

[30] Greenhalgh DG, Housinger TA, Kagan RJ, et al. Maintenance of serum albumin levels in pediatric burn patients: a prospective, randomized trial. J Trauma 1995;39(1):67–73 [discussion 73-64].

[31] Monafo WW, Chuntrasakul C, Ayvazian VH. Hypertonic sodium solutions in the treatment of burn shock. Am J Surg 1973;126(6):778–83.

[32] Warden GD. Burn shock resuscitation. World J Surg 1992;16(1):16–23.

[33] Bulger EM, May S, Kerby JD, et al. Out-of-hospital hypertonic resuscitation after traumatic hypovolemic shock: a randomized, placebo controlled trial. Ann Surg 2011;253(3): 431–41.

[34] Semler MW, Wanderer JP, Ehrenfeld JM, et al. Balanced crystalloids versus saline in the intensive care unit. the SALT randomized trial. Am J Respir Crit Care Med 2017;195(10): 1362–72.

[35] Toporek AH, Semler MW, Self WH, et al. Balanced crystalloids versus saline in critically ill adults with hyperkalemia or acute kidney injury: secondary analysis of a clinical trial. Am J Respir Crit Care Med 2021;203(10):1322–5.

[36] Hammond DA, Lam SW, Rech MA, et al. Balanced crystalloids versus saline in critically ill adults: a systematic review and meta-analysis. Ann Pharmacother 2020;54(1):5–13.

[37] Chaussard M, Depret F, Saint-Aubin O, et al. Physiological response to fluid resuscitation with Ringer lactate versus Plasmalyte in critically ill burn patients. J Appl Physiol (1985) 2020;128(3):709–14.

[38] Greenhalgh DG. Burn resuscitation: the results of the ISBI/ABA survey. Burns 2010;36(2): 176–82.

[39] Moore FD. The body-weight burn budget. Basic fluid therapy for the early burn. Surg Clin North Am 1970;50(6):1249–65.

[40] Evans AJ. Treatment of burns today. Proc Roy Soc Med 1971;64(12):1295–6.

[41] Baxter CR, Shires T. Physiological response to crystalloid resuscitation of severe burns. Ann N Y Acad Sci 1968;150(3):874–94.

[42] Du GB, Slater H, Goldfarb IW. Influences of different resuscitation regimens on acute early weight gain in extensively burned patients. Burns 1991;17(2):147–50.

[43] O'Mara MS, Slater H, Goldfarb IW, et al. A prospective, randomized evaluation of intra-abdominal pressures with crystalloid and colloid resuscitation in burn patients. J Trauma 2005;58(5):1011–8.

[44] Fodor L, Fodor A, Ramon Y, et al. Controversies in fluid resuscitation for burn management: literature review and our experience. Injury 2006;37(5):374–9.

[45] Cochrane Injuries Group Albumin R. Human albumin administration in critically ill patients: systematic review of randomised controlled trials. BMJ 1998;317(7153):235–40.

[46] Finfer S, Bellomo R, Boyce N, et al. A comparison of albumin and saline for fluid resuscitation in the intensive care unit. N Engl J Med 2004;350(22):2247–56.

[47] Charpentier J, Mira JP, Grp ES. Efficacy and tolerance of hyperoncotic albumin administration in septic shock patients: the earss study. Intensive Care Med 2011;37:S115.

[48] Annane D, Siami S, Jaber S, et al. Effects of fluid resuscitation with colloids vs crystalloids on mortality in critically ill patients presenting with hypovolemic shock: the CRISTAL randomized trial. JAMA 2013;310(17):1809–17.

[49] Caironi P, Tognoni G, Masson S, et al. Albumin replacement in patients with severe sepsis or septic shock. N Engl J Med 2014;370(15):1412–21.

[50] Perel P, Roberts I. Colloids versus crystalloids for fluid resuscitation in critically ill patients. Cochrane Database Syst Rev 2012;(6):CD000567.

[51] Recinos PR, Hartford CA, Ziffren SE. Fluid resuscitation of burn patients comparing a crystalloid with a colloid containing solution: a prospective study. J Iowa Med Soc 1975;65(10):426–32.

[52] Jelenko C 3rd, Williams JB, Wheeler ML, et al. Studies in shock and resuscitation, I: use of a hypertonic, albumin-containing, fluid demand regimen (HALFD) in resuscitation. Crit Care Med 1979;7(4):157–67.

[53] Goodwin CW, Dorethy J, Lam V, et al. Randomized trial of efficacy of crystalloid and colloid resuscitation on hemodynamic response and lung water following thermal injury. Ann Surg 1983;197(5):520–31.

[54] Cooper AB, Cohn SM, Zhang HS, et al. Five percent albumin for adult burn shock resuscitation: lack of effect on daily multiple organ dysfunction score. Transfusion 2006;46(1): 80–9.

[55] Blanco-Schweizer P, Sanchez-Ballesteros J, Bendito B, et al. Resuscitation with albumin using BET formula keeps at bay fluid administration in burned patients. An observational study. Burns 2020;46(4):860–7.
[56] Cooper C, Cochran A, Coffey R. Nurses can resuscitate. J Burn Care Res 2021;42(2): 167–70.
[57] Cochran A, Morris SE, Edelman LS, et al. Burn patient characteristics and outcomes following resuscitation with albumin. Burns 2007;33(1):25–30.
[58] Ennis JL, Chung KK, Renz EM, et al. Joint Theater Trauma System implementation of burn resuscitation guidelines improves outcomes in severely burned military casualties. J Trauma 2008;64(2 Suppl):S146–51 [discussion S151-142].
[59] Dulhunty JM, Boots RJ, Rudd MJ, et al. Increased fluid resuscitation can lead to adverse outcomes in major-burn injured patients, but low mortality is achievable. Burns 2008;34(8): 1090–7.
[60] Lawrence A, Faraklas I, Watkins H, et al. Colloid administration normalizes resuscitation ratio and ameliorates "fluid creep". J Burn Care Res 2010;31(1):40–7.
[61] Faraklas I, Lam U, Cochran A, et al. Colloid normalizes resuscitation ratio in pediatric burns. J Burn Care Res 2011;32(1):91–7.
[62] Park SH, Hemmila MR, Wahl WL. Early albumin use improves mortality in difficult to resuscitate burn patients. J Trauma Acute Care Surg 2012;73(5):1294–7.
[63] Muller Dittrich MH, Brunow de Carvalho W, Lopes Lavado E. Evaluation of the "Early" use of albumin in children with extensive burns: a randomized controlled trial. Pediatr Crit Care Med 2016;17(6):e280–6.
[64] Navickis RJ, Greenhalgh DG, Wilkes MM. Albumin in burn shock resuscitation: a meta-analysis of controlled clinical studies. J Burn Care Res 2016;37(3):e268–78.
[65] Eljaiek R, Heylbroeck C, Dubois MJ. Albumin administration for fluid resuscitation in burn patients: A systematic review and meta-analysis. Burns 2017;43(1):17–24.
[66] Comish P, Walsh M, Castillo-Angeles M, et al. Adoption of rescue colloid during burn resuscitation decreases fluid administered and restores end-organ perfusion. Burns 2021;47(8): 1844–50.
[67] Greenhalgh DG, Cartotto R, Taylor SL, et al. Burn Resuscitation Practices in North America: Results of the Acute Burn ResUscitation Multicenter Prospective Trial (ABRUPT). Ann Surg 2023;277(3):512–9.
[68] Mackie DP. Inhalation injury or mechanical ventilation: which is the true killer in burn patients? Burns 2013;39(7):1329–30.
[69] Mackie DP, Spoelder EJ, Paauw RJ, et al. Mechanical ventilation and fluid retention in burn patients. J Trauma 2009;67(6):1233–8 [discussion 1238].
[70] Myburgh JA, Finfer S, Bellomo R, et al. Hydroxyethyl starch or saline for fluid resuscitation in intensive care. N Engl J Med 2012;367(20):1901–11.
[71] Perner A, Haase N, Guttormsen AB, et al. Hydroxyethyl starch 130/0.42 versus Ringer's acetate in severe sepsis. N Engl J Med 2012;367(2):124–34.
[72] Vlachou E, Gosling P, Moiemen NS. Hydroxyethylstarch supplementation in burn resuscitation–a prospective randomised controlled trial. Burns 2010;36(7):984–91.
[73] Bechir M, Puhan MA, Fasshauer M, et al. Early fluid resuscitation with hydroxyethyl starch 130/0.4 (6%) in severe burn injury: a randomized, controlled, double-blind clinical trial. Crit Care 2013;17(6):R299.
[74] Béchir M, Puhan MA, Neff SB, et al. Early fluid resuscitation with hyperoncotic hydroxyethyl starch 200/0.5 (10%) in severe burn injury. Crit Care 2010;14(3):R123.
[75] Thomas-Rueddel DO, Vlasakov V, Reinhart K, et al. Safety of gelatin for volume resuscitation–a systematic review and meta-analysis. Intensive Care Med 2012;38(7):1134–42.
[76] Vigiola Cruz M, Carney BC, Luker JN, et al. Plasma ameliorates endothelial dysfunction in burn injury. J Surg Res 2019;233:459–66.

[77] Lindsey L, Purvis MV, Miles D, et al. An adjusted ideal body weight index formula with fresh frozen plasma (FFP) rescue decreases fluid creep during burn resuscitation. Ann Burns Fire Disasters 2020;33(3):216–23.
[78] Arlati S, Storti E, Pradella V, et al. Decreased fluid volume to reduce organ damage: a new approach to burn shock resuscitation? A preliminary study. Resuscitation 2007;72(3):371–8.
[79] Jeng JC, Jablonski K, Bridgeman A, et al. Serum lactate, not base deficit, rapidly predicts survival after major burns. Burns 2002;28(2):161–6.
[80] Cartotto R, Choi J, Gomez M, et al. A prospective study on the implications of a base deficit during fluid resuscitation. J Burn Care Rehabil 2003;24(2):75–84.
[81] Kaups KL, Davis JW, Dominic WJ. Base deficit as an indicator or resuscitation needs in patients with burn injuries. J Burn Care Rehabil 1998;19(4):346–8.
[82] Cartotto R, Greenhalgh DG, Cancio C. Burn state of the science: fluid resuscitation. J Burn Care Res 2017;38(3):e596–604.
[83] Tanaka H, Matsuda T, Miyagantani Y, et al. Reduction of resuscitation fluid volumes in severely burned patients using ascorbic acid administration: a randomized, prospective study. Arch Surg 2000;135(3):326–31.
[84] Dubick MA, Williams C, Elgjo GI, et al. High-dose vitamin C infusion reduces fluid requirements in the resuscitation of burn-injured sheep. Shock 2005;24(2):139–44.
[85] Kahn SA, Beers RJ, Lentz CW. Resuscitation after severe burn injury using high-dose ascorbic acid: a retrospective review. J Burn Care Res 2011;32(1):110–7.
[86] Lin J, Falwell S, Greenhalgh D, et al. High-dose ascorbic acid for burn shock resuscitation may not improve outcomes. J Burn Care Res 2018;39(5):708–12.
[87] Rizzo JA, Rowan MP, Driscoll IR, et al. Vitamin C in burn resuscitation. Crit Care Clin 2016;32(4):539–46.

Advances in Surgery 58 (2024) 19–34

ADVANCES IN SURGERY

Management of Complications in Crohn's Disease

Dylan Carroll, MD[a], Sandy Kavalukas, MS, MD[b,*]

[a]Department of Surgery, University of Louisville, 550 South Jackson Street, Louisville, KY 40292, USA; [b]Colorectal Surgery, Department of Surgery, University of Louisville, 550 South Jackson Street, Louisville, KY 40292, USA

Keywords

• Crohn's disease • Enterocutaneous fistula • Intestinal stricture • Immunomodulators • Steroids • Kono-S

Key points

- Medical treatment of Crohn's disease should be optimized, when possible, prior to endeavors in the surgical setting.
- Bowel preservation to maintain maximal intestinal length should always be considered during surgery for Crohn's disease given the high likelihood of recurrence.
- Achieving optimal nutrition—be it enteral, parenteral, or both is necessary to avoid surgical complications.
- New anastomotic techniques, such as the Kono-S anastomosis, provide possibilities for decreasing local recurrent disease and need for reoperation.

INTRODUCTION

Inflammatory bowel disease is an autoimmune intestinal disorder, typically subclassified as Crohn's disease or ulcerative colitis. Recently, these 2 diseases have been characterized as more of a "spectrum" and less as "two separate entities", though generally ulcerative colitis has few ongoing complications after colectomy in those patients who progress to surgical treatment. Crohn's disease, however, is known to be persistent and recurrent, with many different presentations. The prevalence of Crohn's disease in North America is 319 per 100,000 people, and is typically higher in industrialized countries compared to underdeveloped nations [1].

*Corresponding author. *E-mail address:* sandy.kavalukas@louisville.edu

https://doi.org/10.1016/j.yasu.2024.04.002

Crohn's disease has a bimodal age distribution–while it is most diagnosed in late adolescence/early adulthood, there is a second uptick in initial disease presentation during the 7th to 8th decade of life. Younger patients have higher incidences of intestinal strictures and small bowel involvement, whereas older patients have more inflammatory and colonic disease [2,3]. These descriptors are key aspects of the Montreal Classification, which is the most commonly used nomenclature [4] (Table 1). Presenting symptoms may include abdominal pain, diarrhea which may or may not have blood, anal fistulas, malnutrition and anemia, or intestinal obstruction from strictures. We briefly highlight the key aspects of medical and surgical management, as these are key basic steps to perform when managing the complications of Crohn's disease.

Medical management

The common mechanism of action of most medications for Crohn's disease is to downregulate inflammatory cytokines. While some providers utilize a "bottom up" approach, in which the less effective but less "potent" medications are used first and progressively advanced with refractory disease, many have shifted to the paradigm of a "top down" approach (Fig. 1). The use of aminosalicylates (ASA) has waned due to their lack of efficacy in maintaining remission in most patients. Other immunomodulators–notably azathioprine and mercaptopurine are also less successful as monotherapy and are most efficacious when added to a biologic (if needed) for maintaining remission [5,6].

Corticosteroids are typically used for severe exacerbations or at the time of initial diagnosis until symptoms have been controlled to transition to other maintenance therapy. The American College of Gastroenterologists (AGA) recommends its use for inducing remission in severe, non-penetrating Crohn's disease [7]. Glucocorticoids result in downregulation of the inflammatory cytokines IL-1β, TNF-α, IL-6, IL-8, and others [8]. Systemic steroids do not have a role in maintenance therapy due to their extensive profile of significant long-term side effects. Other steroids recommended by the AGA include ileal-release budesonide, which has minimal systemic effects and a superior safety profile compared to systemic glucocorticoids and 5-ASA [7,9]. However, there is no significant benefit with the use of budesonide for maintenance therapy after 3 months [10].

Biologic medications have varying specificity in modulating the immune response; this class of medications are preferred as a single agent given their

Table 1
Montreal classification of Crohn's disease

Age	Location	Behavior
A1: <16 y	L1: ileal	B1: nonstricturing, nonpenetrating
A2: 17–40 y	L2: colonic	B2: stricturing
A3: >40 y	L3: ileocolonic	B3: penetrating
	L4: isolated upper disease	p: perianal

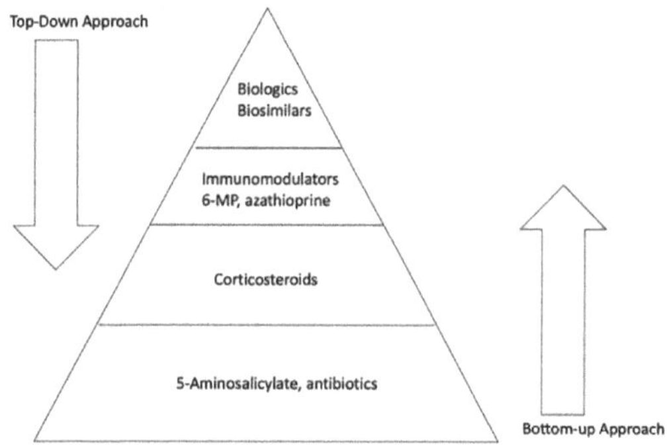

Fig. 1. Medical treatment of Crohn's disease.

success in maintaining long-term remission. Highly specific drugs such as ustekinumab (an IL-12/IL-23 inhibitor) and vedolizumab (a gut-selective anti-integrin) have shown success, and was shown to be equivalent to the anti-TNF inhibitors [11,12]. Since several of these biologic agents have had their patents expire, "biosimilars" have emerged–that have the same efficacy as it is nearly identical in both structure and function to the patented biologic. These started for anti-TNF inhibitors, but more recently there are also biosimilars for the more selective drugs such as ustekinumab.

Surgical intervention

General principles

Nutrition. Malnutrition in Crohn's disease is an independent surgical risk factor for increased morbidity and mortality [13,14]. When dealing with complications of Crohn's disease, it cannot be stressed enough that nutritional status must be optimized. Poor nutritional status and a reduction of more than 10% in the body weight during the 6 months preceding surgery are associated with the worse postoperative outcomes [13]. There are many different types of nutritional therapies: exclusive enteral nutrition (EEN), which is a formula only based on diet, partial enteral nutrition, which is a combination of regular food and formula-based diet, Crohn's disease exclusion diet, which focuses on limiting exposure to certain meats, gluten, and other dietary components, and the Crohn's disease treatment with eating diet, which is a solid food diet that has similar composition to EEN formulas but excludes gluten and lactose [15].

A systematic review conducted in 2021 demonstrated that the current data on use of preoperative EEN trended toward fewer infectious complications and less stoma creations, but the studies were underpowered to demonstrate significance with regard to preoperative EEN [16]. EEN may also be useful as an induction agent, negating the need for steroids in some situations. A meta-analysis comparing the results of 3 randomized controlled trials and 10 observational studies showed no difference in efficacy to induce Crohn's remission in children using EEN rather than steroids [17]. Parenteral nutrition, on the other hand, also continues to play an important role in Crohn's disease. Short-range uses are commonly employed in malnourished patients with the aim of achieving bowel rest in an acute inflammatory phase. Extended uses are for patients with chronic intestinal failure due to short bowel, presence of fistulas, obstruction, or dysfunction at the mucosal level causing malabsorption [18]. Parenteral nutrition will be discussed further sections regarding intestinal failure and short bowel syndrome as a specific complication.

Minimally invasive operative approaches. Patients with Crohn's disease often require reoperative surgery, either due to recurrent disease years apart, or more immediate if complications arise due to the initial surgical procedure. Laparoscopic procedures should be performed whenever possible for the following reasons: faster recovery times, lower rates of incisional hernias, less intra-abdominal adhesive disease, and improved cosmesis. Conventional laparoscopy and robotic approaches are a safe alternative to tradition open surgery with no significant increase in postoperative complication rates, but there is still a conversion to open reported to be 7% to 42% in recurrent Crohn's cases [19]. Specific to our discussion, Crohn's disease also involves inflammation of the mesentery. Mesenteric dissection can be quite difficult due to friability and increased bleeding, which may explain the high conversion rates.

For the younger patient with Crohn's disease who is in their childbearing years, laparoscopy may be advantageous due to lower adhesions with pelvic dissection, though this has not proven to lower fertility rates; it only has shown a decreased time to conceive compared to open procedures [20].

Deep vein thrombosis. Patients with inflammatory bowel disease (IBD) have an increased risk of thromboembolic events–pulmonary embolism and deep venous thrombosis being the most common compared to arterial thrombosis, retinal vein occlusion, and mesenteric or portal venous thrombosis [21]. A retrospective study of 130,000 patients demonstrated that the overall risk of venous thromboembolism (VTE) in patients with IBD is 1.74 times that of patients with non-IBD, and the absolute risk of VTE is doubled with surgery and remains elevated for at least 6 weeks posthospitalization [22]. The pathophysiology of this phenomenon is not clearly defined and likely multifactorial. Many studies have shown elevated homocysteine levels, genetic polymorphisms, vitamin deficiencies, and various regulations in the clotting cascade in patients with IBD [23]. Because of this known risk, it is recommended that patients with IBD undergoing intestinal resection should be considered for extended duration pharmacologic prophylaxis, the length of which is not yet well established [24].

Surgical intervention of Crohn's disease complications

Intestinal strictures

Endoscopic management. Intestinal strictures are classified as inflammatory or noninflammatory/fibrotic. Magnetic resonance enterography is the best cross-sectional imaging tool used to differentiate between these two types, and can evaluate surrounding inflammation and stricture components based on weighted images [25]. Inflammatory strictures may respond with escalation of medical therapy and immunomodulating medications, though this is not the case with fibrotic strictures, which instead may be treated with endoscopic balloon dilation (EBD) or stricturoplasty. Criteria for balloon dilation are the stricture must be endoscopically accessible, less than 5 cm, non-angulated, no associated abscess or fistula, and no suspicions of malignancy. According to the clinical practice guidelines on EBD, it is acceptable to use EBD for de novo and anastomotic strictures based on studies that show similar efficacy and safety profile when using EBD on either type of lesion [26]. In a multivariate analysis, every 1 cm increase in length of a stricture also increased the hazard need for surgery by 8%, where strictures less than 5 cm were associated with avoidance of an operation [27].

Local administration of TNF-alpha antibodies and corticosteroids into a stricture, postdilation, has been described with conflicting results. A randomized, double-blinded controlled trial demonstrated steroid injection into strictures after EBD reduced the need for both re-dilation and subsequent surgery [28]. However, this was performed in a pediatric population and there are a few studies in the adult population with conflicting results [29,30].

Stricturoplasty. Stricturoplasty performed at the time of surgery is indicated in patients with multiple strictures, previous long-segment resections, and those at risk for short bowel syndrome [31]. This technique offers the advantage of preserving small bowel length by avoiding resection. Prior to any stricturoplasty in which no resection is to be performed, one should carefully examine the quality of the bowel wall, the mucosal lumen, and evaluate for any suspicious signs of underlying malignancy. The incidence rate of small bowel adenocarcinoma is 1.5 per 1000 patients with Crohn's disease; 84% of cases are in the terminal ileum, and only 11% had radiographic features of adenocarcinoma [32]. Suspicious features that should prompt the surgeon to perform an intraoperative biopsy during a stricturoplasty are as follows: "hardness" in previous stricturoplasty, chronic fistulizing disease, omental or mesenteric nodularity at the strictured bowel, or encountering a matted small bowel mass [33]. A retrospective study of 68 stricturoplasties with combined small bowel resection showed that 5 cases had intraoperative frozen sections sent for suspicious findings, and all 5 cases were positive for adenocarcinoma.

The various types of stricturoplasties can be visualized in Fig. 2. For strictures less than 10 cm, a Heinike–Mickulicz stricturoplasty can be done by making a longitudinal incision over the stricture and closing the defect in a transverse manner. A Finney stricturoplasty is recommended for strictures 10 to 25 cm. This is performed by looping the intestine on itself, folding the stricture at the middle of the loop. The stricture is then incised, and a common channel is sewn between the 2 folds. For strictures greater than 25 cm, a Michelassi stricturoplasty can be done by transecting the bowel in the middle of the stricture, advancing the 2 limbs and creating an isoperistaltic, side-to-side anastomosis after incising the stricture as the common enterotomy.

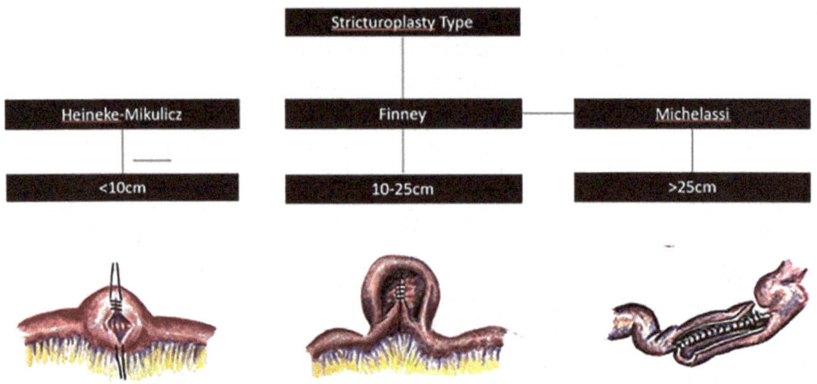

Fig. 2. Types of intestinal stricturoplasty. (Image Courtesy: Drawing by Jessica Masch, MD.)

Historically, colonic stricture has been associated with increased risk of colon adenocarcinoma, though this has been called into question with larger studies [34]. Colonic strictures in ulcerative colitis are associated with malignancy in approximately one-third of cases, while only 6.8% of Crohn's colonic strictures are associated with malignancy [35]. There is no role for colonic stricturoplasty in Crohn's disease, and once the stricture is symptomatic or dysplasia of any type is found on biopsy, an oncologic resection should be performed.

Intestinal resection for strictures, abscess, and fistulas

Anastomotic techniques. About half of patients with Crohn's disease will require a bowel resection, most commonly in the terminal ileum. Unfortunately, about a third of those patients will require repeat resection within 5 years of their initial operation [36]. There are several methods for bowel anastomosis following a resection for Crohn's disease. Traditionally, an end-to-end handsewn anastomosis or side-to-side stapled anastomosis is formed. The CAST trial in 2009 was a multicenter randomized controlled trial comparing handsewn end-to-end with stapled side-to-side anastomosis resulting in endoscopically similar recurrence rates for Crohn's disease at 1 year follow up surveillance [37]. A 2019 Cochrane review demonstrated significantly higher leak rates with handsewn compared to stapled ileocolic anastomoses, though a subgroup analysis specifically in Crohn's disease was not performed [38].

The mesentery has been identified as an active participant in the pathogenesis of Crohn's inflammation [39,40]. The mesentery and creeping fat have been shown to contain increased populations of macrophages, T and B cells, and proinflammatory chemokines [41,42]. A recent change in surgical technique is to ensure extended mesenteric excision given this understanding of the mesentery's contribution to recurrent disease and inflammation. This involves a high ligation of the vascular pedicle and "wedging out" the mesentery with the surgical specimen as one would harvest the lymph node basin for an oncologic resection.

Given this newly understood role of the mesentery, another corresponding advancement in surgical technique is the advent of the Kono-S anastomosis, which excludes the mesentery from the anastomosis. The Kono-S anastomosis positions the anastomosis on the antimesenteric border while maintaining the natural orientation of the bowel's blood supply and peristaltic direction(Fig. 3). The benefit of the Kono-S is a supporting column that prevents distortion of the bowel, an endoscopically accessible end-to-end anastomosis, and less stasis at the anastomosis [43]. A meta-analysis comparing outcomes Kono-S to traditional anastomoses showed a lower incidence of anastomotic leak as well as a lower 5 year disease recurrence rate [44]. Though outcomes have yet to be reported, a totally stapled version of the Kono-S that would theoretically allow for shorter operative times compared to the handsewn version has been described [45]. A Cochrane review of 9 studies (896 patients) showed the Kono-S to be associated with lower incidence of Crohn's disease recurrence and a lower rate of anastomotic leak when incorporated into an operation versus an extended mesenteric excision [46]. A technical feasibility and safety study was performed of dual mesenteric excision and anastomotic exclusion procedure (extended mesenteric excision combined with a Kono-S anastomosis), in which no anastomotic leaks were reported in a small series of 22 patients [47].

Surgical treatment for perianal Crohn's disease

Anorectal stricture. Anorectal strictures may be functional due to stenosis. Chronic diarrhea can cause a functional stricture due to anal spasm whereas

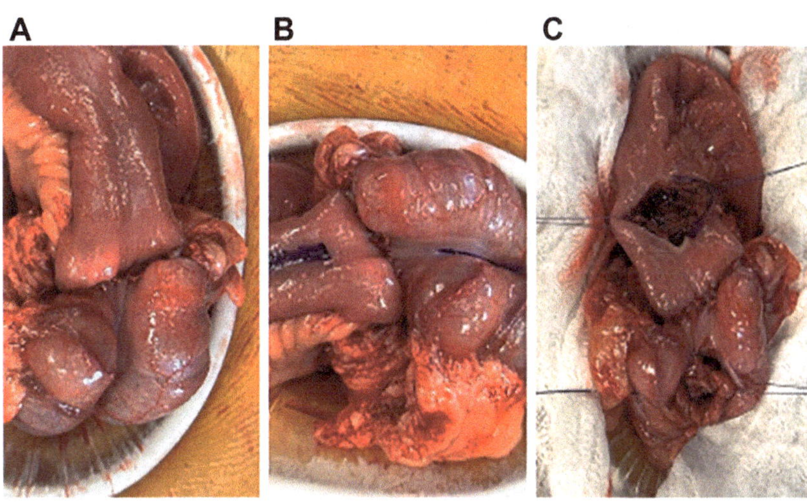

Fig. 3. Technique of the Kono S anastomosis: (*A*) End-to-end configuration of an ileo-colic anastomosis; the staple lines of each end have been sewn together to create a supporting column. (*B*) Markings for the enterotomies which are made perpendicular to the supporting column. (*C*) Anastomosis in a transverse manner by placing corner stitches mid-way on either side of the enterotomy.

stenosis develops because of healing and remodeling from episodes of perianal inflammation [48]. Topical therapies may be helpful in the setting of acute inflammation in anal strictures. 5-ASA and corticosteroids can be used separately to induce proctitis remission, though the combination of the two may have a synergistic effect [49]. Biologic therapy is often helpful for management even in isolated perianal Crohn's disease. Yearly surveillance and directed biopsy are necessary to rule out underlying malignancy (either squamous or adenocarcinoma), and often these patients require repeated dilations–either EBD or with Hegar dilators, and if progressive may ultimately require proctectomy. A systematic review of perianal strictures in Crohn's disease concluded that most patients will undergo total proctocolectomy in the setting of concurrent perianal fistulizing disease, though fecal diversion can also allow for symptomatic relief [50].

Perianal fistula. The pathophysiology of anal fistulas in Crohn's disease is attributed to the penetrating, full thickness inflammation of the bowel wall (the hallmark of Crohn's disease) within the anal canal and rectum. Symptoms of pain, purulent drainage, and fecal incontinence markedly affect quality of life. While antibiotics such as ciprofloxacin or metronidazole may be used for minor flares, biologic therapy is often necessary as maintenance therapy for fistulizing perianal disease. Adalimumab is associated with a complete fistula closure at a rate of 33%, and newer biologic therapies such as Vedolizumab and Ustekinumab are also associated with at least partial fistula response [51].

A major potential complication of this is prolonged immunosuppression in a population of patients that is known to have higher rates of HPV infection. The combination of immunosuppression, HPV infection, and difficulty of routine examination due to the presence of fistulizing disease or anal stricture raises concern for promoting the risk of anal squamous cell carcinoma (SCC). Women with IBD have been shown to have a higher incidence of abnormal cervical pap smears compared to patients with non-IBD and those on immunomodulators had a higher association with concordant HPV infection [52]. A study performed to demonstrate the association between Crohn's disease and anal SCC suggested long-standing perianal fistulizing Crohn's disease is an independent risk factor for SCC, as over half this cohort had perianal fistulizing disease for over 10 years [53]. This finding is supported by a systematic review finding a mean duration of fistulizing disease of 10 to 11 years between fistulizing perianal Crohn's disease and diagnosis of anal SCC [54].

Surgical management depends on the type of fistula and the presence of active proctitis as shown in Fig. 4. The primary goal of surgery is control of infection/sepsis and seton placement for drainage may be the only intervention. Draining setons can often be removed following initiation of a biologic therapy after inflammation has subsided, though there is not a consensus for the optimal timing of removal (often after >6 months). In the absence of proctitis, an endorectal advancement flap or ligation of inter-sphincteric fistula tract can be considered for higher trans-sphincteric fistulas.

Fistula type	Description	Proctitis?	Medical therapy	Surgical options
Simple	Inter-sphincteric, Low trans-sphincteric, Single opening	Yes	Antibiotics Immunomodulators Biologic	Non-cutting seton
		No		Fistulotomy
Complex	Multiple openings, Atypical location High trans-sphincteric, Perianal abscess, Adjacent structure involved, Horseshoe configuration	Yes	Antibiotics Immunomodulators Biologic	Non-cutting seton Fecal Diversion Proctectomy
		No		Endorectal advancement flap Ligation of Intersphincteric Fistula Tract (LIFT) Acellular fistula plug Stem cell based therapy

Fig. 4. The surgical approach to perianal fistula management based on fistula type and presence of proctitis. (*From*: Pogacnik JS, Salgado G. Perianal Crohn's Disease. Clin Colon Rectal Surg. 2019;32(5):377 to 385. https://doi.org/10.1055/s-0039-1687834).

A recent innovative approach in the treatment of perianal Crohn's disease is the use of mesenchymal stem cells. The largest study to date on this is the Adipose Derived Mesenchymal Stem Cells of Induction of Remission of Perianal Fistulizing Crohn's Disease trial. This randomized controlled trial demonstrated the use of stem cells to produce combined clinical and radiographic remission in 50% of patients treated with stem cells versus 34% in the control group. Clinical remission was observed in 57% versus 41%, and closure of at least 50% of external fistula openings was observed in 71% of patients receiving mesenchymal stem cell treatment versus 53% of the control patients [55]. In contrast to hematopoietic stem cell-based therapy, mesenchymal stem cell therapy shows a milder side effect profile and is associated with lower infection risk and immunogenicity [56].

Postoperative complications

Enterocutaneous fistulas

Enterocutaneous fistulas (ECFs) in Crohn's disease result from penetrating inflammation from the epithelialized lining of the gut that forms a mature tract with the epithelialized lining of the skin. As intestinal contents are expelled on the skin surface, consequences of skin excoriation, sepsis, malnutrition, and poor quality of life ensue. Following ECF formation, 3 phases can be expected: a hypersecretory phase characterized by large volume intestinal losses lasting for 1 to 2 months, an adaptation phase characterized by decreasing fistula output lasting for up to 12 months, and a stabilization phase in which the fistula output further decreases and becomes predictable [57]. Similarly, the management of ECFs can be considered in 4 phases: control of sepsis, management of effluent, protection of skin, and nutritional support [58].

After control of sepsis by ensuring adequate drainage of any intra-abdominal or abdominal wall abscess and antibiotic administration, the nutritional status of the patient should be accurately assessed. This can be done by obtaining serum levels of albumin, transferrin, pre-albumin, and C-reactive protein (CRP) (Fig. 5). While no one laboratory value is the gold standard, these nutritional markers are most useful in combination with each other. The CRP: pre-albumin ratio can be used as a prognostic marker in patients with multiple organ dysfunction [59]. The route of nutritional supplementation is an important consideration as enteral nutrition may increase the ECF output leading to paradoxic dehydration. Total parenteral nutrition, nil per os status, proton pump inhibitors or H2 blockers, and antidiarrheal medications may reduce gastrointestinal secretions to promote spontaneous fistula closure and may be necessary in a high output ECF (>500 mL per day).

Ninety percent of all ECFs (not related to Crohn's disease) will close spontaneously within 5 weeks and do not require operative intervention [60]. However, this number drastically drops to 30% in patients with Crohn's disease [61]. Octreotide can be incorporated for patients who have fistula outputs of greater than 1 L per day, but should be discontinued after 72 hours if there is no significant decrease in fistula output [60]. The continued inflammatory state in Crohn's disease contributes to fistula patency and can be addressed with a biologic agent, though this should only be initiated after sepsis control and intestinal stenosis excluded (ruling out an obstructive etiology) [61].

Endoscopic suturing to promote closure of a chronic fistula has a 23% success rate; however, acute fistulas associated with a recent operation had higher clinical success rates of 79% [62]. Other endoscopic techniques such as through the scope clipping and over the scope clipping have been used to manage iatrogenic perforations less than 2 cm [63]. In light of these findings, the utility of these endoscopic techniques for Crohn's disease may be best suited for post-operative complications, such as a leak from an ileocolic or colonic resection once the underlying disease has been addressed. In clinically stable patients in which intra-abdominal sepsis can be managed with percutaneous drainage,

Nutritional marker	Half Life	Interpretation	Disadvantage
Albumin	14-20 days	Hypoalbuminemia is associated with increased morbidity and mortality in hospitalized patients	Falsely elevated in ECF patients due to GI fluid losses
Pre-albumin	2 days	Low levels predict inflammation and catabolic states	Falsely elevated as a sign of recent intake rather than overall nutrition
Transferrin	8-10 days	Decreased with anemia, folate deficiency, over hydration, catabolic state	False elevation in iron deficiency, dehydration, pregnancy, medications
C- reactive protein	19 hours	Elevated in acute and chronic inflammation	Use alone is non-specific

Fig. 5. Common markers used to assess nutrition and their relative ability to interpret clinical status.

these endoscopic methods may allow for bowel preservation and prevention stoma formation.

Intestinal failure/short bowel syndrome

Patients with Crohn's disease are at particular risk for intestinal failure due to repeated resections from recurrent disease, presence of proximal ECFs, and loss of absorptive capacity due to inflammation and scarring. Given these mechanisms, it is possible to have intestinal failure with an adequate length of bowel. Intestinal failure is determined by inability to maintain growth or homeostasis, and signs are typically ongoing weight loss and a myriad of vitamin deficiencies. While this may typically be considered with less than 180 cm of small bowel remaining, instead it is highly variable depending on the segment of bowel lost/affected, presence of an ileocecal valve, and bowel motility rates.

There are 3 types of short bowel syndrome: Type 1–end jejunostomy, Type 2–jejunocolic anastomosis, and Type 3–jejunoileal anastomosis [64]. Type 2 is the most common type in patients with Crohn's disease given that the terminal ileum is most commonly affected and repeat ileocolic resections may be necessary, with loss of the ileocecal valve at the first operation. This type is characterized by weight loss, diarrhea, and micronutrient deficiencies. With previous discussions highlighting the importance of nutritional status, parenteral nutrition is usually necessary.

Antimotility agents are important to slow down bowel transit time to allow more time for absorption. The recent progress in management of this complication is the glucagon-like peptide 2 (GLP-2) analogs; the most widely studied being teduglutide. This medication has a trophic effect on the small bowel mucosa, primarily by increasing its absorptive capacity. A small study of 13 patients with Crohn's disease had a decrease in their need for parenteral nutrition (69%–8%) after 2 years of therapy [65]. Furthermore, all patients were on intravenous (IV) hydration; 46% of the patients no longer had need for additional hydration and those that still were on IV fluids had their requirement decrease by a median of 3100 mL/wk. Similar studies have supported its use for intestinal failure specifically in patients with Crohn's disease [66,67]. It should be noted that since this is an intestinotropic hormone, frequent monitoring for intestinal neoplasia must be performed and the drug discontinued if neoplasms are found.

Stoma complications

Patients with Crohn's disease may have a temporary or permanent ostomy depending on the location and extent of disease. Following stoma creation, patients may have issues with skin excoriation, leakage form around the ostomy appliance, and foul smells. Preoperative marking and counseling by a trained wound ostomy nurse have been proven to prevent many of these pouching issues [68]. Specifically related to Crohn's disease, pyoderma gangrenosum occurs in less than 1.5% of patients with IBD and may be the result of repeated skin trauma during the removal and application of ostomy devices. A meta-analysis concluded that the presence of a permanent stoma is an independent risk factor and

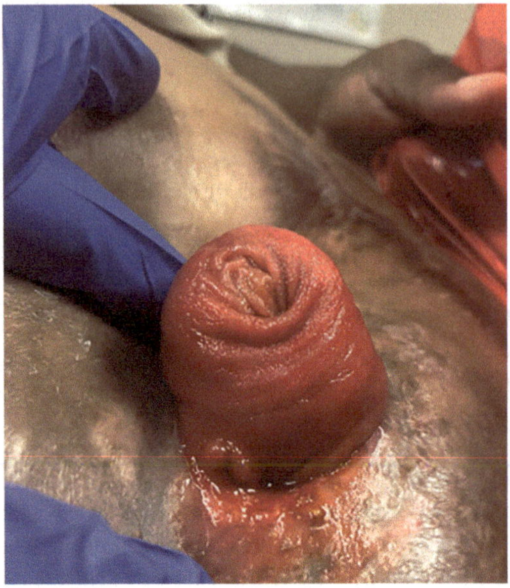

Fig. 6. Peristomal fistula. In this particular case, the effluent from the stoma is entirely from the fistula site, creating a difficult case for pouching.

identified female gender, autoimmune disease, and elevated body mass index (BMI) as additional risk factors for pyoderma [69]. Treatment of pyoderma gangrenosum includes oral steroids, immunomodulators (tacrolimus or cyclosporine), anti-TNF antibodies (infliximab or adalimumab), or topical tacrolimus for small lesions [70].

Peristomal fistulas (Fig. 6) may occur as a manifestation of local disease recurrence in patients with fistulizing disease. This may present as a peristomal abscess or ulceration that drains feculent material. Though the majority of patients with Crohn's disease who undergo revisional stoma procedures due to common complications seemingly unrelated to their disease, examination of many of the pathologic specimens show evidence of active ileal Crohn's disease [68]. After adjusting medical therapy to attempt spontaneous resolution, local surgical revision of the stoma to include resection of the fistulous tract and rematuration of the stoma is necessary. Preoperative ileoscopy may be helpful in assessing the degree of inflammation of the ileum to direct escalation of medical therapy.

SUMMARY

Management of patients with Crohn's disease is often complicated by recurrent disease, malnutrition, and need for chronic immunosuppression. The underlying principles continue to include optimization of nutritional status, controlling the disease process with biologics and avoidance of corticosteroids, and preservation of bowel length when possible. However, there have been several recent advances in both the medical and surgical management of the disease. Medically, more gut-specific biologic agents are available, and biosimilar medications are now available as more accessible and cost-effective strategies. GLP-2 analogues are a new addition in the management of intestinal failure and have decreased the need for parenteral nutrition and its associated complications. Understanding the contribution of the mesentery to inflammation, new surgical techniques such as the Kono-S anastomosis and extended mesenteric resection have been shown to decrease surgical recurrence rates at the anastomosis and decreasing the need for repeated resections.

The clinician taking care of Crohn's disease must consider the increased risk of malignancy related to longstanding chronic inflammation–either in fistula tracts, intestinal strictures, or the anal canal. Many of the immunomodulating medications for the disease can have serious adverse effects including other malignancies. These patients are also at risk for thrombotic events that may only be detected with clinical suspicion.

CLINICS CARE POINTS

- It is imperative to biopsy inflammatory strictures to rule out malignancy.
- All surgical treatments for Crohn's disease should be limited and tailored to the individual problem, with foresight that repeated resections may be necessary.
- Management of Crohn's disease should involve interventions to palliate acute issues (phlegmons, abscess, etc) with drainage in order to start biologic treatment that may allow interal resection and avoid stoma creation.

Disclosure

The authors have nothing to disclose.

References

[1] Ng SC, Shi HY, Hamidi N, et al. Worldwide incidence and prevalence of inflammatory bowel disease in the 21st century: a systematic review of population-based studies. Lancet 2017;390(10114):2769–78.

[2] Polito JM 2nd, Childs B, Mellits ED, et al. Crohn's disease: influence of age at diagnosis on site and clinical type of disease. Gastroenterology 1996;111(3):580–6.

[3] Elloumi H, Sfar S, Ben Abdelaziz A, et al. [Crohn's disease: influence of age at diagnosis on clinical type of disease]. Tunis Med 2007;85(10):862–5.

[4] Silverberg MS, Satsangi J, Ahmad T, et al. Toward an integrated clinical, molecular and serological classification of inflammatory bowel disease: report of a Working Party of the 2005 Montreal World Congress of Gastroenterology. Can J Gastroenterol 2005;19(Suppl A): 5A–36A.

[5] Cosnes J, Bourrier A, Laharie D, et al. Early administration of azathioprine vs conventional management of Crohn's Disease: a randomized controlled trial. Gastroenterology 2013;145(4):755–8.

[6] Feuerstein JD, Cheifetz AS. Crohn Disease: Epidemiology, Diagnosis, and Management. Mayo Clin Proc 2017;92(7):1088–103.
[7] Blackwell J, Selinger C, Raine T, et al. Steroid use and misuse: a key performance indicator in the management of IBD. Frontline Gastroenterol 2021;12(3):207–13.
[8] Dorrington AM, Selinger CP, Parkes GC, et al. The Historical Role and Contemporary Use of Corticosteroids in Inflammatory Bowel Disease. J Crohns Colitis 2020;14(9):1316–29.
[9] Claytor J, Kumar P, Ananthakrishnan AN, et al. Mild Crohn's Disease: Definition and Management. Curr Gastroenterol Rep 2023;25(3):45–51.
[10] Kuenzig ME, Rezaie A, Kaplan GG, et al. Budesonide for the Induction and Maintenance of Remission in Crohn's Disease: Systematic Review and Meta-Analysis for the Cochrane Collaboration. J Can Assoc Gastroenterol. 2018;1(4):159–73.
[11] Sandborn WJ, Gasink C, Gao L-L, et al. Ustekinumab induction and maintenance therapy in refractory Crohn's disease. N Engl J Med 2012;367(16):1519–28.
[12] Sandborn WJ, Feagan BG, Rutgeerts P, et al. Vedolizumab as induction and maintenance therapy for Crohn's disease. N Engl J Med 2013;369(8):711–21.
[13] Caio G, Lungaro L, Caputo F, et al. Nutritional Treatment in Crohn's Disease. Nutrients 2021;13(5):1628.
[14] Traiki TA Bin, Alshammari SA, Aljomah NA, et al. The impact of preoperative total parenteral nutrition on the surgical complications of Crohn's disease: A retrospective cohort study. Saudi J Gastroenterol Off J Saudi Gastroenterol Assoc. 2023;29(3):158–63.
[15] Verburgt CM, Ghiboub M, Benninga MA, et al. Nutritional Therapy Strategies in Pediatric Crohn's Disease. Nutrients 2021;13(1):212.
[16] Gordon-Dixon A, Gore-Rodney J, Hampal R, et al. The role of exclusive enteral nutrition in the pre-operative optimisation of adult patients with Crohn's disease. A systematic review. Clin Nutr ESPEN 2021;46:99–105.
[17] Yu Y, Chen K-C, Chen J. Exclusive enteral nutrition versus corticosteroids for treatment of pediatric Crohn's disease: a meta-analysis. World J Pediatr. 2019;15(1):26–36.
[18] Aksan A, Farrag K, Blumenstein I, et al. Chronic intestinal failure and short bowel syndrome in Crohn's disease. World J Gastroenterol 2021;27(24):3440–65.
[19] Ford MM. Crohn's Disease Obstructions. Clin Colon Rectal Surg 2021;34(4):227–32.
[20] Gorgun E, Cengiz TB, Aytac E, et al. Does laparoscopic ileal pouch-anal anastomosis reduce infertility compared with open approach? Surgery 2019;166(4):670–7.
[21] Coremans L, Strubbe B, Peeters H. Venous thromboembolism in patients with inflammatory bowel disease: review of literature and practical algorithms. Acta Gastroenterol Belg 2021;84(1):79–85.
[22] Chu TPC, Grainge MJ, Card TR. The risk of venous thromboembolism during and after hospitalisation in patients with inflammatory bowel disease activity. Aliment Pharmacol Ther 2018;48(10):1099–108.
[23] Giannotta M, Tapete G, Emmi G, et al. Thrombosis in inflammatory bowel diseases: what's the link? Thromb J 2015;13:14.
[24] Patel SV, Liberman SA, Burgess PL, et al. The American Society of Colon and Rectal Surgeons Clinical Practice Guidelines for the Reduction of Venous Thromboembolic Disease in Colorectal Surgery. Dis Colon Rectum 2023;66(9):1162–73.
[25] Sleiman J, El Ouali S, Qazi T, et al. Prevention and Treatment of Stricturing Crohn's Disease - Perspectives and Challenges. Expet Rev Gastroenterol Hepatol 2021;15(4):401–11.
[26] Yamamoto H, Yano T, Araki A, et al. Guidelines for endoscopic balloon dilation in treating Crohn's disease-associated small intestinal strictures (supplement to the Clinical Practice Guidelines for Enteroscopy). Dig Endosc 2022;34(7):1278–96.
[27] Bettenworth D, Gustavsson A, Atreja A, et al. A Pooled Analysis of Efficacy, Safety, and Long-term Outcome of Endoscopic Balloon Dilation Therapy for Patients with Stricturing Crohn's Disease. Inflamm Bowel Dis 2017;23(1):133–42.

[28] Di Nardo G, Oliva S, Passariello M, et al. Intralesional steroid injection after endoscopic balloon dilation in pediatric Crohn's disease with stricture: a prospective, randomized, double-blind, controlled trial. Gastrointest Endosc 2010;72(6):1201–8.
[29] Brooker JC, Beckett CG, Saunders BP, et al. Long-acting steroid injection after endoscopic dilation of anastomotic Crohn's strictures may improve the outcome: a retrospective case series. Endoscopy 2003;35(4):333–7.
[30] East JE, Brooker JC, Rutter MD, et al. A pilot study of intrastricture steroid versus placebo injection after balloon dilatation of Crohn's strictures. Clin Gastroenterol Hepatol 2007;5(9): 1065–9.
[31] Chandrasinghe P. Surgical Management of Small Bowel Crohn's Disease. Front Surg 2022;9:759668; https://doi.org/10.3389/fsurg.2022.759668.
[32] Chin YH, Jain SR, Lee MH, et al. Small bowel adenocarcinoma in Crohn's disease: a systematic review and meta-analysis of the prevalence, manifestation, histopathology, and outcomes. Int J Colorectal Dis 2022;37(1):239–50.
[33] Hussain T, Jeganathan NA, Karagkounis G, et al. Small bowel adenocarcinoma in Crohn's disease: a rare but devastating complication. Tech Coloproctol 2020;24(10):1055–62.
[34] Shah SC, Itzkowitz SH. Colorectal Cancer in Inflammatory Bowel Disease: Mechanisms and Management. Gastroenterology 2022;162(3):715–30.e3.
[35] Coviello LC, Stein SL. Surgical management of nonpolypoid colorectal lesions and strictures in colonic inflammatory bowel disease. Gastrointest Endosc Clin N Am 2014;24(3): 447–54.
[36] Click B, Merchea A, Colibaseanu DT, et al. Ileocolic Resection for Crohn Disease: The Influence of Different Surgical Techniques on Perioperative Outcomes, Recurrence Rates, and Endoscopic Surveillance. Inflamm Bowel Dis 2022;28(2):289–98.
[37] McLeod RS, Wolff BG, Ross S, et al, Investigators of the CAST Trial. Recurrence of Crohn's disease after ileocolic resection is not affected by anastomotic type: results of a multicenter, randomized, controlled trial. Dis Colon Rectum 2009;52(5):919–27.
[38] Luglio G, Corcione F. Stapled versus handsewn methods for ileocolic anastomoses. Tech Coloproctol 2019;23(11):1093–5.
[39] Turri G, Carvello M, Ben David N, et al. Intriguing Role of the Mesentery in Ileocolic Crohn's Disease. Clin Colon Rectal Surg 2022;35(4):321–7.
[40] Becker MAJ, Does de Willebois EMLV, Bemelman WA, et al. Role of the Mesentery in Crohn's Terminal Ileitis. Clin Colon Rectal Surg 2022;35(4):316–20.
[41] Peyrin-Biroulet L, Gonzalez F, Dubuquoy L, et al. Mesenteric fat as a source of C reactive protein and as a target for bacterial translocation in Crohn's disease. Gut 2012;61(1):78–85.
[42] da Silva FAR, Pascoal LB, Dotti I, et al. Whole transcriptional analysis identifies markers of B, T and plasma cell signaling pathways in the mesenteric adipose tissue associated with Crohn's disease. J Transl Med 2020;18(1):44.
[43] Kono T, Fichera A. Surgical Treatment for Crohn's Disease: A Role of Kono-S Anastomosis in the West. Clin Colon Rectal Surg 2020;33(6):335–43.
[44] Ng CH, Chin YH, Lin SY, et al. Kono-S anastomosis for Crohn's disease: a systemic review, meta-analysis, and meta-regression. Surg Today 2021;51(4):493–501.
[45] Bislenghi G, Devriendt S, Wolthuis A, et al. Totally stapled Kono-S anastomosis for Crohn's disease. Tech Coloproctol 2022;26(3):213–6.
[46] Alshantti A, Hind D, Hancock L, et al. The Role of Kono-S Anastomosis and Mesenteric Resection in Reducing Recurrence after Surgery for Crohn's Disease: A Systematic Review. Colorectal Dis 2021;23:7–17.
[47] Holubar SD, Gunter RL, Click BH, et al. Mesenteric Excision and Exclusion for Ileocolic Crohn's Disease: Feasibility and Safety of an Innovative, Combined Surgical Approach With Extended Mesenteric Excision and Kono-S Anastomosis. Dis Colon Rectum 2022;65(1):e5–13.
[48] Pogacnik JS, Salgado G. Perianal Crohn's Disease. Clin Colon Rectal Surg 2019;32(5): 377–85.

[49] Lightner AL, Regueiro M. Anorectal Strictures in Complex Perianal CD: How to Approach? Clin Colon Rectal Surg 2022;35(1):44–50.
[50] Lightner AL, Click B, Yamamoto T, et al. Management of Isolated Anal Strictures in Crohn's Disease. Dis Colon Rectum 2020;63(12):1639–47.
[51] Parian AM, Obi M, Fleshner P, et al. Management of Perianal Crohn's Disease. Am J Gastroenterol 2023;118(8):1323–31.
[52] Kane S, Khatibi B, Reddy D. Higher incidence of abnormal Pap smears in women with inflammatory bowel disease. Am J Gastroenterol 2008;103(3):631–6.
[53] Lightner AL, Moncrief SB, Smyrk TC, et al. Long-standing Crohn's disease and its implication on anal squamous cell cancer management. Int J Colorectal Dis 2017;32(5):661–6.
[54] Kotsafti A, Scarpa M, Angriman I, et al. Fistula-Related Cancer in Crohn's Disease: A Systematic Review. Cancers 2021;13(6); https://doi.org/10.3390/cancers13061445.
[55] Panés J, García-Olmo D, Van Assche G, et al. Expanded allogeneic adipose-derived mesenchymal stem cells (Cx601) for complex perianal fistulas in Crohn's disease: a phase 3 randomised, double-blind controlled trial. Lancet 2016;388(10051):1281–90.
[56] Wang R, Yao Q, Chen W, et al. Stem cell therapy for Crohn's disease: systematic review and meta-analysis of preclinical and clinical studies. Stem Cell Res Ther 2021;12(1):463.
[57] Ghimire P. Management of Enterocutaneous Fistula: A Review. JNMA J Nepal Med Assoc 2022;60(245):93–100.
[58] Kennedy GD. Expert Commentary on the Management of Enterocutaneous Fistula. Dis Colon Rectum 2019;62(8):910–1.
[59] Badrasawi M, Shahar S, Sagap I. Nutritional Management in Enterocutaneous Fistula. What is the evidence? Malays J Med Sci 2015;22(4):6–16.
[60] Cowan K.B. and Cassaro S., *Enterocutaneous Fistula*, In: *StatPearls*. 2023: Treasure Island, FL.
[61] Papa A, Lopetuso LR, Minordi LM, et al. A modern multidisciplinary approach to the treatment of enterocutaneous fistulas in Crohn's disease patients. Expet Rev Gastroenterol Hepatol 2020;14(9):857–65.
[62] Sharaiha RZ, Kumta NA, DeFilippis EM, et al. A Large Multicenter Experience With Endoscopic Suturing for Management of Gastrointestinal Defects and Stent Anchorage in 122 Patients: A Retrospective Review. J Clin Gastroenterol 2016;50(5):388–92.
[63] Singh RR, Nussbaum JS, Kumta NA. Endoscopic management of perforations, leaks and fistulas. Transl Gastroenterol Hepatol 2018;3:85.
[64] Buchman AL, Scolapio J, Fryer J. AGA technical review on short bowel syndrome and intestinal transplantation. Gastroenterology 2003;124(4):1111–34.
[65] Kochar B, Long MD, Shelton E, et al. Safety and Efficacy of Teduglutide (Gattex) in Patients With Crohn's Disease and Need for Parenteral Support Due to Short Bowel Syndrome-associated Intestinal Failure. J Clin Gastroenterol 2017;51(6):508–11.
[66] Jeppesen PB, Gabe SM, Seidner DL, et al. Factors Associated With Response to Teduglutide in Patients With Short-Bowel Syndrome and Intestinal Failure. Gastroenterology 2018;154(4):874–85.
[67] Al Draiweesh S, Ma C, Gregor JC, et al. Teduglutide in Patients With Active Crohn's Disease and Short Bowel Syndrome. Inflamm Bowel Dis 2019;25(9):e109.
[68] Aboulian A. Ostomy Complications in Crohn's Disease. Clin Colon Rectal Surg 2019;32(4):314–22.
[69] States V, O'Brien S, Rai JP, et al. Pyoderma Gangrenosum in Inflammatory Bowel Disease: A Systematic Review and Meta-Analysis. Dig Dis Sci 2020;65(9):2675–85.
[70] Rogler G, Singh A, Kavanaugh A, et al. Extraintestinal Manifestations of Inflammatory Bowel Disease: Current Concepts, Treatment, and Implications for Disease Management. Gastroenterology 2021;161(4):1118–32.

Advances in Surgery 58 (2024) 35–47

ADVANCES IN SURGERY

Poverty and Its Impact on Surgical Care

Adrian Diaz, MD, MPH,
Timothy M. Pawlik, MD, PhD, MPH, MTS, MBA*

Division of Surgical Oncology, Department of Surgery, The Ohio State University Wexner Medical Center, James Comprehensive Cancer Center, Columbus, OH 43210, USA

Keywords

• Surgery • Poverty • Access • Outcomes • Social determinants

Key points

- There is a profound relationship between poverty, access to surgical care, and quality of post-operative outcomes.
- It is critical to understand the multifaceted nature of poverty and how poverty extends beyond financial constraints to encompass barriers to healthcare access, limited health literacy, nutritional challenges, and the complex interplay of social factors.
- Recognizing and addressing these disparities is not only an ethical obligation but also an urgent imperative for the entire healthcare community.

INTRODUCTION

Often a life-saving and transformative medical intervention, surgery is a cornerstone of modern healthcare that contributes significantly to the health and well-being of individuals. Today, there are at least 50 million operations performed annually in the United States [1] with the average American expected to undergo 7 operations during their lifetime [2]. Surgery-related spending now accounts for more than half the annual budget of the Centers for Medicare & Medicaid Services, underscoring the substantial financial and resource commitment within the healthcare system [3]. A growing body of evidence suggests, however, that the surgical realm is not immune to the

*Corresponding author. Department of Surgery, The Ohio State University Wexner Medical Center, 395 West 12th Avenue, Suite 670, Columbus, OH 43210. *E-mail address:* tim.pawlik@osumc.edu

https://doi.org/10.1016/j.yasu.2024.04.003

pervasive influence of socioeconomic disparities, particularly the insidious grip of poverty.

Despite advances in surgical care over the last decade, disparities in access to high-quality care continue to contribute to inequitable outcomes. In fact, a growing body of literature has highlighted the role of social determinants of health (SDoH) such as patient-level socioeconomic status, sex, race/ethnicity, and insurance status, among others, in dictating surgical care processes and outcomes [4–6]. For example, patients in the poorest 1% of the income distribution have a 14.6-year reduction in life expectancy compared with individuals in the richest 1% strata [7]. Several studies have suggested that, alongside patient sociodemographic factors, community characteristics may also play a critical role in determining access to health care [5,8–10]. For example, areas characterized by financial insecurity and limited social services are more likely to have poor access to health care resources and facilities [11–13].

The authors herein provide an overview of the existing body of evidence concerning poverty and its repercussions on surgical care access and outcomes. The authors offer a definition of poverty and note its multifaceted nature, acknowledging the various dimensions it encompasses. Subsequently, the intricate interplay between poverty and surgical care relative to SDoH, barriers impeding access, and the complex web of social factors influencing surgical outcomes are explored. In addition to highlighting how poverty contributes to surgical complications, recovery delays, and the perpetuation of disparities in healthcare, the authors propose strategies aimed at enhancing access to surgical care and improving surgical outcomes across the entire economic spectrum.

DEFINING POVERTY AND ITS MULTIFACETED NATURE

Poverty is a complex and multifaceted social issue that has far-reaching implications for individuals and communities. To effectively understand its impact on surgical patients, it is crucial to define poverty and characterize its many dimensions. Poverty is not limited to the absence of financial resources; rather, poverty encompasses a wide range of factors that influence an individual's well-being, health, and access to medical care. At its core, poverty is often defined as the state of lacking financial resources and material possessions required to meet basic human needs such as food, clothing, shelter, and access to healthcare. However, this definition belies a much deeper and multifaceted problem. In the context of healthcare and surgery, poverty extends beyond the financial aspect and manifests in several dimensions.

The most common association with poverty is income, or lack thereof. In this sense, poverty refers to a person or household's inability to meet their basic needs because of insufficient income. In impoverished communities, patients may lack the financial means to access quality healthcare or afford surgical procedures that can lead to delayed diagnoses and treatments. Poverty also limits access to healthcare services, creating barriers to essential medical and surgical interventions. Individuals in impoverished areas often experience inadequate healthcare infrastructure [14,15], long travel distances [16–18], and limited availability of surgical facilities [16,19]. Geographic isolation and limited access to healthcare facilities are common in impoverished areas. Patients may have to travel long distances to reach a surgical center, increasing the challenges to obtain timely care.

Lack of insurance or financial resources makes seeking surgical care a challenging endeavor. Educational poverty is a critical aspect of understanding the impact of poverty on surgical outcomes. Limited access to quality education can result in low health literacy among patients, making it difficult for individuals to comprehend medical recommendations, adhere to postoperative care instructions, and make informed decisions regarding surgical procedures. Poverty can take a significant toll on mental and emotional well-being. The stress, anxiety, and depression associated with economic hardships can hinder a patient's ability to cope with surgery, adhere to treatment plans, and engage effectively in the rehabilitation process. Poverty is intrinsically linked to a range of SDoH, including housing conditions, employment opportunities, and exposure to environmental hazards [20–22]. Patients living in impoverished communities often face greater health risks, including higher rates of chronic diseases, which can complicate surgical outcomes. Fig. 1 is an example of a conceptual model attempting to explain how SDoH, including poverty, may ultimately impact their access to and outcomes after surgery.

ACCESS TO HEALTHCARE SERVICES

Despite advances in surgical care over the last decade, disparities in access to high-quality care continue to contribute to inequitable outcomes. Specifically, patients residing in persistently poor counties are at a disproportionately increased risk of worse access to surgical care. A study that analyzed hospitals

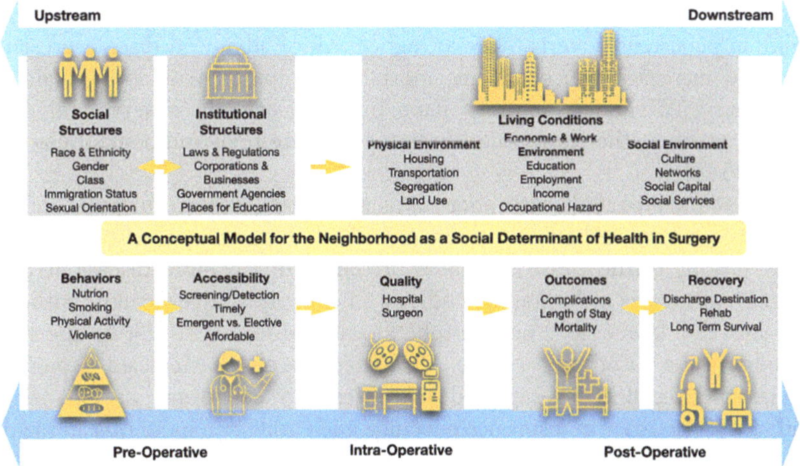

Fig. 1. Conceptual model of neighborhoods and surgical care delivery.

with surgical capacity from 2005 to 2015 reported that hospital closures resulted in a 16% increase in the number of individuals who had to travel greater than 30 minutes to the nearest hospital that offered adult inpatient surgical services [16]. Of note, most of these individuals with worsening access to surgical services live in areas with higher levels of poverty. A separate study demonstrated similar patterns for cancer care [18]. In yet another study, 1 in 10 Americans were noted to have limited geographic access to any hospital with emergency surgical capabilities, and 1 in 4 had limited access to any hospital with advanced clinical resources. Regions characterized by a preponderance of uninsured individuals, publicly insured populations, as well as racial and ethnic minority groups in micropolitan and rural areas had the highest likelihood of limited access to healthcare services [23].

Concerns about decreasing access to surgical care have been raised broadly but more specifically among access-sensitive surgical conditions. Access-sensitive surgical conditions are diagnoses requiring surgery that preferably is planned (ie, elective) but, when access is limited, may be delayed until worsening symptoms require riskier and costlier unplanned (ie, emergency, or urgent) surgery. For example, in a study of patients who underwent colon resection for a primary diagnosis of either diverticulitis or colon cancer (ie, access-sensitive surgical conditions), patients residing in vulnerable communities characterized by high social vulnerability were more likely to undergo an unplanned (ie, emergency or urgent) operation [24]. In a different study of unplanned surgery, patients residing in communities with the least social vulnerability more often had an elective operation. In contrasts, individuals from areas with higher vulnerability were not only more likely to undergo unplanned procedures but also had worse outcomes, characterized by increased mortality and a higher incidence of additional surgeries within a month [9]. For cancer specifically, Papageorge and colleagues reported on patients with non-small cell lung, breast, and colorectal cancer, and noted that individuals living in persistent poverty were at higher risk of advanced disease presentation and increased cancer-specific mortality compared with individuals not in poverty [25]. These findings have been consistently observed in other settings and for other cancers, including gastrointestinal and hepatobiliary tumors [26–29].

Beyond poverty itself, insurance status can affect access to surgical care. For example, patients without insurance or with inadequate insurance more often delay seeking medical care and often present with advanced disease across a range of diagnoses including appendicitis, cholecystitis, diverticulitis, aortic aneurysms, and lower extremity peripheral artery disease [30–33]. In one study examining the association of the Affordable Care Act Medicaid expansion, Loehrer and colleagues reported that Medicaid expansion was associated with a 7.5% increase in insurance coverage and earlier receipt of care in the disease course [34]. In a separate study, Zhao and colleagues compared patients with private insurance with individuals who were uninsured or Medicaid-insured. Of note, uninsured or Medicaid-insured patients were significantly more likely to be diagnosed with late-stage cancer, leading to worse short- and long-term outcomes including death [35].

The issue of access to healthcare services remains a critical concern, with profound implications for surgical care and outcomes. Despite notable advancements in surgical practices, disparities in access persist, creating inequities in healthcare delivery. Patients in persistently poor counties face heightened barriers to access surgical care, particularly in rural and micropolitan areas, where healthcare facilities may be scarce. Concerns surrounding decreased access to surgical care are particularly prominent in access-sensitive surgical conditions in which timely elective procedures can be postponed until symptoms worsen, necessitating more urgent and costlier interventions. Poverty, insurance status, and geographic factors play intricate roles in access to surgical care, exacerbating disparities, and impacting outcomes, especially for patients with cancer. Medicaid expansion under the Affordable Care Act has improved insurance coverage and facilitated earlier access to care, but challenges persist. In turn, there is a need for ongoing efforts to address disparities in surgical care access and enhance patient outcomes.

SURGICAL OUTCOMES AND POVERTY

An evolving body of literature has consistently demonstrated a connection between SDoH, especially poverty, and surgical outcomes. For example, Lima and colleagues reported on over 300,000 patients who underwent either a lung resection, a colectomy, coronary artery bypass graft, or a lower extremity joint replacement [36]. In this article, patients who resided in areas of persistent poverty were at increased risk of serious postoperative complications, 30-day readmission, 30-day mortality, and higher expenditures (Fig. 2) [36]. Similarly, Azap and colleagues demonstrated that among patients undergoing cardiac surgery, including aortic and mitral valve repair, Medicare care beneficiaries residing in counties with persistent poverty had a higher odds of undergoing

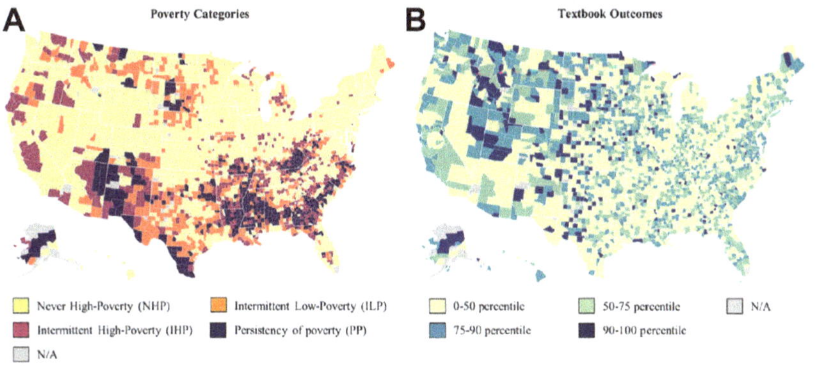

Fig. 2. County-level PP categories across the US (*A*), county-level rates of postoperative TO achievement (*B*).

a nonelective operation, as well as an increased odds of 30- and 90-day mortality after surgery [37].

The neighborhood in which one lives has an close relationship with poverty and therefore, this "lived environment" impacts patient outcomes related to surgery [5,38,39]. In addition, patient social vulnerability, as a whole, has a strong association the risk of unfavorable post-operative outcomes following procedures such as colon or lung resection, coronary artery bypass, and hip and knee replacement [40]. In particular, individuals living in communities characterized by high social vulnerability tend to experience more adverse post-operative outcomes. Of note, the impact of social vulnerability is particularly pronounced among Black and minority patients, as opposed to their White counterparts. Hyer and colleagues reported that individuals residing in communities characterized by a high social vulnerability index had a reduced likelihood of undergoing high-risk cancer surgery at high-volume hospitals [41,42]. This trend was particularly evident among patients who lived in high social vulnerability areas, resulting in an increased incidence of postoperative complications and mortality.

Of note, some of the increased risk of adverse outcomes among patients living in poverty could be mitigated by undergoing surgery at high-volume hospitals [42,43]. For example, in assessing colon resection for conditions like diverticulitis or cancer, patients hailing from high social vulnerability areas more frequently underwent non-elective operations versus individuals from low social vulnerability regions [24]. Carmicheal and colleagues demonstrated that patients originating from high social vulnerability areas were more likely to undergo emergent cholecystectomies versus individuals from low social vulnerability areas [40]. Additionally, Azap and colleagues reported an association between the social vulnerability index and decreased likelihood to undergo resection or transplantation for early-stage hepatocellular carcinoma (HCC). These data collectively suggest that individuals living in highly vulnerable communities encountered barriers in accessing surgical care and receiving appropriate interventions for early-stage HCC [44]. In turn, these studies underscore how patients from areas with high vulnerability and lower socioeconomic status face significant challenges to obtain timely, high-quality surgical care. These challenges, in turn, contribute to the widening disparities in surgical outcomes and overall health.

Understanding the effect of poverty on surgical outcomes is complex and intertwined with other factors. Specifically, poverty and race and ethnicity are closely related, and the intersection of race, poverty, and surgical outcomes is notable. Specifically, Black patients have worse outcomes compared with White patients following a myriad of different elective and emergent operations. For example, Black patients have an estimated 20% to 50% higher risk of mortality following a wide range of common operations versus White patients [45–49]. Although the mechanisms for racial disparities related to surgical care are complicated and multifactorial, emerging data have suggested that Black patients are more likely to present later in the course of their care and have higher odds of needing an emergent operation [50–52]. Additionally, other data suggest that Black patients are more likely to undergo an operation at centers that have worse quality of care [10,53].

Overall, there is an intricate connection between SDoH, particularly poverty, and surgical outcomes. As noted, data have consistently demonstrated that patients residing in persistently impoverished areas are at increased risk of facing serious postoperative complications, readmissions, and higher healthcare expenditures. Social vulnerability plays a significant role in influencing surgical outcomes, with patients from communities characterized by high social vulnerability experiencing a greater likelihood of adverse postoperative results. This impact is particularly pronounced among Black and minority patients, highlighting disparities in surgical care. While the challenges posed by poverty and social vulnerability are undeniable, some risks appear to be mitigated when surgery is performed at high-volume hospitals. Addressing disparities and the complex interplay with other factors is needed to ensure equitable access to high-quality surgical care and improve surgical outcomes for all patients, regardless of their socioeconomic circumstances. Efforts in this direction hold the potential to reduce disparities and enhance the overall healthcare equity.

STRATEGIES FOR IMPROVING SURGICAL OUTCOMES

Given the disparities in access to surgical care, as well as the differences in outcomes related to SDoH and poverty, practical approaches to address and alleviate surgical disparities are needed. In particular, pragmatic strategies are needed for healthcare professionals, policymakers, and advocates to drive initiatives to improve surgical care for all, irrespective of socioeconomic circumstances. To this point, several state and federal interventions have been implemented to combat poverty. To date, perhaps the most notable national policy intervention aimed at addressing the intersection of poverty and healthcare has been Medicaid expansion. Medicaid expansion under the Affordable Care Act (ACA) sought to extend Medicaid eligibility to more low-income adults, providing these individuals with access to essential healthcare services. By increasing income thresholds, Medicaid Expansion has reduced the number of individuals who are uninsured in those states that adopted the ACA; in turn, this adoption of Medicaid expansion has helped millions of Americans gain vital health coverage and improve overall healthcare access and outcomes [54].

Medicaid expansion has had profound effects on mitigating the effect of poverty on access to and outcomes related to surgery [55]. For example, the proportion of uninsured among trauma patients in states that expanded Medicaid decreased by 16% points [56]. Similarly, albeit less pronounced trends, have been observed among emergency general surgery and vascular surgery patients [34]. Beyond insurance coverage, Medicaid expansion has also been associated with more timely access to surgery. Specifically, in states that expanded Medicaid, patients with cancer were more likely to be diagnosed with early or localized disease following Medicaid expansion [57,58]. In a separate study of acute general and vascular surgery conditions, expansion was associated with an increased likelihood of patients presenting with early uncomplicated disease, such as unruptured appendicitis or diverticulitis without perforation [34].

In addition to improved access to surgery, Medicaid expansion has driven improvements in quality of care. For example, in states that have expanded Medicaid, patients were more likely to undergo minimally invasive versus open surgery for acute conditions like appendicitis and cholecystitis. Moreover, patients in Medicaid expansion states experienced fewer amputations for acute limb ischemia [34]. Patients with complex cancers, such as pancreatic and esophageal tumors, who reside in Medicaid expansion state, were more likely to undergo surgery at high-volume and high-quality hospitals [59–61]. While evidence on reduced inpatient mortality is somewhat inconclusive, an emerging body of research has suggested a possible decline in mortality among patients undergoing surgery in Medicaid expansion states. For example, recent population-level analyses of low-income adults pre- and post-Medicaid expansion indicated an overall mortality reduction of approximately 10% among eligible Medicaid beneficiaries [62,63].

In addition to clinical outcomes, Medicaid expansion may be associated with lower financial pressures on patients undergoing surgical procedures. Notably, earlier presentation of disease (eg, appendicitis before perforation) may be related to lower cost-related delays [34,57,58]. Additionally, the improved financial risk protection afforded to patients by Medicaid expansion has resulted in lower out-of-pocket costs and thereby, a lower likelihood of catastrophic health expenditure [64–67]. Liu and colleagues conducted an analysis using the Medical Expenditure Panel Survey to assess the impact of ACA on the financial stability of injured patients [66]. Before ACA implementation, over 20% of patients–regardless of income level or insurance type–who were admitted to the hospital for traumatic injuries faced catastrophic healthcare expenses [66]. Notably, among injured patients with income levels eligible for Medicaid expansion, there was a 30% decrease in out-of-pocket costs and a nearly 40% risk reduction experiencing catastrophic healthcare expenses following ACA implementation [66].

To enhance outcomes for at-risk populations, a comprehensive approach that considers each step in a patient's healthcare journey is essential. Certain high-risk individuals living near high-quality hospitals may not access these centers, highlighting the need to better understand how barriers such as health literacy, insurance limitations, or personal preferences impede access to high volume care [41,68]. Triaging patients to nearby, high-quality hospitals within small geographic areas could serve as a model to enhance the quality of surgical care [69]. For individuals residing farther from such hospitals, overcoming the burden of travel to access higher-quality care will be critical. Health systems need to explore innovative solutions like coordinating transportation, establishing patient navigator programs, as well as collaborating with local community and business stakeholders to ensure complex operations for high-risk patients occur at centers of excellence [70]. Beyond merely reporting disparate care, the authors must move toward measuring and demonstrating equity in outcomes by race and socioeconomic status. Providers and hospitals should be held accountable for the equity of healthcare that is delivered, similar to how other quality metrics are scrutinized. To this end, many payers and providers have begun to issue "equity reports" which demonstrate quality outcomes stratified by race, ethnicity, sex, and socioeconomic status [71–74].

SUMMARY

There is profound relationship between poverty, access to surgical care, and quality of post-operative outcomes. As the US population ages and the socio-economic divide widens, the impact of poverty on surgical care should be priority among surgeons, researchers, and policy makers. It is critical to understand the multifaceted nature of poverty and how poverty extends beyond financial constraints to encompass barriers to healthcare access, limited health literacy, nutritional challenges, and the complex interplay of social factors. Poverty not only increases the likelihood of surgical complications but also contributes to delayed recovery, perpetuating a cycle of disparity that adversely affects individuals living in impoverished circumstances. Recognizing and addressing these disparities is not only an ethical obligation but also an urgent imperative for the entire healthcare community. The solutions are complex, requiring collaborative efforts among healthcare professionals, policy-makers, and the community at large to ensure equitable surgical care for all. The path ahead is challenging, but it is one that must be taken, as every patient deserves the opportunity for a healthier and more equitable future.

CLINICS CARE POINTS

- Poverty worsens access to healthcare and surgery and also increases the likelihood of surgical complications contributing to delayed recovery and increase morbidity.
- Recognizing and addressing these disparities is not only an ethical obligation but also an urgent imperative for the entire healthcare community.

References

[1] Hall MJ. Ambulatory surgery data from hospitals and ambulatory surgery centers: United States, 2010. Natl Health Stat Report 2017;(102):15.

[2] Lee PHU, Gawande AA. The number of surgical procedures in an American lifetime in 3 states. J Am Coll Surg 2008;207(3):S75.

[3] Kaye DR, Luckenbaugh AN, Oerline M, et al. Understanding the Costs Associated With Surgical Care Delivery in the Medicare Population. Ann Surg 2020;271(1):23–8.

[4] Zogg CK, Scott JW, Jiang W, et al. Differential access to care: The role of age, insurance, and income on race/ethnicity-related disparities in adult perforated appendix admission rates. Surgery 2016;160(5):1145–54.

[5] Diaz A, Hyer JM, Barmash E, et al. County-level Social Vulnerability is Associated With Worse Surgical Outcomes Especially Among Minority Patients. Ann Surg 2021;274(6):881–91.

[6] De Oliveira GS, McCarthy RJ, Wolf MS, et al. The impact of health literacy in the care of surgical patients: a qualitative systematic review. BMC Surg 2015;15(1):86.
[7] Chetty R, Stepner M, Abraham S, et al. The Association Between Income and Life Expectancy in the United States, 2001-2014. JAMA 2016;315(16):1750.
[8] Kind AJH, Buckingham WR. Making Neighborhood-Disadvantage Metrics Accessible — The Neighborhood Atlas. N Engl J Med 2018;378(26):2456–8.
[9] Zhang Y, Kunnath N, Dimick JB, et al. Social Vulnerability And Outcomes For Access-Sensitive Surgical Conditions Among Medicare Beneficiaries. Health Aff 2022;41(5): 671–9.
[10] Diaz A, Lindau ST, Obeng-Gyasi S, et al. Association of Hospital Quality and Neighborhood Deprivation With Mortality After Inpatient Surgery Among Medicare Beneficiaries. JAMA Netw Open 2023;6(1):e2253620; https://doi.org/10.1001/jamanetworkopen.2022.53620.
[11] Chan L, Hart LG, Goodman DC. Geographic access to health care for rural Medicare beneficiaries. J Rural Health 2006;22(2):140–6.
[12] Hung P, Henning-Smith CE, Casey MM, et al. Access To Obstetric Services In Rural Counties Still Declining, With 9 Percent Losing Services, 2004–14. Health Aff 2017;36(9): 1663–71.
[13] McGinnis JM. Income, Life Expectancy, and Community Health: Underscoring the Opportunity. JAMA 2016;315(16):1709–10.
[14] Balasubramanian S, Jones E. Hospital closures and the current healthcare climate: the future of rural hospitals in the USA. Rural Rem Health 2016;16(3):3935.
[15] Chaudhary MA, Shah AA, Zogg CK, et al. Differences in rural and urban outcomes: a national inspection of emergency general surgery patients. J Surg Res 2017;218:277–84.
[16] Diaz A, Schoenbrunner A, Pawlik TM. Trends in the Geospatial Distribution of Inpatient Adult Surgical Services across the United States. Ann Surg 2021;273(1):121–7.
[17] Diaz A, Schoenbrunner A, Cloyd J, et al. Geographic distribution of adult inpatient surgery capability in the USA. J Gastrointest Surg 2019;23(8):1652–60.
[18] Diaz A, Schoenbrunner A, Pawlik TM. Trends in the Geospatial Distribution of Adult Inpatient Surgical Cancer Care Across the United States. J Gastrointest Surg 2020;24(9): 2127–34.
[19] Kaufman BG, Thomas SR, Randolph RK, et al. The Rising Rate of Rural Hospital Closures. J Rural Health 2016;32(1):35–43.
[20] Adler NE, Glymour MM, Fielding J. Addressing Social Determinants of Health and Health Inequalities. JAMA 2016;316(16):1641–2.
[21] Artiga S, Hinton E. Beyond health care: the role of social determinants in Promoting health and health equity. KFF; 2018. Available at: https://www.kff.org/disparities-policy/issue-brief/beyond-health-care-the-role-of-social-determinants-in-promoting-health-and-health-equity/. [Accessed 24 June 2020].
[22] Bharmal N, Derose KP, Felician MF, et al. Understanding the upstream social determinants of health. RAND Corporation; 2015. Available at: https://www.rand.org/pubs/working_papers/WR1096.html.
[23] McCrum ML, Wan N, Han J, et al. Disparities in Spatial Access to Emergency Surgical Services in the US. JAMA Health Forum 2022;3(10):e223633; https://doi.org/10.1001/jamahealthforum.2022.3633.
[24] Diaz A, Barmash E, Azap R, et al. Association of County-Level Social Vulnerability with Elective Versus Non-elective Colorectal Surgery. J Gastrointest Surg 2021;25(3):786–94.
[25] Papageorge MV, Woods AP, de Geus SWL, et al. The Persistence of Poverty and its Impact on Cancer Diagnosis, Treatment and Survival. Ann Surg 2022; https://doi.org/10.1097/SLA.0000000000005455.
[26] Rawicz-Pruszyński K, Woldesenbet S, Endo Y, et al. Persistent poverty impacts access to minimally invasive surgery among patients with hepatopancreatobiliary cancer. J Surg Oncol 2023;128(5):823–30.

[27] Munir MM, Woldesenbet S, Endo Y, et al. Association of Race/Ethnicity, Persistent Poverty, and Opioid Access Among Patients with Gastrointestinal Cancer Near the End of Life. Ann Surg Oncol 2023;30(13):8548–58.
[28] Shaikh CF, Munir MM, Woldesenbet S, et al. Association of persistent poverty and U.S. News and World Report hospital rankings among patients undergoing major surgery. Am J Surg 2023;228:11–9.
[29] Neroda P, Hsieh MC, Wu XC, et al. Racial Disparity and Social Determinants in Receiving Timely Surgery Among Stage I-IIIA Non-small Cell Lung Cancer Patients in a U.S. Southern State. Front Public Health 2021;9:662876; https://doi.org/10.3389/fpubh.2021.662876.
[30] Scott JW, Havens JM, Wolf LL, et al. Insurance status is associated with complex presentation among emergency general surgery patients. Surgery 2017;161(2):320–8.
[31] Greenstein AJ, Moskowitz A, Gelijns AC, et al. Payer Status and Treatment Paradigm for Acute Cholecystitis. Arch Surg 2012;147(5):453–8.
[32] Giacovelli JK, Egorova N, Nowygrod R, et al. Insurance status predicts access to care and outcomes of vascular disease. J Vasc Surg 2008;48(4):905–11.e1.
[33] Andersen ND, Hanna JM, Ganapathi AM, et al. Insurance status predicts acuity of thoracic aortic operations. J Thorac Cardiovasc Surg 2014;148(5):2082–6.
[34] Loehrer AP, Chang DC, Scott JW, et al. Association of the Affordable Care Act Medicaid Expansion With Access to and Quality of Care for Surgical Conditions. JAMA Surg 2018;153(3):e175568; https://doi.org/10.1001/jamasurg.2017.5568.
[35] Zhao J, Han X, Nogueira L, et al. Health insurance status and cancer stage at diagnosis and survival in the United States. CA Cancer J Clin 2022;72(6):542–60.
[36] Lima HA, Moazzam Z, Woldesenbet S, et al. Persistence of Poverty and its Impact on Surgical Care and Postoperative Outcomes. Ann Surg 2023;278(3):347.
[37] Azap L, Woldesenbet S, Lima H, et al. The Association of Persistent Poverty and Outcomes Among Patients Undergoing Cardiac Surgery. J Surg Res 2023;292:30–7.
[38] Hyer JM, Tsilimigras DI, Diaz A, et al. High Social Vulnerability and "Textbook Outcomes" after Cancer Surgery. J Am Coll Surg 2020;232(4):351–9.
[39] Diaz A, O'Reggio R, Norman M, et al. Association of Historic Housing Policy, Modern Day Neighborhood Deprivation and Outcomes After Inpatient Hospitalization. Ann Surg 2021;274(6):985–91.
[40] Carmichael H, Moore A, Steward L, et al. Using the Social Vulnerability Index to Examine Local Disparities in Emergent and Elective Cholecystectomy. J Surg Res 2019;243:160–4.
[41] Diaz A, Chavarin D, Paredes AZ, et al. Association of Neighborhood Characteristics with Utilization of High-Volume Hospitals Among Patients Undergoing High-Risk Cancer Surgery. Ann Surg Oncol 2021;28(2):617–31.
[42] Diaz A, Hyer JM, Azap R, et al. Association of social vulnerability with the use of high-volume and Magnet recognition hospitals for hepatopancreatic cancer surgery. Surgery 2021;170(2):571–8.
[43] Diaz A, Beane JD, Hyer JM, et al. Impact of hospital quality on surgical outcomes in patients with high social vulnerability: Association of textbook outcomes and social vulnerability by hospital quality. Surgery 2021;171(6):1612–8.
[44] Azap RA, Hyer JM, Diaz A, et al. Association of County-Level Vulnerability, Patient-Level Race/Ethnicity, and Receipt of Surgery for Early-Stage Hepatocellular Carcinoma. JAMA Surgery 2021;156(2):197–9.
[45] Rangrass G, Ghaferi AA, Dimick JB. Explaining Racial Disparities in Outcomes After Cardiac Surgery: The Role of Hospital Quality. JAMA Surgery 2014;149(3):223–7.
[46] Osborne NH, Upchurch GR, Mathur AK, et al. Explaining racial disparities in mortality after abdominal aortic aneurysm repair. J Vasc Surg 2009;50(4):709–13.
[47] Morris AM, Rhoads KF, Stain SC, et al. Understanding Racial Disparities in Cancer Treatment and Outcomes. J Am Coll Surg 2010;211(1):105.

[48] Haider AH, Scott VK, Rehman KA, et al. Racial Disparities in Surgical Care and Outcomes in The United States: A Comprehensive Review of Patient, Provider and Systemic Factors. J Am Coll Surg 2013;216(3):482–92.e12.
[49] Lucas FL, Stukel TA, Morris AM, et al. Race and Surgical Mortality in the United States. Ann Surg 2006;243(2):281–6.
[50] Tsai TC, Joynt KE, Orav EJ, et al. Variation in surgical-readmission rates and quality of hospital care. N Engl J Med 2013;369(12):1134–42.
[51] Birkmeyer JD, Dimick JB. Understanding and reducing variation in surgical mortality. Annu Rev Med 2009;60:405–15.
[52] Scarborough JE, Bennett KM, Pietrobon R, et al. Trends in the utilization of high-volume hospitals by minority and underinsured surgical patients. Am Surg 2010;76(5):529–38.
[53] Dimick J, Ruhter J, Sarrazin MV, et al. Black patients more likely than whites to undergo surgery at low-quality hospitals in segregated regions. Health Aff 2013;32(6):1046–53.
[54] Patient protection and affordable care act. Vol 18031.; 2010:974.
[55] Scott JW, Ayanian JZ, Dimick JB. Medicaid Expansion and Surgical Care—Evaluating the Evidence. JAMA Surgery 2021;156(1):7–8.
[56] Zogg CK, Scott JW, Metcalfe D, et al. Association of Medicaid Expansion With Access to Rehabilitative Care in Adult Trauma Patients. JAMA Surgery 2019;154(5):402–11.
[57] Sineshaw HM, Ellis MA, Yabroff KR, et al. Association of Medicaid Expansion Under the Affordable Care Act With Stage at Diagnosis and Time to Treatment Initiation for Patients With Head and Neck Squamous Cell Carcinoma. JAMA Otolaryngology–Head & Neck Surgery 2020;146(3):247–55.
[58] Takvorian SU, Oganisian A, Mamtani R, et al. Association of Medicaid Expansion Under the Affordable Care Act With Insurance Status, Cancer Stage, and Timely Treatment Among Patients With Breast, Colon, and Lung Cancer. JAMA Netw Open 2020;3(2):e1921653; https://doi.org/10.1001/jamanetworkopen.2019.21653.
[59] Diaz A, Chavarin D, Paredes AZ, Pawlik TM. Utilization of High-Volume Hospitals for High-Risk Cancer Surgery in California Following Medicaid Expansion. J Gastrointest Surg 2021;25(7):1875–84.
[60] Aliu O, Auger KA, Sun GH, et al. The effect of pre-Affordable Care Act (ACA) Medicaid eligibility expansion in New York State on access to specialty surgical care. Med Care 2014;52(9):790–5.
[61] Graves JA, Swartz K. Effects of Affordable Care Act Marketplaces and Medicaid Eligibility Expansion on Access to Cancer Care. Cancer J 2017;23(3):168–74.
[62] Miller S, Altekruse S, Johnson N, et al. Medicaid and mortality: new evidence from linked Survey and administrative data. National Bureau of Economic Research; 2019; https://doi.org/10.3386/w26081.
[63] Miller S, Wherry LR. Health and Access to Care during the First 2 Years of the ACA Medicaid Expansions. N Engl J Med 2017;376(10):947–56.
[64] Liu C, Rahman AS, Chao TE. Catastrophic expenditures in trauma patients after the Affordable Care Act: Reduced financial risk and racial disparities. Am J Surg 2020; https://doi.org/10.1016/j.amjsurg.2020.04.012.
[65] Scott JW, Neiman PU, Scott KW, et al. High Deductibles are Associated With Severe Disease, Catastrophic Out-of-Pocket Payments for Emergency Surgical Conditions. Ann Surg 2023;278(4):e667–74.
[66] Scott KW, Scott JW, Sabbatini AK, et al. Assessing Catastrophic Health Expenditures Among Uninsured People Who Seek Care in US Hospital-Based Emergency Departments. JAMA Health Forum 2021;2(12):e214359; https://doi.org/10.1001/jamahealthforum.2021.4359.
[67] Neiman PU, Mouli VH, Taylor KK, et al. The Impact of Medicare Coverage on Downstream Financial Outcomes for Adults Who Undergo Surgery. Ann Surg 2022;275(1):99–105.

[68] Diaz A, Burns S, Paredes AZ, et al. Accessing surgical care for pancreaticoduodenectomy: Patient variation in travel distance and choice to bypass hospitals to reach higher volume centers. J Surg Oncol 2019;120(8):1318–26.
[69] Smith ME, Shubeck SP, Nuliyalu U, et al. Local Referral of High-risk Patients to High-quality Hospitals: Surgical Outcomes, Cost Savings, and Travel Burdens. Ann Surg 2020;271(6): 1065–71.
[70] Ibrahim A, Dimick JB. Redesigning the Delivery of Specialty Care Within Newly Formed Hospital Networks. Catalyst Carryover 2017;3(2); https://doi.org/10.1056/CAT.17.0503.
[71] Humana Highlights Commitment to Addressing Health Equity in 2020 Corporate Responsibility Report. Available at: https://press.humana.com/news/news-details/2021/Humana-Highlights-Commitment-to-Addressing-Health-Equity-in-2020-Corporate-Responsibility-Report/default.aspx. [Accessed 15 November 2021].
[72] Equity in Health Care Quality I Disparities Solutions Center. DSC. Available at: https://www.mghdisparitiessolutions.org/equity-in-health-care-quality. [Accessed 15 November 2021].
[73] WHO Commission on Social Determinants of Health, World Health Organization, eds Closing the Gap in a Generation: Health Equity through Action on the Social Determinants of Health: Commission on Social Determinants of Health Final Report. World Health Organization, Commission on Social Determinants of Health; 2008.
[74] Health Equity Report I Blue cross blue shield of Massachusetts. Available at: https://www.bluecrossma.org/myblue/equity-in-health-care/health-equity-report. [Accessed 15 November 2021].

Advances in Surgery 58 (2024) 49–64

ADVANCES IN SURGERY

Is Hyperthermic Intraperitoneal Chemotherapy Appropriate for Colon Cancer?

Nolan M. Winicki, MS[a], Jonathan B. Greer, MD[b,*]

[a]Department of Surgery, Johns Hopkins University School of Medicine, Baltimore, MD 21287, USA; [b]Division of Gastrointestinal Surgical Oncology, Peritoneal Surface Malignancy Program, Johns Hopkins University School of Medicine, 600 North Wolfe Street, Halsted 614, Baltimore, MD 21287, USA

Keywords

• Colorectal cancer • Peritoneal carcinomatosis • Peritoneal metastasis
• Cytoreductive surgery • Hyperthermic intraperitoneal chemotherapy • HIPEC

Key points

- Colorectal cancer (CRC) with peritoneal metastases is a complex disease and its management presents significant clinical challenges.
- Based on the results of recent randomized controlled trials, HIPEC using oxaliplatin after CRS with shortened perfusion periods (30 minutes) is no longer recommended.
- There is a movement toward utilizing mitomycin C as a first-line intraperitoneal agent with extended perfusion times (90–120 minutes); however, there is currently little prospective evidence to support its widespread use.
- The use of CRS and HIPEC as prophylactic therapy in high-risk patients does not appear to be effective with oxaliplatin but a recent trial has demonstrated a benefit in local control with mitomycin C.

CLINICAL BACKGROUND

Colorectal cancer (CRC) is a major global health problem, representing the third most common cancer and second leading cause of cancer-related mortality worldwide [1]. In 2023, there were approximately 153,000 new cases of CRC and 52,550 deaths in the United States [2]. Upon initial diagnosis, up to 20% of patients were found to have metastatic CRC, whereas 40% of

*Corresponding author. *E-mail address:* jgreer13@jhmi.edu

https://doi.org/10.1016/j.yasu.2024.04.004
0065-3411/24/

patients presented with recurrence after previously treated localized disease [3]. The liver, lung, and peritoneal cavity are the most common sites of metastasis [4]. However, the incidence of peritoneal metastases (PM) is likely to be underreported, as the size of individual peritoneal tumor nodules is often below the detection level of conventional computed tomography (CT) or PET imaging [5]. The prognosis of patients with PM is poor, with a 5 year survival rate of less than 20% [6].

The peritoneal environment, including the extracellular matrix, growth factors, and resident cells, provides a fertile soil for metastasis development. The process of PM occurs via transcoelomic metastasis, with free cancer cells detaching from the primary tumor and spreading within the peritoneal cavity [7,8]. This process occurs via direct invasion, intraoperative seeding, or hematogenous/lymphatic spread [8]. Direct adhesion to the peritoneal mesothelium, invasion of the submesothelial extracellular matrix, and proliferation are key steps in PM formation [9]. As such, upregulation of adhesion molecules, such as CD44 and integrins, and the cytokines and growth factors IL-6, IL-8, and VEGF have been shown to promote the formation of PM [10]. Additionally, exfoliated colorectal cancer cells in the peritoneal cavity tend to aggregate and form spheroids, thereby enhancing their survival and metastatic capabilities [11].

Patients with PM can present with abdominal pain, distension, weight loss, and rapidly declining performance status; however, the majority of patients are asymptomatic [3]. Risk factors associated with the development of PMs from colorectal adenocarcinoma include advanced tumor stage, lymph node metastases, synchronous ovarian metastases, poor tumor differentiation, left-sided primary origin, incomplete resection of the index tumor, mucinous adenocarcinoma, signet ring cell histology, emergency surgery at the time of diagnosis, and younger age [12].

The 8th edition of the AJCC Cancer Staging Manual introduced a new M1c substage (compared to M1a, defined as metastasis to one organ, and M1b, metastasis to more than one organ) specifically for CRC patients with PM [13]. In the presence of PM from CRC, the overall stage becomes 4C [13]. The EVOCAPE 1 study in 2000 demonstrated that patients with a larger burden of PM had the shortest survival [14]. Mean survival for patients with localized less than 5 mm peritoneal implants was 14.3 months; those with diffusely distributed less than 5 mm implants had a mean survival of 8.4 months; patients with implants between 5 mm and 2 cm had a mean survival of 6 months; and patients with large malignant cakes (>2 cm in size) had a mean survival of 4.4 months [14]. To quantify the degree of disease burden, the peritoneal carcinomatosis index (PCI) was established to describe lesion size and location by defined region in the abdomen (Fig. 1) [15]. Increasing levels of PCI have been demonstrated to be an independent predictor of poor survival after cytoreductive surgery (CRS) and hyperthermic intraperitoneal chemotherapy (HIPEC; Fig. 2) [15–18]. For patients with a PCI greater than 20, several studies have recommended against proceeding

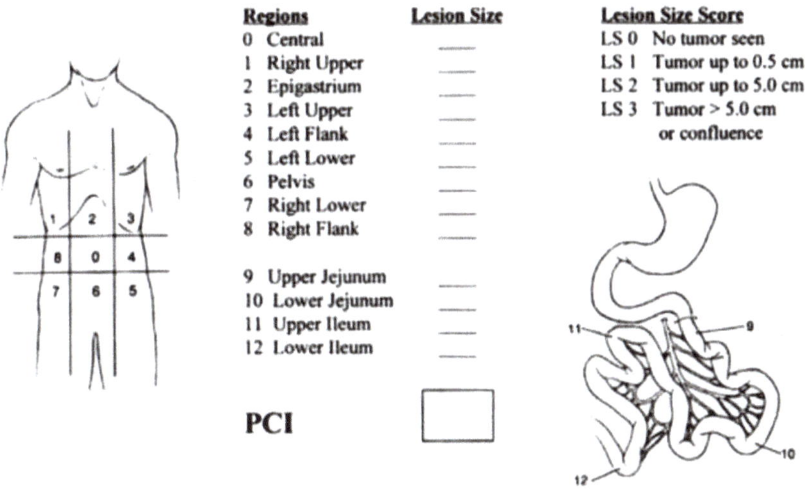

Fig. 1. Visual representation of calculation of the peritoneal cancer index. The abdomen and the pelvis are divided into 13 regions. The lesion size of the largest sizes of the largest implants is scored (0 through 3) in each abdominopelvic region. Each regional score is summed to generate a summary score. (*From* Glehen O, Kwiatkowski F, Sugarbaker PH, et al. Cytoreductive surgery combined with perioperative intraperitoneal chemotherapy for the management of peritoneal carcinomatosis from colorectal cancer: a multi-institutional study. J Clin Oncol. Aug 15 2004;22(16):3284-92. https://doi.org/10.1200/jco.2004.10.012.)

with CRS/HIPEC due to a significantly lower overall survival (OS) (3 year OS of 56% for PCI 1–10 vs 15% for PCI >20) and disease-free survival (DFS; median DFS of 13 months for PCI $\leq$ 20 vs 7 months for PCI > 20) [10,19,20]. To further stratify patients with PM and help guide appropriate

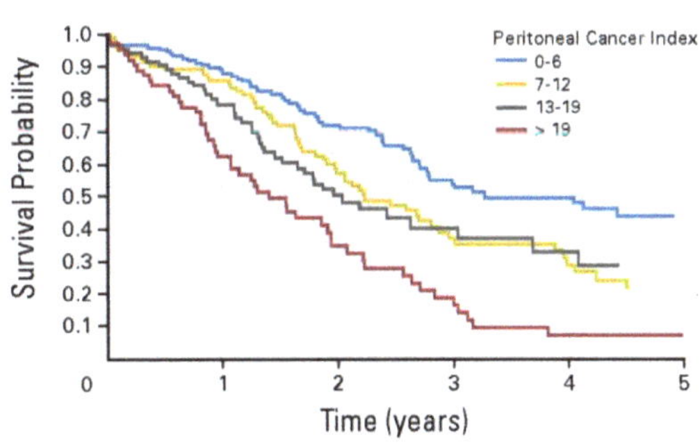

Fig. 2. Prognostic impact of the extent of carcinomatosis, quantified by the peritoneal carcinomatosis index, on 5 year overall survival. (*From* Elias D, Gilly F, Boutitie F, et al. Peritoneal colorectal carcinomatosis treated with surgery and perioperative intraperitoneal chemotherapy: retrospective analysis of 523 patients from a multicentric French study. J Clin Oncol. Jan 1 2010;28(1):63-8. https://doi.org/10.1200/jco.2009.23.9285.)

therapy, the Peritoneal Surface Disease Severity Score (PSDSS) was developed to include (1) symptoms (weight loss, abdominal pain, and ascites); (2) extent of peritoneal dissemination (PCI); and (3) primary tumor histology (Table 1) [21,22]. PSDSS also has been shown in retrospective studies to correspond to survival outcomes with each increase in PSDSS stage corresponding to a stepwise worsening of median and long-term survival (5 year OS, Stage I: 47%–65%, Stage II: 18%–47%, Stage III: 0%–18%, Stage IV: 0%) [19,23].

CYTOREDUCTIVE SURGERY AND HYPERTHERMIC INTRAPERITONEAL CHEMOTHERAPY TECHNIQUE

CRS consists of extensive surgical resection of visible tumor deposits from the peritoneal surfaces and affected organs in patients with PM with the goal of removing all macroscopic disease. The completeness of cytoreduction (CC) score was developed to quantify the residual tumor burden after CRS and is scored from CC-0 to CC-3, with lower scores indicating less residual disease [24]. A CC-0 (no macroscopic residual disease) resection is associated with best survival outcomes with a stepwise survival decline for CC-1 (residual nodules $\leq$ 2.5 mm), CC-2 (residual nodules 2.5 mm–2.5 cm), and CC-3 (residual nodules >2.5 cm or confluent tumor) resections (Fig. 3) [24]. The ability to achieve CC-0/1 resection is recommended as a selection criterion for CRS and is an important prognostic factor [15]. Large, multicenter studies have demonstrated significant survival advantages for patients with complete cytoreduction (an R0 resection) [25]. However, specific organ and tissue resection during CRS must be tailored to the individual patient as practice varies significantly by primary histology [26–29].

Following CRS, HIPEC is performed to treat any microscopic disease that may remain. The process involves the chemotherapy solution to be heated (40–43°C) and circulated (30–120 min) throughout the peritoneal cavity, inducing direct cytotoxicity against tumor cells not removed during CRS

Table 1
Calculation of the peritoneal surface disease severity score

Peritoneal carcinomatosis index	Tumor grade/histopathology/ nodal status	Clinical symptoms
PCI <10 = 1 point	Well-moderately differentiated, N0 = 1 point	Asymptomatic = 0 points
PCI 10–20 = 3 points	Moderately differentiated, N1–N2 = 3 points	Mild symptoms = 1 point
PCI >20 = 7 points	Poorly differentiated or signet ring = 9 points	Severe symptoms = 6 points

Data from Glehen O, Kwiatkowski F, Sugarbaker PH, et al. Cytoreductive surgery combined with perioperative intraperitoneal chemotherapy for the management of peritoneal carcinomatosis from colorectal cancer: a multi-institutional study. J Clin Oncol. Aug 15 2004;22(16):3284-92. doi:10.1200/jco.2004.10.012.

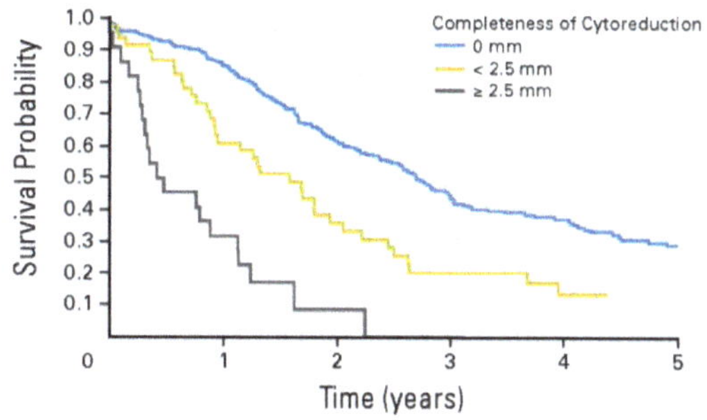

Fig. 3. Prognostic impact of the completeness of cytoreduction on 5 year overall survival. (*From* Elias D, Gilly F, Boutitie F, et al. Peritoneal colorectal carcinomatosis treated with surgery and perioperative intraperitoneal chemotherapy: retrospective analysis of 523 patients from a multicentric French study. J Clin Oncol. Jan 1 2010;28(1):63-8. https://doi.org/10.1200/jco.2009.23.9285.)

(Fig. 4). The procedural rationale is based on (1) CRS exposes residual tumor cells that may not be reached by the diffusion of intravenous or even intraperitoneal chemotherapy; (2) direct local administration of chemotherapy to the peritoneal cavity allows for homogeneous drug distribution; (3) the cytotoxicity and diffusive ability of chemotherapy is potentiated by heat; and (4) limited systemic penetration allows for higher regional doses than when given intravenously [30]. Mitomycin-C, cisplatin, and oxaliplatin are the most common chemotherapy agents utilized for HIPEC due to the direct cytotoxic effects but low systemic absorption through the peritoneum [31,32]. The optimal regimen for PM from CRC remains debated; however, the majority of global

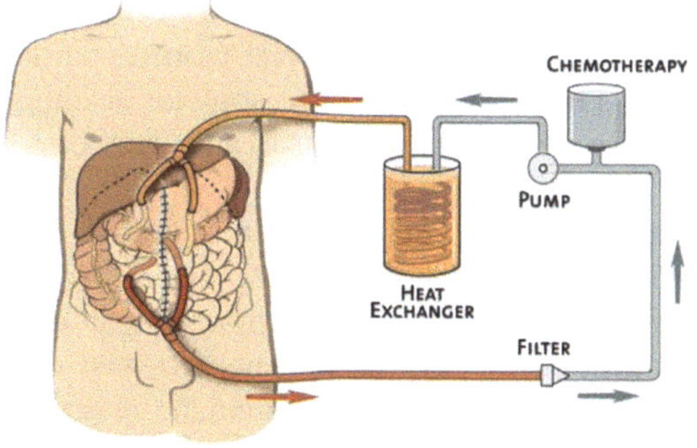

Fig. 4. Schematic of an intraperitoneal hyperthermic chemotherapy circuit. (*From* Shen P, Thai K, Stewart JH, et al. Peritoneal Surface Disease from Colorectal Cancer: Comparison with the Hepatic Metastases Surgical Paradigm in Optimally Resected Patients. Annals of Surgical Oncology. 2008/12/01 2008;15(12):3422-3432. https://doi.org/10.1245/s10434-008-0127-4.)

experts consider mitomycin-C the first-line agent [33,34]. Perfusion time also varies by center, but extended durations of 60 to 90 minutes have become the prevalent time frames [34]. The technique of performing HIPEC, either via an open or closed abdomen, has been shown not to be independently associated with relevant postoperative or long-term outcomes, and thus, can be left to the discretion of the operating surgeon [35]. Early postoperative intraperitoneal chemotherapy has additionally been utilized at some centers, but this has not been widely adopted [36,37]. The results of the ICARuS trial will be informative [38].

MORBIDITY ASSOCIATED WITH CYTOREDUCTIVE SURGERY AND HYPERTHERMIC INTRAPERITONEAL CHEMOTHERAPY

Despite advances in surgical techniques, CRS/HIPEC remains a challenging operation, associated with substantial morbidity. Postoperative complication rates range from 16% to 42%, resulting in reoperations and readmissions, as well as decreased survival [39–42]. Ileus, abdominal abscesses, wound infection, pleural effusion, and acute kidney injury are the most cited complications following CRS/HIPEC [39,43,44]. The high incidence of pulmonary complications (ventilator use >48 h, pneumonia, and unplanned reintubation) post-CRS/HIPEC has been attributed to the massive resuscitation required during the procedure, leading to postoperative fluid shifts, which affects postoperative pulmonary function [45]. However, when compared to other high-risk oncologic procedures such as right hepatic lobectomy or trisegmentectomy, pancreaticoduodenectomy, and esophagectomy, CRS/HIPEC was found to be safer across the spectrum of NSQIP safety metrics [45].

A multicenter study from the US HIPEC Collaborative in 2020 demonstrated that preoperative functional status and individual cytoreductive procedures predicted readmission, whereas neoadjuvant chemotherapy, PCI, and CC did not [40]. Notably, the preoperative and intraoperative factors that were predictive of readmission were an ECOG score of 3 or higher, depression, preoperative TPN, splenectomy, low anterior resection or partial colectomy, and stoma creation [40]. The most common reasons for readmission were failure to thrive, infection, inadequate pain control, and ileus or bowel obstructions [40,46].

Given the complexity of the index operation and disease, several groups have investigated postoperative quality of life. Two studies presented congruent findings that there was a consistent decline in quality of life during the first 3 months postoperatively, but patients returned to their preoperative baseline by 6 months [47,48]. A recent systematic review of 14 studies that used 12 different questionnaires to measure quality of life after CRS/HIPEC showed that patients experienced a diminished quality of life within 3 months after surgery, but recovered to baseline or greater by 12 months [49]. Quality of life was negatively affected by older age, female sex, prolonged operation time, extensive disease, residual disease, adjuvant chemotherapy, complications, stoma placement, and recurrent disease [49].

CURRENT STATUS OF CYTOREDUCTIVE SURGERY AND HYPERTHERMIC INTRAPERITONEAL CHEMOTHERAPY IN COLORECTAL CANCER PERITONEAL METASTASIS

Currently, there are several areas of debate in the field of CRS and HIPEC for patients with CRC PM. These include the therapeutic contribution of HIPEC after CRS, the use of mitomycin C versus oxaliplatin as first-choice chemotherapeutic agent in HIPEC, the optimal timing and duration of systemic chemotherapy, if any, around CRS and HIPEC, and the role of prophylactic HIPEC in high-risk patients.

THERAPEUTIC CONTRIBUTION OF HYPERTHERMIC INTRAPERITONEAL CHEMOTHERAPY TO CYTOREDUCTIVE SURGERY IN COLORECTAL CANCER

The phase III, multicenter, PRODIGE 7 study was the first prospective, randomized, controlled trial that attempted to establish whether HIPEC confers additional survival benefit when administered in combination with complete CRS [33]. Patients with a PCI of less than 25 were randomly assigned to undergo CRS with or without IV fluorouracil and folinic acid and 30 minutes of oxaliplatin-based HIPEC. After a median follow-up of 63 months, there were no significant differences in OS (41 months [95% CI 36–53] vs 41 months [35–49]; $P = .99$) or relapse-free survival (13 months [12–15] vs 11 months [9–12]; $P = .43$) between the CRS/HIPEC and the CRS-alone groups. Furthermore, the proportion of patients who were recurrence-free at 5 years was similar between the two groups, but those treated with HIPEC experienced a higher number of postoperative complications within 60 days. Additionally, in subgroup analysis, HIPEC over CRS alone for patients with a PCI of 11 to 15 was favored, leading some centers to choose CRS-alone for patients with a PCI less than 10, HIPEC for PCI 11 to 15, and no surgery for PCI greater than 16. The conclusions from the original study are as follows: (1) High-dose oxaliplatin-based HIPEC administered over a short duration should no longer be used for CRC with PM, and (2) macroscopically complete CRS should be considered the mainstay of treatment for peritoneal metastases.

Given that the major finding was that adjuvant HIPEC after complete CRS did not increase OS compared with complete CRS alone, there was criticism that in this patient population, the whole rationale for HIPEC was disproven, regardless of the intraperitoneal drug regimen, HIPEC duration, selection of patients, or origin of peritoneal disease [50]. A follow-up survey study of CRS/HIPEC experts from 19 countries on the impact of PRODIGE 7 showed that there was a switch toward mitomycin C-based HIPEC regimens and prolongation of HIPEC perfusion time, a reduction in the number of referrals from non-HIPEC centers for colorectal PM, a reduction in national consensus, the removal of HIPEC from national guidelines, and a reduced reimbursement rate [34]. However, the results of the PRODIGE 7 trial had little impact on the personal opinions of the responding experts regarding the value of HIPEC, with the vast majority of experts still considering HIPEC to be indicated for

PM from CRC [34]. In 2020, the national consensus regarding PM from CRC deemed CRS/HIPEC to be the standard of care in 3 countries, whereas the majority reported an ambiguous role for CRS/HIPEC and stated that it was sometimes indicated [34].

MITOMYCIN C VERSUS OXALIPLATIN

One majorly debated aspect of HIPEC is the use of mitomycin C versus oxaliplatin-based regimens as the superior chemotherapeutic agent. Both agents interfere with DNA synthesis as cell-cycle alkylating agents, have limited systemic absorption owing to their large molecular weight, and offer similar tissue penetration of 2 mm with hyperthermia. Oxaliplatin typically has a shorter perfusion time (30 min vs 90 min) and does not induce neutropenia, like mitomycin C [51,52]. Previous retrospective studies have compared outcomes between mitomycin C and oxaliplatin, with varying results. Although oxaliplatin is internationally recommended as one of the first-line systemic regimens for the treatment of PM from CRC, recent investigations utilizing organoid technology have demonstrated that oxaliplatin may not be the ideal intraperitoneal chemotherapy [53]. These findings and the fact that the cytotoxicity of chemotherapeutic agents is dependent on exposure time and temperature may have contributed to the suboptimal oncologic activity during the 30 min HIPEC perfusion time with oxaliplatin during PRODIGE 7. Furthermore, the vast majority of patients in the PRODIGE 7 trial were treated with neoadjuvant oxaliplatin-based therapy, raising the specter of clonal selection, meaning that oxaliplatin intraperitoneally may not be effective against the remaining oxaliplatin-resistant clones [33] (Fig. 5).

The current consensus is a movement toward mitomycin C-based regimens with an extended perfusion time (90–120 minutes). Several retrospective cohort studies have demonstrated that mitomycin C is relatively safe and achieves good long-term results [54]. Since oxaliplatin was the only intraperitoneal chemotherapy used during the PRODIGE 7 trial, it is important to consider mitomycin C-based regimens as a potential option for patients with PM from CRC. Efforts to run an American PRODIGE 7-like trial have been unsuccessful [55].

SYSTEMIC CHEMOTHERAPY AND CYTOREDUCTIVE SURGERY WITH HYPERTHERMIC INTRAPERITONEAL CHEMOTHERAPY

Currently, there is a lack of consensus regarding the benefits of systemic therapy for resectable PM from CRC. As a result, the timing of systemic therapy between HIPEC centers varies from neoadjuvant to adjuvant, both, or none [56].

There have been mixed results regarding the survival benefit of neoadjuvant chemotherapy. The CAIRO6 phase II study is the first randomized controlled trial to investigate the use of perioperative chemotherapy and has demonstrated that perioperative systemic therapy seems feasible and safe, although the benefit remains unconfirmed [57]. A recent systematic review and meta-

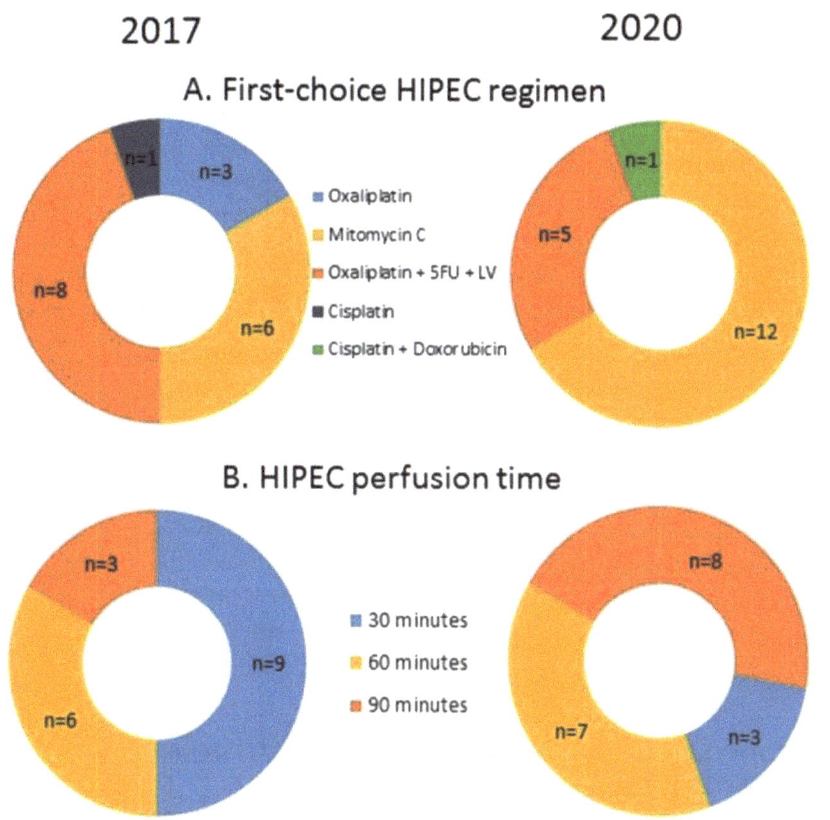

Fig. 5. Changes in first choice HIPEC regimen and HIPEC perfusion time before (2017) and after the results of PRODIGE (2020). (*From* van de Vlasakker VCJ, Lurvink RJ, Cashin PH, et al. The impact of PRODIGE 7 on the current worldwide practice of CRS-HIPEC for colorectal peritoneal metastases: A web-based survey and 2021 statement by Peritoneal Surface Oncology Group International (PSOGI). European Journal of Surgical Oncology. 2021/11/01/ 2021;47(11):2888-2892. doi:https://doi.org/10.1016/j.ejso.2021.05.023.)

analysis of 12 studies reported that there was no apparent difference in major perioperative morbidity and mortality between patients who underwent surgery first and those who received neoadjuvant systemic chemotherapy [58]. There was also no significant difference in OS or DFS at 3 years; however, at 5 years, neoadjuvant chemotherapy patients had superior OS (P=.001) [58]. In a single-center retrospective study, Ceelen and colleagues demonstrated a significant increase in the median survival with neoadjuvant bevacizumab versus no neoadjuvant bevacizumab, although there was no significant benefit between neoadjuvant chemotherapy and none [59]. However, a recent global propensity matched study of 354 patients in each arm (neoadjuvant vs none) showed no difference in median OS 37.0 months (95% CI: 32.6–42.7) versus 34.7 months (95% CI: 31.2–38.8, P=.46) [60].

Several studies have demonstrated that adjuvant chemotherapy is associated with increased median survival. The phase 2 COMBATAC trial displayed safety in perioperative systemic chemotherapy and possible improvement in progression-free survival; however, the trial was terminated early owing to slow recruitment [61]. In one of the larger retrospective studies (N = 506), the median survival significantly increased from 15.6 to 25.2 months, and 3 smaller studies demonstrated improved survival in both univariate and multivariable analyses [25,62,63]. A propensity matched Dutch study with 142 patients in each group (CRS/HIPEC and adjuvant systemic chemotherapy group vs CRS/HIPEC alone) reported a survival benefit for adjuvant systemic chemotherapy [64]. The median OS was significantly higher in the adjuvant group, 39.2 months (IQR 21.1–111.1) versus 24.8 months (IQR 15.0–58.4) (P=.006). The difference remained significant when accounting for patients who died within 6 months postoperatively and after adjusting for major postoperative morbidity. Another global propensity-matched study with 389 patients in each arm (no adjuvant therapy vs adjuvant therapy) exhibited a significant increase in median OS for patients who received adjuvant chemotherapy, 37.0 months (95% CI: 32.9–41.8) versus 45.7 months (95% CI: 38.8–56.2) (P=.022) [60]. Recurrence-free survival was also significantly longer in the adjuvant group (HR 0.83; 95% CI: 0.70–0.98; P=.03). The most common systemic regimen was oxaliplatin ± irinotecan (63%) followed by mitomycin C (37%) [60].

PROPHYLACTIC HYPERTHERMIC INTRAPERITONEAL CHEMOTHERAPY IN HIGH-RISK PATIENTS

The rate of PM from T4 CRCs is reported to be over 15% at 12 months and 25% to 36% at 36 months postsurgical resection. Thus, prophylactic HIPEC has been proposed for patients with T4 colorectal tumors [52].

The COLOPEC study was a multicenter, phase III randomized controlled trial conducted in specialized HIPEC centers in the Netherlands [65]. The trial evaluated adjuvant and prophylactic HIPEC in patients with advanced colon cancer (T4NxM0) or perforated disease without PM. The intraperitoneal chemotherapy regimen chosen was oxaliplatin (460 mg/m^2) perfused over 30 minutes. In the intention-to-treat analysis, there was no statistically significant difference in 18 month PM-free survival between groups (80.9% [95% CI: 73.3–88.5] for the experimental arm vs 76.2% [95% CI: 68–84.4] for the control arms; P=.28). However, there was a higher incidence of major complications in the simultaneous HIPEC-treated group (37.5% of cases [3 of 8 patients], with an overall complication rate of 88%) compared to the staged HIPEC cohort (6% overall morbidity).

The PROPHYLOCHIP-PRODIGE 15 trial was another open-label, randomized, phase III study performed in France that investigated the role of second-look surgery with HIPEC in patients with CRC considered at high risk of PM [66]. Inclusion criteria included patients considered at high risk for peritoneal relapse, such as those with synchronous PM or ovarian metastases radically resected at the time of treatment of primary or perforated tumors. All patients (N = 150) received 6 months of adjuvant systemic chemotherapy and then were randomized to either a second-look operation with HIPEC or surveillance. The intraperitoneal regimens perfused for 30 minutes were as follows: (1) oxaliplatin 460 mg/m^2, (2) oxaliplatin 300 mg/m^2 plus irinotecan 200 mg/m^2, plus intravenous fluorouracil 400 mg/m^2, or (3) mitomycin C (mitomycin 35 mg/m^2). The primary outcome of 3 year DFS was not significantly different between the cohorts (44% vs 53%, respectively; *P*=.82). There was also no significant difference in 5 year OS (68% and 72%, respectively). Similar to the COLOPEC trial, the incidence of postoperative morbidity was significantly higher in the second-look HIPEC cohort, with a major postoperative complication rate (grades 3–4) of 41% (29 of 71 patients).

The most recent randomized controlled trial, HIPECT4, investigated the locoregional control rate at 3 years in patients with cT4NxM0 CRC after CRS/HIPEC versus CRS alone [67]. A total of 184 patients were enrolled and randomized into either cohort. Notably, the intraperitoneal chemotherapy regimen was mitomycin C (30 mg/m2 perfused over 60 minutes) and both cohorts were treated with adjuvant systemic chemotherapy. The 3 year locoregional control rate was higher in the CRS/HIPEC group (97.6%) than in the CRS group (87.6%) (*P* = .03). However, there was no significant difference in the 3 year DFS or OS (DFS: 81.2% vs 78.0%, *P* = .22; OS: 91.7% vs 92.9%, *P*=.68). Contrary to the COLOPEC and the PROPHYLOCHIP-PRODIGE 15 trials, there was no difference in postoperative morbidity between the two cohorts.

SUMMARY

CRC with PM is a complex disease and its management presents significant clinical challenges. In well-selected patients at experienced centers, CRS/HIPEC can be performed with acceptable morbidity and is associated with prolonged survival. Based on the results of recent randomized controlled trials, HIPEC using oxaliplatin after CRS with shortened perfusion periods (30 minutes) is no longer recommended. There is a movement toward utilizing mitomycin C as a first-line intraperitoneal agent with extended perfusion times (90–120 minutes); however, there is currently little prospective evidence to support its widespread use. There may be an emerging role for neoadjuvant and/or adjuvant systemic chemotherapy based on retrospective analyses, but the optimal sequencing and duration has yet to be established. The use of CRS and HIPEC as prophylactic therapy in high-risk patients does not appear to be effective with oxaliplatin but a recent trial has demonstrated a benefit in local control with mitomycin C.

CLINICS CARE POINTS

- Patients with CRC and PM are best treated with CRS/HIPEC in high-volume centers experienced in the treatment of peritoneal carcinomatosis.

- CRS/HIPEC offers survival benefits in selected patients with CRC and PM.
- Oxaliplatin, with a shortened perfusion time, is no longer recommended as a first-line intraperitoneal chemotherapy regimen. Mitomycin C, with an extended perfusion time, is regarded as the current consensus; however, there is limited prospective evidence.
- HIPEC with oxaliplatin should not be used as prophylactic therapy in high-risk patients. Results with mitomycin C have shown improved locoregional control but lacks survival benefit.

Disclosure

None.

References

[1] Baidoun F, Elshiwy K, Elkeraie Y, et al. Colorectal cancer epidemiology: recent trends and impact on outcomes. Curr Drug Targets 2021;22(9):998–1009.
[2] Siegel RL, Wagle NS, Cercek A, et al. Colorectal cancer statistics, 2023. CA A Cancer J Clin 2023;73(3):233–54.
[3] Biller LH, Schrag D. Diagnosis and treatment of metastatic colorectal cancer: a review. JAMA 2021;325(7):669–85.
[4] Riihimäki M, Hemminki A, Sundquist J, et al. Patterns of metastasis in colon and rectal cancer. Sci Rep 2016;6:29765.
[5] Koh JL, Yan TD, Glenn D, et al. Evaluation of preoperative computed tomography in estimating peritoneal cancer index in colorectal peritoneal carcinomatosis. Ann Surg Oncol 2009;16(2):327–33.
[6] Franko J, Shi Q, Meyers JP, et al. Prognosis of patients with peritoneal metastatic colorectal cancer given systemic therapy: an analysis of individual patient data from prospective randomised trials from the Analysis and Research in Cancers of the Digestive System (ARCAD) database. Lancet Oncol 2016;17(12):1709–19.
[7] Lemoine L, Sugarbaker P, Van der Speeten K. Pathophysiology of colorectal peritoneal carcinomatosis: Role of the peritoneum. World J Gastroenterol 2016;22(34):7692–707.
[8] Kawasaki M, Kameyama M, Kobayashi H, et al. Investigation of the Japanese Classification of Peritoneal Metastasis from Colorectal Cancer Referring to the Correlation with PCI. J Anus Rectum Colon 2020;4(4):157–64.
[9] Kim CH. Molecular analyses in peritoneal metastasis from colorectal cancer: a review-an english version. J Anus Rectum Colon 2022;6(4):197–202.
[10] Mendoza-Moreno F, Diez-Alonso M, Matías-García B, et al. Prognostic factors of survival in patients with peritoneal metastasis from colorectal cancer. J Clin Med 2022;11(16).
[11] Zajac O, Raingeaud J, Libanje F, et al. Tumour spheres with inverted polarity drive the formation of peritoneal metastases in patients with hypermethylated colorectal carcinomas. Nat Cell Biol 2018;20(3):296–306.
[12] Sánchez-Hidalgo JM, Rodríguez-Ortiz L, Arjona-Sánchez Á, et al. Colorectal peritoneal metastases: Optimal management review. World J Gastroenterol 2019;25(27):3484.
[13] Weiser MR. AJCC 8th edition: colorectal cancer. Ann Surg Oncol 2018/06/01 2018;25(6):1454–5.
[14] Sadeghi B, Arvieux C, Glehen O, et al. Peritoneal carcinomatosis from non-gynecologic malignancies: results of the EVOCAPE 1 multicentric prospective study. Cancer 2000;88(2):358–63.
[15] Glehen O, Kwiatkowski F, Sugarbaker PH, et al. Cytoreductive surgery combined with perioperative intraperitoneal chemotherapy for the management of peritoneal carcinomatosis from colorectal cancer: a multi-institutional study. J Clin Oncol 2004;22(16):3284–92.

[16] Nizam W, Fackche N, Pessoa B, et al. Prognostic significance of preoperative tumor markers in pseudomyxoma peritonei from low-grade appendiceal mucinous neoplasm: a study from the US HIPEC Collaborative. J Gastrointest Surg 2022;26(2):414–24.

[17] Engbersen MP, Aalbers AGJ, Van't Sant-Jansen I, et al. Extent of peritoneal metastases on preoperative DW-MRI is predictive of disease-free and overall survival for CRS/HIPEC candidates with colorectal cancer. Ann Surg Oncol 2020;27(9):3516–24.

[18] Burnett A, Lecompte MA, Trabulsi N, et al. Peritoneal carcinomatosis index predicts survival in colorectal patients undergoing HIPEC using oxaliplatin: a retrospective single-arm cohort study. World J Surg Oncol 2019;17(1):83.

[19] Arjona-Sanchez A, Rodriguez-Ortiz L, Baratti D, et al. RAS mutation decreases overall survival after optimal cytoreductive surgery and hyperthermic intraperitoneal chemotherapy of colorectal peritoneal metastasis: a modification proposal of the peritoneal surface disease severity score. Ann Surg Oncol 2019;26(8):2595–604.

[20] da Silva RG, Sugarbaker PH. Analysis of prognostic factors in seventy patients having a complete cytoreduction plus perioperative intraperitoneal chemotherapy for carcinomatosis from colorectal cancer. J Am Coll Surg 2006;203(6):878–86.

[21] Ng JL, Ong WS, Chia CS, et al. Prognostic relevance of the peritoneal surface disease severity score compared to the peritoneal cancer index for colorectal peritoneal carcinomatosis. Int J Surg Oncol 2016;2016:2495131.

[22] Pelz JO, Stojadinovic A, Nissan A, et al. Evaluation of a peritoneal surface disease severity score in patients with colon cancer with peritoneal carcinomatosis. J Surg Oncol 2009;99(1):9–15.

[23] Hentzen J, Rovers KP, Kuipers H, et al. Impact of synchronous versus metachronous onset of colorectal peritoneal metastases on survival outcomes after cytoreductive surgery (CRS) with hyperthermic intraperitoneal chemotherapy (HIPEC): a multicenter, retrospective, observational study. Ann Surg Oncol 2019;26(7):2210–21.

[24] Neuwirth MG, Alexander HR, Karakousis GC. Then and now: cytoreductive surgery with hyperthermic intraperitoneal chemotherapy (HIPEC), a historical perspective. J Gastrointest Oncol 2016;7(1):18–28.

[25] Elias D, Gilly F, Boutitie F, et al. Peritoneal colorectal carcinomatosis treated with surgery and perioperative intraperitoneal chemotherapy: retrospective analysis of 523 patients from a multicentric French study. J Clin Oncol 2010;28(1):63–8.

[26] Florissi IS, Radomski SN, Winicki NM, et al. Prophylactic hysterectomy during cytoreductive surgery and hyperthermic intraperitoneal chemotherapy for high grade tumors is associated with fewer pelvic recurrences. Ann Surg Oncol 2023/08/01 2023;30(8):4576–8.

[27] Farrell R, Liauw WS, Morris DL. Cytoreductive surgery and hyperthermic intraperitoneal chemotherapy (HIPEC) for ovarian cancer in an Australian institution: lessons from 20 years' experience. BMC Surg 2022;22(1):338.

[28] Sugarbaker PH, Chang D. Extent of disease on visceral peritoneal surfaces of mucinous appendiceal neoplasms controls survival. Ann Surg Open 2022;3(3):e193.

[29] Istl AC, Gage MM, Esquivel J, et al. Management of Low-Grade Appendiceal Mucinous Neoplasms (LAMN): An International Survey of Surgeons Performing CRS and HIPEC. Ann Surg Oncol 2021;28(7):3831–7.

[30] Yurttas C, Hoffmann G, Tolios A, et al. Systematic Review of Variations in Hyperthermic Intraperitoneal Chemotherapy (HIPEC) for Peritoneal Metastasis from Colorectal Cancer. J Clin Med 2018;7(12).

[31] Valente MA, Moran BJ. Cytoreductive surgery and hyperthermic intraperitoneal chemotherapy. In: Steele SR, Hull TL, Hyman N, et al, editors. The ASCRS Textbook of colon and rectal surgery. Springer International Publishing; 2022. p. 605–17.

[32] Braam HJ, Hoogwater FJH. Selection of chemotherapy in hyperthermic intraperitoneal chemotherapy. In: Canbay E, editor. Unusual cases in peritoneal surface malignancies. Springer International Publishing; 2017. p. 11–22.

[33] Quénet F, Elias D, Roca L, et al. Cytoreductive surgery plus hyperthermic intraperitoneal chemotherapy versus cytoreductive surgery alone for colorectal peritoneal metastases (PRODIGE 7): a multicentre, randomised, open-label, phase 3 trial. Lancet Oncol 2021;22(2): 256–66.
[34] van de Vlasakker VCJ, Lurvink RJ, Cashin PH, et al. The impact of PRODIGE 7 on the current worldwide practice of CRS-HIPEC for colorectal peritoneal metastases: A web-based survey and 2021 statement by Peritoneal Surface Oncology Group International (PSOGI). Eur J Surg Oncol 2021/11/01/2021;47(11):2888–92.
[35] Leiting JL, Cloyd JM, Ahmed A, et al. Comparison of open and closed hyperthermic intraperitoneal chemotherapy: Results from the United States hyperthermic intraperitoneal chemotherapy collaborative. World J Gastrointest Oncol 2020;12(7):756–67.
[36] Soucisse ML, Liauw W, Hicks G, et al. Early postoperative intraperitoneal chemotherapy for lower gastrointestinal neoplasms with peritoneal metastasis: a systematic review and critical analysis. Pleura and peritoneum 2019;4(3):20190007.
[37] Maillet M, Glehen O, Lambert J, et al. Early postoperative chemotherapy after complete cytoreduction and hyperthermic intraperitoneal chemotherapy for isolated peritoneal carcinomatosis of colon cancer: a multicenter study. Ann Surg Oncol 2016;23:863–9.
[38] ClinicalTrials.gov. ICARuS Post-operative Intraperitoneal Chemotherapy (EPIC) and Hyperthermic Intraperitoneal Chemotherapy (HIPEC) After Optimal Cytoreductive Surgery (CRS) for Neoplasms of the Appendix, Colon or Rectum With Isolated Peritoneal Metastasis (Icarus. Available at: https://clinicaltrials.gov/study/NCT01815359. [Accessed 23 January 2024].
[39] Zhou S, Feng Q, Zhang J, et al. High-grade postoperative complications affect survival outcomes of patients with colorectal Cancer peritoneal metastases treated with Cytoreductive surgery and Hyperthermic Intraperitoneal chemotherapy. BMC Cancer 2021;21(1):41.
[40] Lee TC, Wima K, Sussman JJ, et al. Readmissions after cytoreductive surgery and hyperthermic intraperitoneal chemotherapy: a US HIPEC collaborative study. J Gastrointest Surg 2020;24(1):165–76.
[41] Bartlett EK, Meise C, Roses RE, et al. Morbidity and mortality of cytoreduction with intraperitoneal chemotherapy: outcomes from the ACS NSQIP database. Ann Surg Oncol 2014;21:1494–500.
[42] Schneider MA, Eshmuminov D, Lehmann K. Major postoperative complications are a risk factor for impaired survival after CRS/HIPEC. Ann Surg Oncol 2017;24:2224–32.
[43] Baratti D, Kusamura S, Iusco D, et al. Postoperative complications after cytoreductive surgery and hyperthermic intraperitoneal chemotherapy affect long-term outcome of patients with peritoneal metastases from colorectal cancer: a two-center study of 101 patients. Dis Colon Rectum 2014;57(7):858–68.
[44] Tan JW-S, Tan GHC, Ng WY, et al. High-grade complication is associated with poor overall survival after cytoreductive surgery and hyperthermic intraperitoneal chemotherapy. Int J Clin Oncol 2020;25(5):984–94.
[45] Foster JM, Sleightholm R, Patel A, et al. Morbidity and mortality rates following cytoreductive surgery combined with hyperthermic intraperitoneal chemotherapy compared with other high-risk surgical oncology procedures. JAMA Netw Open 2019;2(1):e186847.
[46] Martin AS, Abbott DE, Hanseman D, et al. Factors associated with readmission after cytoreductive surgery and hyperthermic intraperitoneal chemotherapy for peritoneal carcinomatosis. Ann Surg Oncol 2016;23:1941–7.
[47] Tsilimparis N, Bockelmann C, Raue W, et al. Quality of life in patients after cytoreductive surgery and hyperthermic intraperitoneal chemotherapy: is it worth the risk? Ann Surg Oncol 2013;20(1):226–32.
[48] Steffens D, Koh C, Ansari N, et al. Quality of life after cytoreductive surgery and hyperthermic intraperitoneal chemotherapy: early results from a prospective cohort study of 115 patients. Ann Surg Oncol 2020;27(10):3986–94.

[49] Leimkühler M, Hentzen JEKR, Hemmer PHJ, et al. Systematic review of factors affecting quality of life after cytoreductive surgery with hyperthermic intraperitoneal chemotherapy. Ann Surg Oncol 2020/10/01 2020;27(10):3973–83.
[50] Evrard S. Autopsy of an expert consensus: end of hyperthermic intraperitoneal chemotherapy in colorectal carcinomatosis. Eur J Surg Oncol 2018;44(12):1845–6.
[51] Prada-Villaverde A, Esquivel J, Lowy AM, et al. The American Society of Peritoneal Surface Malignancies evaluation of HIPEC with Mitomycin C versus Oxaliplatin in 539 patients with colon cancer undergoing a complete cytoreductive surgery. J Surg Oncol 2014;110(7):779–85.
[52] Arjona-Sánchez A, Barrios P, Boldo-Roda E, et al. HIPECT4: multicentre, randomized clinical trial to evaluate safety and efficacy of Hyperthermic intra-peritoneal chemotherapy (HIPEC) with Mitomycin C used during surgery for treatment of locally advanced colorectal carcinoma. BMC Cancer 2018/02/13 2018;18(1):183.
[53] Ubink I, Bolhaqueiro A, Elias S, et al. Organoids from colorectal peritoneal metastases as a platform for improving hyperthermic intraperitoneal chemotherapy. J Br Surg 2019;106(10):1404–14.
[54] Kuijpers AM, Mirck B, Aalbers AG, et al. Cytoreduction and HIPEC in the Netherlands: nationwide long-term outcome following the Dutch protocol. Ann Surg Oncol 2013;20:4224–30.
[55] Foster JM, Alexander HR, Zhang C. Regional therapy trials in peritoneal metastases: The path to standardization of care: Introduction. J Surg Oncol 2022;125(1):55–6.
[56] Rovers KP, Simkens GA, Punt CJ, et al. Perioperative systemic therapy for resectable colorectal peritoneal metastases: Sufficient evidence for its widespread use? A critical systematic review. Crit Rev Oncol-Hematol 2017/06/01/2017;114:53–62.
[57] Rovers KP, Bakkers C, Nienhuijs SW, et al. Perioperative systemic therapy vs cytoreductive surgery and hyperthermic intraperitoneal chemotherapy alone for resectable colorectal peritoneal metastases: a phase 2 randomized clinical trial. JAMA Surgery 2021;156(8):710–20.
[58] Flood MP, Kong JCH, Wilson K, et al. The impact of neoadjuvant chemotherapy on the surgical management of colorectal peritoneal metastases: a systematic review and meta-analysis. Ann Surg Oncol 2022/10/01 2022;29(11):6619–31.
[59] Ceelen W, Van Nieuwenhove Y, Putte DV, et al. Neoadjuvant chemotherapy with bevacizumab may improve outcome after cytoreduction and hyperthermic intraperitoneal chemoperfusion (HIPEC) for colorectal carcinomatosis. Ann Surg Oncol 2014;21:3023–8.
[60] Cashin PH, Esquivel J, Larsen SG, et al. Perioperative chemotherapy in colorectal cancer with peritoneal metastases: a global propensity score matched study. eClinicalMedicine 2023;55.
[61] Glockzin G, Zeman F, Croner RS, et al. Perioperative systemic chemotherapy, cytoreductive surgery, and hyperthermic intraperitoneal chemotherapy in patients with colorectal peritoneal metastasis: results of the prospective multicenter phase 2 COMBATAC Trial. Clin Colorectal Cancer 2018;17(4):285–96.
[62] Adachi T, Hinoi T, Egi H, et al. Oxaliplatin and molecular-targeted drug therapies improved the overall survival in colorectal cancer patients with synchronous peritoneal carcinomatosis undergoing incomplete cytoreductive surgery. Surg Today 2015/08/01 2015;45(8):986–92.
[63] Elias D, Glehen O, Pocard M, et al. A comparative study of complete cytoreductive surgery plus intraperitoneal chemotherapy to treat peritoneal dissemination from colon, rectum, small bowel, and nonpseudomyxoma appendix. Ann Surg 2010;251(5).
[64] Rovers KP, Bakkers C, van Erning FN, et al. Adjuvant systemic chemotherapy vs active surveillance following up-front resection of isolated synchronous colorectal peritoneal metastases. JAMA Oncol 2020;6(8):e202701.

[65] Klaver CE, Wisselink DD, Punt CJ, et al. Adjuvant hyperthermic intraperitoneal chemotherapy in patients with locally advanced colon cancer (COLOPEC): a multicentre, open-label, randomised trial. The lancet Gastroenterology & hepatology 2019;4(10):761–70.
[66] Goéré D, Glehen O, Quenet F, et al. Second-look surgery plus hyperthermic intraperitoneal chemotherapy versus surveillance in patients at high risk of developing colorectal peritoneal metastases (PROPHYLOCHIP–PRODIGE 15): A randomised, phase 3 study. Lancet Oncol 2020;21(9):1147–54.
[67] Arjona-Sánchez A, Espinosa-Redondo E, Gutiérrez-Calvo A, et al. Efficacy and safety of intraoperative hyperthermic intraperitoneal chemotherapy for locally advanced colon cancer: a phase 3 randomized clinical trial. JAMA Surgery 2023;158(7):683–91.

Advances in Surgery 58 (2024) 65–77

ADVANCES IN SURGERY

Prevention and Treatment of Lymphedema in Breast Cancer

Maureen P. McEvoy, MD*, Sheldon Feldman, MD

Department of Surgery, Division of Breast Surgery, Montefiore Medical Center, Montefiore Breast Care Center, 1250 Waters Place, Tower 1, 7th Floor, Bronx, NY 10461, USA

Keywords

• Breast cancer related lymphedema • Lymphedema prevention
• Lymphedema treatment • Axillary reverse mapping • LyMPHA

Key points

- Breast cancer related lymphedema requires surveillance in order to detect it early and provide a chance for early intervention.
- Surgical de-escalation of the axilla is critical in prevention of breast cancer related lymphedema.
- Numerous treatments for breast cancer related lymphedema are available, both surgical and nonsurgical.

INTRODUCTION

Breast cancer mortality is decreasing due to improved diagnostics and treatments. As survival is increased, the long-term sequalae of treatment and quality of life are relevant. Breast cancer related lymphedema (BCRL) affects about 3 to 5 million patients worldwide. The financial impact is profound. A recent study found that patients with BCRL were estimated to have an average of $2306 in out-of-pocket costs per year, compared to $1090 for those without lymphedema, a 112% difference [1].

PATHOPHYSIOLOGY

BCRL results from the disruption of the lymphatic system. This prevents adequate drainage allowing the lymph fluid to accumulate in the interstitial space [2–4] (Fig. 1). The fluid transport mechanism within the lymphatic system consists of the lymphatic transport capacity and the lymphatic load [5].

*Corresponding author. *E-mail address:* mmcevoy@montefiore.org

https://doi.org/10.1016/j.yasu.2024.04.005
0065-3411/24/

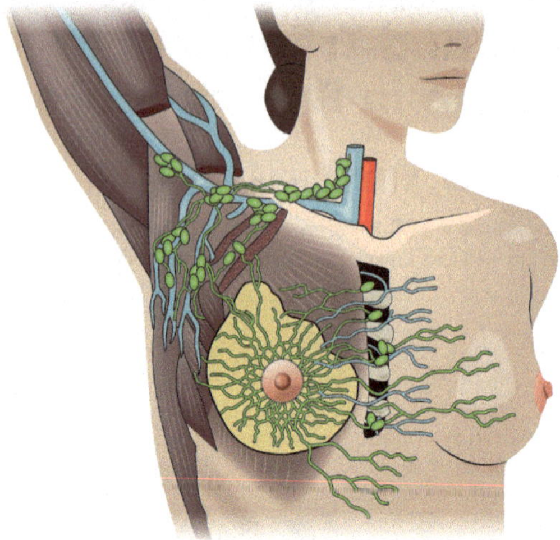

Fig. 1. Breast lymphatic drainage. The breast drains to several lymph node basins, including the internal mammary, and levels 1, 2, and 3 of the axilla.

DEFINITION

BCRL is defined as a 2 cm increase in limb circumference, a 200 mm increase in limb volume, or a 5% to 10% change in limb volume compared to the unaffected arm [4,6,7]. Patients with no symptoms are classified as subclinical lymphedema.

ASSESSMENT/SURVEILLANCE

BCRL assessment and management are part of breast cancer survivorship by major organizations including National Comprehensive Cancer Network. The guidelines state that early detection/diagnosis of lymphedema is key for optimal management. They recommend pre-treatment measurement of both arms as a baseline and establish a program of regular follow-up using an objective, reproducible tool such as bioimpedance spectroscopy (BIS). There are several methods to detect and monitor lymphedema (Table 1).

There is 1 randomized trial comparing BIS to tape measurement. This study randomized 879 patients, with those patients requiring early intervention using a compression sleeve and gauntlet for 4 weeks. The primary endpoint was progression to clinical lymphedema requiring complex decongestive physiotherapy (CPD) with 3 years follow-up. They found BIS had a lower rate of CPD (7.9% versus 19.2%) [8].

The Prospective Surveillance Model is a comprehensive approach to survivorship health care for women with breast cancer [9,10]. It provides time points for assessments and education from diagnosis through long-term survivorship, emphasizing identification and management of impairments (including BCRL)

Table 1
Assessment tools for BCRL

Method	Features measured	Advantages	Disadvantages
Tape measure circumference	Circumferential difference using tape measure	• Simple	• Not precise • Operator variability
Water displacement	Water overflow	• Reliable • Validated • Includes hand	• Not localized • No open wound
Perometry	IR scanning with calculation of multiple limb area volumes	• Fast • Bilateral • Localize	• High upfront cost
Bioimpedance spectroscopy	Impedance ratio between limbs L-Dex ratio	• Rapid • Painless • Early detection	• Limited to arm and leg • Limited bilateral • Upfront cost
3D laser scanning	Real-time digital 3D images	• Sensitive	• Large upfront cost • Not localized easily
Lymphoscintigraphy	Axillary/elbow lymph nodes Lymphatic ducts Dermal backflow	• Gold standard for diagnosis • Shows lymphatic obstruction • Shows deep lymph flow	• Not standardized
ICG Lymphography	Superficial lymphatic ducts Dermal backflow	• Detailed visualization • No radiation exposure	• Limited to lymphatics 2.0 cm into subcutaneous tissue • Technically demanding
MR Lymphangiography	Lymphatics Fat deposition Precise limb volume	• Gives information on function • No radiation	• Costly • Technically demanding

From Pappalardo M, Starnoni M, Franceschini G, Baccarani A, De Santis G. Breast Cancer-Related Lymphedema: Recent Updates on Diagnosis, Severity and Available Treatments. Journal of personalized medicine. 2021;11(5).

and health-promoting behaviors. There are several studies showing benefit to BCRL surveillance in reducing long-term effects.

Patient-reported symptoms are an important assessment as well. A recent study compared the BREAST-Q reconstruction module score of patients with lymphedema matched to patients without lymphedema. There were 322 patients per group who recorded BREAST-Q scores between 1 and 3 years post-surgery. Patients with BCRL reported significantly lower scores in all aspects of physical well-being of the chest, satisfaction with breasts, sexual well-being, and psychosocial well-being at the various time points [11].

PREDICTIVE MODEL

The next step beyond assessment is simple and accurate prediction models. There have been several in the literature, the most recent one looking at preoperative and postoperative models. Rochlin and colleagues conducted a study of 1882 patients of a diverse background undergoing sentinel node biopsy (SLNB) or axillary node dissection (ALND). The preoperative model identified high-risk patients who require close monitoring or prevention measures, while the postoperative model was able to screen for high-risk patients and decrease the need for frequent clinical visits and arm measurements. The models will not only serve to tailor monitoring, but perhaps inform preventive surgical measures as well [12].

RISK FACTORS

Both patient specific and treatment specific factors play a role in BCRL (Table 2).

AXILLARY SURGERY

The extent of axillary surgery had direct effect on BCRL. ALND causes a fourfold increase in BCRL compared to SLNB [13] (Fig. 2). Kilbreath and colleagues demonstrated that in patients with more than 5 lymph nodes removed the rate of BCRL was 18.2% compared to 3.3% in those with less than 5 nodes removed [14].

NODAL RADIATION

Regional lymph node radiation (RLNR) can have a significant increase in BCRL. Compared to breast/chest wall irradiation, RLNR has a hazard ratio of 1.70 [15] (Table 3).

SURGICAL RISK REDUCTION

There is a strong trend toward de-escalation of axillary surgery, and more data reveal minimal benefit.

NO AXILLARY SURGERY

- Choosing Wisely Campaign
  - Not required in women ≥ 70 y/o with ≤ T2N0 hormone positive breast cancer undergoing breast conserving surgery (BCS) [16]
  - Pure DCIS undergoing BCS [17].
  - Prophylactic mastectomy
- SOUND Trial
  - Not required in women with ≤ T2N0 with negative axillary ultrasound [18]

Table 2
Risk factors for BCRL

Patient specific factors	Treatment specific factors
BMI	Axillary surgery
Race	Nodal radiation
Genetics	

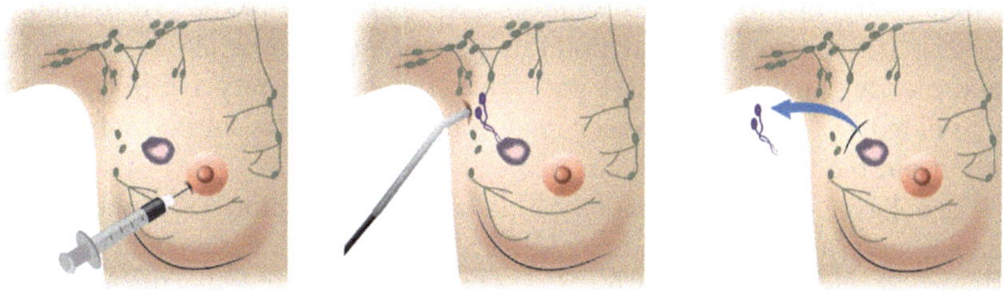

Fig. 2. Sentinel node biopsy. Sentinel node biopsy is performed by lymphatic mapping of the breast to the nodes in the axilla. The axilla is opened and using a gamma probe, or visualization of dye, the sentinel nodes are identified and removed.

CLINICALLY NODE NEGATIVE

- SLNB only, ALND not required [19].

PATHOLOGICALLY NODE POSITIVE (cN0)

- $\leq$ T2N0 undergoing BCS with $\leq$ 2 positive nodes on SLNB undergoing whole breast radiation does not need further axillary surgery [20]
- $\leq$ T2N0 undergoing BCS or mastectomy with $\leq$ 2 positive nodes on SLNB radiation therapy is not inferior to ALND [21]

CLINICALLY NODE POSITIVE AND PATHOLOGICALLY NODE POSITIVE

- SLNB is safe and accurate after neoadjuvant systemic therapy (NAST) if 3 or more nodes are removed and dual tracer is utilized [22].
- Targeted axillary dissection can reduce the false negative rate after neoadjuvant chemotherapy [23].

Prediction of pathologic complete response rate (pCR) in patients receiving NAST is correlated with the tumor subtype [24].

SURGICAL PREVENTION TECHNIQUE

Axillary reverse mapping

Axillary reverse mapping (ARM) is a technique to distinguish the lymphatic drainage of the arm from that of the breast coursing through the axilla,

Table 3
Rate of BCRL based on surgery and radiation

Type of surgery	BCRL rate at 5 y
SLNB	8.0%
SLNB + RLNR	10.7%
ALND	24.9%
ALND + RLNR	30.1%

Abbreviations: ALND, axillary lymph node dissection; RLNR, regional lymph node radiation; SLNB, sentinel lymph node biopsy.

enabling surgeons to minimize unnecessary disruption of the arm lymphatics [25–27]. It is based on the hypothesis that because the axilla and the breast have mostly separate drainage pathways, upper extremity lymphedema can be avoided by removal of tracer identified lymph nodes and lymphatics that only drain the axilla. Fig. 3.

There have been incidences of the SLN coinciding with the ARM node in some patients, and studies have reported ARM/SLN crossover rates anywhere between 0% and 28% [26–35]. In a small fraction of patients, it is possible that the ARM (blue) node will also be the SLN (hot) node [35]. Reapproximation via anastomosis can be performed in these cases. Tummel and colleagues found that crossover (SLN hot and blue) occurred in 3.8% and 5.6% of SLNB and ALND procedures, respectively. At 14 months of follow-up, the overall lymphedema rate was 18.7% when an identified blue lymphatic channel was transected without a corrective reanastomosis procedure; this rate fell to 0% when reanastomosis was performed [32].

The ALLIANCE Trial NCT0392702, Axillary Reverse Mapping in Preventing Lymphedema in Patients with Breast Cancer Undergoing Axillary Lymph Node Dissection [36], is a prospective trial to determine the occurrence of post-surgery lymphedema in patients undergoing ALND randomized to ARM versus no ARM.

LYMPHATIC MICROSURGICAL PREVENTIVE HEALING APPROACH (LyMPHA)

In those cases where the malignant node is found to be draining the arm, a lympha-vascular anastomosis can prevent secondary lymphedema. The blue

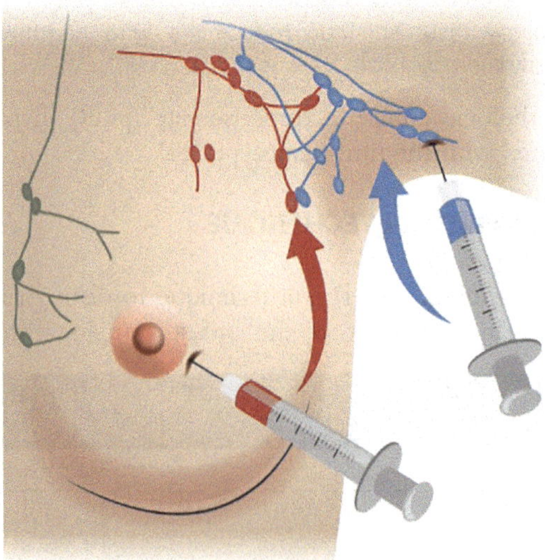

Fig. 3. Axillary reverse mapping. Axillary reverse mapping technique uses dual tracer, one to map the nodes draining the breast and a second to map the nodes draining the upper extremity.

arm node is removed and the blue lymphatic vessel can then be anastomosed in an end-to-end fashion to a branch of the axillary vein with a competent valve via 8-0 non-absorbable suture (Fig. 4).

In a 2011 randomized study, Boccardo and colleagues showed that in 46 patients undergoing complete ALND, lymphedema was reported in 1 LyMPHA patient (4.34%) versus 7 control patients (30.43%) at 6 months [37]. Long-term follow-up at 4 years showed no sign of lymphedema in 71 of 74 (96%) of patients who underwent LyMPHA [38]. Feldman and colleagues found that the lymphedema rate was 3 (12.5%) of 24 in successfully completed and 4 (50%) of 8 in unsuccessfully treated patients. They found it was feasible, safe, and effective for the primary prevention of BCRL [39].

Ozman and colleagues [40] evaluated Simplified Lymphatic Microsurgical Preventing Healing Approach (S-LyMPHA). This procedure is a slightly modified and simplified version of LyMPHA. It is performed by the operating surgeon performing the ALND. During the ALND, transected blue lymphatic channels are identified and at the completion of the dissection those channels are carefully dissected and invaginated using a sleeve technique into the cut end of a neighboring vein with two 7-0 non-absorbable stitches. The microscope is not used in any part of this surgery. They evaluated 380 patients who underwent ALND and found a significantly lower rate of lymphedema among patients who received S-LyMPHA (3%) than those who did not

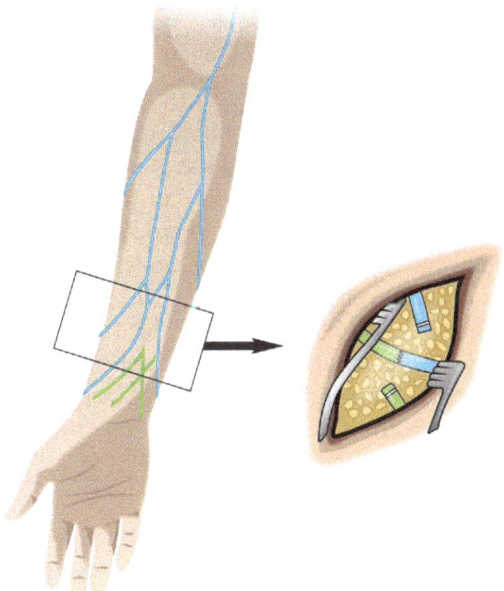

Fig. 4. Lymphatic venous anastomosis lymphatic channels are identified, a recipient vein is identified, and microsurgical anastomosis is created between the two.

(19%), a relationship that is statistically significant in both univariate and multivariate analysis ($P = .001$ and $P = .003$, respectively).

SELECTIVE AXILLARY DISSECTION

With evidence to show that ALND does not change survival in positive SLNB, extrapolation can be made for which nodes can be left behind during ALND. Selective axillary dissection (SAD) refers to a less aggressive approach to ALND, taking obviously positive nodes, targeted positive nodes, and leaving nodes that are draining the extremity based on ARM if they are not suspicious. Data from AMAROS demonstrate that regional lymph node radiation is non inferior to ALND, with less BCRL, and therefore selective dissection should be strongly considered [21]. There is growing evidence to show the oncologic safety of SAD, with studies of 130 patients with 51 months of follow-up, showing an axillary failure rate of 1.63% and improved BCRL when randomized to ALND versus SAD [41,42].

ADJUVANT THERAPY PREVENTION TECHNIQUE

- Partial breast irradiation (PBI)
  - PBI external beam radiation (EBRT) is as effective as whole breast radiation (WBI) [43–45].
  - Intraoperative radiation therapy (IORT) is as effective as WBI [46].
- Hypofractionated radiation
  - 3 weeks is non inferior to 5 weeks [47].
- Omit radiation in particular cases
  - ≥70 y/o with ≤T2N0 hormone positive patients [16].
  - ≥55 y/o with T1N0 grade 1 or 2 luminal A and Ki67≤13.5% with endocrine therapy [48].

Quality of life parameters for IORT have been reported [49]. They found that patients treated with IORT alone reported less general pain and arm symptoms as well as better role functioning than those in the EBRT group. The most common issues were pain in the arm or shoulder and difficulty moving or raising the arm sideways. The frequencies of moderate or severe symptoms reported by patients in each group for swelling in the arm or hand were 8% and 4% with IORT versus 9% and 7% with WBI. The TARGIT-A trial has not yet reported specifically on breast cancer related lymphedema; however, one may extrapolate from the arm pain and swelling data. Since radiotherapy to the axilla is totally avoided with IORT, the BCRL rate would likely be lower compared with EBRT on formal analysis.

LYMPHEDEMA TREATMENT

Nonsurgical

The mainstay of nonoperative treatment is complete decongestive therapy, complex decongestive therapy, combined physical therapy, complex decongestive physiotherapy, or complex lymphedema treatment [50]. This is the universal first-line therapy. There are two phases consisting of reduction and maintenance. The reduction phase includes manual lymph drainage, sequential gradient pump, exercises, low-stretch bandages, and skin care. The maintenance phase consists of compression garment, exercises, and skin care.

Physical therapy by lymphedema trained therapists has been shown to be more beneficial than just patient education and physical therapy alone [51,52].

Photobiomodulation (PBM), also known as low-level laser therapy (LLLT), is a type of phototherapy that uses light of wavelengths between 650 and 1000 nm delivered at low irradiance to the target site [53]. PBM has been shown to reduce inflammation, promote lymphatic mobility and regeneration, and prevent/manage fibrosis [53,54].

Drug therapy

Studies on the use of pharmacotherapy agents are based on tissue modulation or anti-inflammatory drugs. All are in the experiment phases currently.

Surgical management

Surgical management is another option, especially in patients who have no response to non-invasive treatment. The two surgical strategies are ablative and physiologic procedures.

Ablative procedures remove edematous tissue thus reducing limb volume. Liposuction or suction-assisted protein lipectomy (SAPL) are preferred over debulking procedures that require skin grafting. Liposuction/SAPL has been shown to have significant volume reductions [55–57].

Physiologic procedures work by rebuilding and directing axillary lymphatic drainage. This is done with re-anastomosis of lymphatics to distal tissue or veins.

Procedures utilizing distal tissues generally involve lymphatic grafts or vascularized flaps containing lymphatic soft tissue. The lymphaticolymphatic bypass procedure involves an anastomosis between healthy lymphatic tissue of the lower extremity to the affected arm's axillary lymphatics and supraclavicular lymphatics. This has been shown to produce long-term patency and reduce upper extremity volume [58,59].

Lymphatic venous anastomosis (LVA) is a method of diverting lymph into the venous system, bypassing proximal obstruction. Lymphatic channels are identified, a recipient vein is identified, and microsurgical techniques are used to create an anastomosis between the two [60] (Fig. 4). In patients with BCRL, studies have associated LVA with symptom improvement, arm volume reduction, and, notably, fewer episodes of cellulitis. More recently, a study of LVA side-to-end anastomoses in early grade lymphedema reported that it eliminated the need for compression garments later [61].

Rather than bypass obstructions in existing lymph node drainage, in vascular lymph node transfer (VLNT) an autologous lymph node flap microsurgically harvested from a distant donor site is transplanted to the target area with its blood supply preserved by anastomosing artery and vein in the graft to vessels at the receptor site, which may be axilla, elbow, or wrist. Donor sites include jejunal mesenteric, groin, lateral thoracic, omental, and submental [62,63].

A meta-analysis compared the outcome of VLNT and LVA and showed that both were efficient in short-term outcomes but patients with VLNT had better improvement in the long term with a better chance of discontinuing the wearing of compression garments [64].

There are no randomized clinical trials yet to fully compare and evaluate the benefits of these surgical procedures.

SUMMARY

BCRL is a significant quality of life detriment to breast cancer survivors. Surveillance, prevention, and treatment are critical to address this issue.

CLINICS CARE POINTS

- BCRL surveillance is important for early detection-prevention measures should be considered to decress the chances of BCRL-various treatment modalities exist for established BCRL.

Disclosure

The authors have nothing to disclose.

References

[1] Dean LT, Moss SL, Ransome Y, et al. "It still affects our economic situation": long-term economic burden of breast cancer and lymphedema. Support Care Cancer 2019;27(5):1697–708.

[2] Chowdhry M, Rozen WM, Griffiths M. Lymphatic mapping and preoperative imaging in the management of post-mastectomy lymphoedema. Gland Surg 2016;5(2):187–96.

[3] Hespe GENM, Mehrara BJ. Pathophysiology of lymphedema. Springer; 2015.

[4] McEvoy MP, Ravetch E, Patel G, et al. Prevention of breast cancer-related lymphedema. Clin Breast Cancer 2021;21(2):128–42.

[5] Division of Plastic H, Microsurgery Depart of Surgery Ludwig Maximilians University. Pathophysiology of lymphedemas with respect to surgery. Available at: https://plasticsurgerykey.com/pathophysiology-of-lymphedemas-with-respect-to-surgery/.

[6] Veronesi U, Paganelli G, Viale G, et al. A randomized comparison of sentinel-node biopsy with routine axillary dissection in breast cancer. N Engl J Med 2003;349(6):546–53.

[7] McLaughlin SA, Wright MJ, Morris KT, et al. Prevalence of lymphedema in women with breast cancer 5 years after sentinel lymph node biopsy or axillary dissection: patient perceptions and precautionary behaviors. J Clin Oncol 2008;26(32):5220–6.

[8] Ridner SH, Dietrich MS, Boyages J, et al. A Comparison of bioimpedance spectroscopy or tape measure triggered compression intervention in chronic breast cancer lymphedema prevention. Lymphatic Res Biol 2022;20(6):618–28.

[9] Stout NL, Binkley JM, Schmitz KH, et al. A prospective surveillance model for rehabilitation for women with breast cancer. Cancer 2012;118(8 Suppl):2191–200.

[10] McLaughlin SA, Stout NL, Schaverien MV. Avoiding the swell: advances in lymphedema prevention, detection, and management. Am Soc Clin Oncol Educ Book 2020;40:1–10.

[11] Coriddi M, Kim LN, Haglich K, et al. The impact of lymphedema on patient-reported outcomes after breast reconstruction: a preliminary propensity score-matched analysis. Ann Surg Oncol 2023;30(5):3061–71.

[12] Rochlin DH, Barrio AV, McLaughlin S, et al. Feasibility and clinical utility of prediction models for breast cancer-related lymphedema incorporating racial differences in disease incidence. JAMA Surg 2023;158(9):954–64.
[13] DiSipio T, Rye S, Newman B, et al. Incidence of unilateral arm lymphoedema after breast cancer: a systematic review and meta-analysis. Lancet Oncol 2013;14(6):500–15.
[14] Kilbreath SL, Refshauge KM, Beith JM, et al. Risk factors for lymphoedema in women with breast cancer: A large prospective cohort. Breast 2016;28:29–36.
[15] Warren LE, Miller CL, Horick N, et al. The impact of radiation therapy on the risk of lymphedema after treatment for breast cancer: a prospective cohort study. Int J Radiat Oncol Biol Phys 2014;88(3):565–71.
[16] Hughes KS, Schnaper LA, Berry D, et al. Lumpectomy plus tamoxifen with or without irradiation in women 70 years of age or older with early breast cancer. N Engl J Med 2004;351(10):971–7.
[17] Early Breast Cancer Trialists' Collaborative G, Correa C, McGale P, Taylor C, et al. Overview of the randomized trials of radiotherapy in ductal carcinoma in situ of the breast. J Natl Cancer Inst Monogr 2010;2010(41):162–77.
[18] Gentilini OD, Botteri E, Sangalli C, et al. Sentinel lymph node biopsy vs no axillary surgery in patients with small breast cancer and negative results on ultrasonography of axillary lymph nodes: the SOUND randomized clinical trial. JAMA Oncol 2023.
[19] Ashikaga T, Krag DN, Land SR, et al. Morbidity results from the NSABP B-32 trial comparing sentinel lymph node dissection versus axillary dissection. J Surg Oncol 2010;102(2): 111–8.
[20] Giuliano AE, Ballman KV, McCall L, et al. Effect of axillary dissection vs no axillary dissection on 10-year overall survival among women with invasive breast cancer and sentinel node metastasis: The ACOSOG Z0011 (Alliance) randomized clinical trial. JAMA 2017;318(10):918–26.
[21] Donker M, van Tienhoven G, Straver ME, et al. Radiotherapy or surgery of the axilla after a positive sentinel node in breast cancer (EORTC 10981-22023 AMAROS): a randomised, multicentre, open-label, phase 3 non-inferiority trial. Lancet Oncol 2014;15(12):1303–10.
[22] Boughey JC, McCall LM, Ballman KV, et al. Tumor biology correlates with rates of breast-conserving surgery and pathologic complete response after neoadjuvant chemotherapy for breast cancer: findings from the ACOSOG Z1071 (Alliance) Prospective Multicenter Clinical Trial. Ann Surg 2014;260(4):608–14 [discussion 14-6].
[23] Caudle AS, Yang WT, Krishnamurthy S, et al. Improved axillary evaluation following neoadjuvant therapy for patients with node-positive breast cancer using selective evaluation of clipped nodes: implementation of targeted axillary dissection. J Clin Oncol 2016;34(10):1072–8.
[24] Pilewskie M, Zabor EC, Mamtani A, et al. The optimal treatment plan to avoid axillary lymph node dissection in early-stage breast cancer patients differs by surgical strategy and tumor subtype. Ann Surg Oncol 2017;24(12):3527–33.
[25] Klimberg VS. A new concept toward the prevention of lymphedema: axillary reverse mapping. J Surg Oncol 2008;97(7):563–4.
[26] Thompson M, Korourian S, Henry-Tillman R, et al. Axillary reverse mapping (ARM): a new concept to identify and enhance lymphatic preservation. Ann Surg Oncol 2007;14(6): 1890–5.
[27] Boneti C, Korourian S, Bland K, et al. Axillary reverse mapping: mapping and preserving arm lymphatics may be important in preventing lymphedema during sentinel lymph node biopsy. J Am Coll Surg 2008;206(5):1038–42 [discussion 42-4].
[28] Ahmed M, Rubio IT, Kovacs T, et al. Systematic review of axillary reverse mapping in breast cancer. Br J Surg 2016;103(3):170–8.
[29] Britton TB, Solanki CK, Pinder SE, et al. Lymphatic drainage pathways of the breast and the upper limb. Nucl Med Commun 2009;30(6):427–30.

[30] Noguchi M, Noguchi M, Nakano Y, et al. Axillary reverse mapping using a fluorescence imaging system in breast cancer. J Surg Oncol 2012;105(3):229–34.
[31] Noguchi M, Yokoi M, Nakano Y. Axillary reverse mapping with indocyanine fluorescence imaging in patients with breast cancer. J Surg Oncol 2010;101(3):217–21.
[32] Tummel E, Ochoa D, Korourian S, et al. Does axillary reverse mapping prevent lymphedema after lymphadenectomy? Ann Surg 2017;265(5):987–92.
[33] Ochoa D, Korourian S, Boneti C, et al. Axillary reverse mapping: five-year experience. Surgery 2014;156(5):1261–8.
[34] Connor C, McGinness M, Mammen J, et al. Axillary reverse mapping: a prospective study in women with clinically node negative and node positive breast cancer. Ann Surg Oncol 2013;20(10):3303–7.
[35] Boneti C, Korourian S, Diaz Z, et al. Scientific Impact Award: Axillary reverse mapping (ARM) to identify and protect lymphatics draining the arm during axillary lymphadenectomy. Am J Surg 2009;198(4):482–7.
[36] Institute NC. Axillary reverse mapping in preventing lymphedema in patients with breast cancer undergoing axillary lymph node dissection. 2019. Available at: https://classic.clinicaltrials.gov/ct2/show/NCT03927027.
[37] Boccardo FM, Casabona F, Friedman D, et al. Surgical prevention of arm lymphedema after breast cancer treatment. Ann Surg Oncol 2011;18(9):2500–5.
[38] Boccardo F, Valenzano M, Costantini S, et al. LYMPHA Technique to Prevent Secondary Lower Limb Lymphedema. Ann Surg Oncol 2016;23(11):3558–63.
[39] Boccardo F, Casabona F, De Cian F, et al. Lymphatic microsurgical preventing healing approach (LYMPHA) for primary surgical prevention of breast cancer-related lymphedema: over 4 years follow-up. Microsurgery 2014;34(6):421–4.
[40] Ozmen T, Lazaro M, Zhou Y, et al. Evaluation of simplified lymphatic microsurgical preventing healing approach (S-LYMPHA) for the prevention of breast cancer-related clinical lymphedema after axillary lymph node dissection. Ann Surg 2019;270(6):1156–60.
[41] Gennaro M, Listorti C, Mariani L, et al. Oncological safety of selective axillary dissection after axillary reverse mapping in node-positive breast cancer. Eur J Surg Oncol 2021;47(7):1606–10.
[42] Gennaro M, Maccauro M, Mariani L, et al. Occurrence of breast-cancer-related lymphedema after reverse lymphatic mapping and selective axillary dissection versus standard surgical treatment of axilla: A two-arm randomized clinical trial. Cancer 2022;128(24):4185–93.
[43] Meattini I, Marrazzo L, Saieva C, et al. Accelerated partial-breast irradiation compared with whole-breast irradiation for early breast cancer: long-term results of the randomized phase III APBI-IMRT-florence trial. J Clin Oncol 2020;38(35):4175–83.
[44] Ganz PA, Cecchini RS, White JR, et al. Patient-reported outcomes (PROs) in NRG oncology/NSABP B-39/RTOG 0413: A randomized phase III study of conventional whole breast irradiation (WBI) versus partial breast irradiation (PBI) in stage 0, I, or II breast cancer. J Clin Oncol 2019;37(15_suppl):508.
[45] Vicini FA, Cecchini RS, White JR, et al. Long-term primary results of accelerated partial breast irradiation after breast-conserving surgery for early-stage breast cancer: a randomised, phase 3, equivalence trial. Lancet 2019;394(10215):2155–64.
[46] Vaidya JS, Bulsara M, Baum M, et al. Long term survival and local control outcomes from single dose targeted intraoperative radiotherapy during lumpectomy (TARGIT-IORT) for early breast cancer: TARGIT-A randomised clinical trial. BMJ 2020;370:m2836.
[47] Whelan TJ, Pignol JP, Levine MN, et al. Long-term results of hypofractionated radiation therapy for breast cancer. N Engl J Med 2010;362(6):513–20.
[48] Whelan TJ, Smith S, Parpia S, et al. Omitting radiotherapy after breast-conserving surgery in luminal a breast cancer. N Engl J Med 2023;389(7):612–9.

[49] Welzel G, Boch A, Sperk E, et al. Radiation-related quality of life parameters after targeted intraoperative radiotherapy versus whole breast radiotherapy in patients with breast cancer: results from the randomized phase III trial TARGIT-A. Radiat Oncol 2013;8:9.
[50] Lasinski BB, McKillip Thrift K, Squire D, et al. A systematic review of the evidence for complete decongestive therapy in the treatment of lymphedema from 2004 to 2011. PM & R 2012;4(8):580–601.
[51] Torres Lacomba M, Yuste Sanchez MJ, Zapico Goni A, et al. Effectiveness of early physiotherapy to prevent lymphoedema after surgery for breast cancer: randomised, single blinded, clinical trial. BMJ 2010;340:b5396.
[52] Box RC, Reul-Hirche HM, Bullock-Saxton JE, et al. Physiotherapy after breast cancer surgery: results of a randomised controlled study to minimise lymphoedema. Breast Cancer Res Treat 2002;75(1):51–64.
[53] Baxter GD, Liu L, Petrich S, et al. Low level laser therapy (Photobiomodulation therapy) for breast cancer-related lymphedema: a systematic review. BMC Cancer 2017;17(1):833.
[54] Mayrovitz HN, Davey S. Changes in tissue water and indentation resistance of lymphedematous limbs accompanying low level laser therapy (LLLT) of fibrotic skin. Lymphology 2011;44(4):168–77.
[55] Granzow JW, Soderberg JM, Kaji AH, et al. An effective system of surgical treatment of lymphedema. Ann Surg Oncol 2014;21(4):1189–94.
[56] Greene AK, Maclellan RA. Operative treatment of lymphedema using suction-assisted lipectomy. Ann Plast Surg 2016;77(3):337–40.
[57] Boyages J, Kastanias K, Koelmeyer LA, et al. Liposuction for advanced lymphedema: a multidisciplinary approach for complete reduction of arm and leg swelling. Ann Surg Oncol 2015;22(Suppl 3):S1263–70.
[58] Baumeister RG, Siuda S, Bohmert H, et al. A microsurgical method for reconstruction of interrupted lymphatic pathways: autologous lymph-vessel transplantation for treatment of lymphedemas. Scand J Plast Reconstr Surg 1986;20(1):141–6.
[59] Baumeister RG, Mayo W, Notohamiprodjo M, et al. Microsurgical lymphatic vessel transplantation. J Reconstr Microsurg 2016;32(1):34–41.
[60] Chang EI, Skoracki RJ, Chang DW. Lymphovenous anastomosis bypass surgery. Semin Plast Surg 2018;32(1):22–7.
[61] AlJindan FK, Lin CY, Cheng MH. Comparison of outcomes between side-to-end and end-to-end lymphovenous anastomoses for early-grade extremity lymphedema. Plast Reconstr Surg 2019;144(2):486–96.
[62] Schaverien MV, Asaad M, Selber JC, et al. Outcomes of vascularized lymph node transplantation for treatment of lymphedema. J Am Coll Surg 2021;232(6):982–94.
[63] Granzow JW, Soderberg JM, Kaji AH, et al. Review of current surgical treatments for lymphedema. Ann Surg Oncol 2014;21(4):1195–201.
[64] Basta MN, Gao LL, Wu LC. Operative treatment of peripheral lymphedema: a systematic meta-analysis of the efficacy and safety of lymphovenous microsurgery and tissue transplantation. Plast Reconstr Surg 2014;133(4):905–13.

Advances in Surgery 58 (2024) 79–85

ADVANCES IN SURGERY

Are Antibiotics of Value for a Whipple Procedure?

Jonah D. Thomas, MD, MS[a],
Carlos Fernández-del Castillo, MD[a,b,*]

[a]Department of Surgery, Massachusetts General Hospital, Harvard Medical School, 55 Fruit Street, Boston, MA 02114, USA; [b]GI Cancer Center, Pancreas and Biliary Surgery Program

Keywords

• Pancreatoduodenectomy • Surgical prophylaxis • Perioperative antibiotics
• Piperacillin-tazobactam • Zosyn • SSI

Key points

- Pancreatoduodenectomy (Whipple procedure) has a high rate of surgical-site infections (SSIs), which lead to prolonged hospital stays, readmissions, delays in adjuvant therapies, and significant financial burden.
- Preoperative instrumentation of the biliary system leads to contamination and is one of the leading risk factors for the development of SSI.
- Common organisms leading to SSIs include *Enterococcus faecalis, Escherichia coli, Klebsiella pneumoniae, Enterobacter cloacae, Klebsiella oxytoca, Pseudomonas aeruginosa, Staphylococcus spp,* and *Streptococcus spp.*
- Piperacillin-tazobactam has been shown to decrease 30 day SSI rates, compared to cefoxitin, following pancreatoduodenectomy in patients without a penicillin allergy.

Surgical-site infections (SSIs) are one of the leading causes of postoperative morbidity following pancreatoduodenectomy (Whipple procedure). Multiple studies have reported the incidence of wound infection following pancreatoduodenectomy to be greater than 10%, even at high-volume referral centers [1,2]. The etiology of these infections is often complex, and they pose a significant clinical and economic burden. As related to

*Corresponding author. Department of Surgery, Massachusetts General Hospital, Harvard Medical School, 55 Fruit Street, Boston, MA 02114. *E-mail address:* cfernandez@mgh.harvard.edu
Twitter: @_JonahT (J.D.T.)

https://doi.org/10.1016/j.yasu.2024.04.006
0065-3411/24/

pancreatoduodenectomy, patients suffering from SSIs face decreased chances of receiving adjuvant therapy and are more prone to encountering delays in this treatment, ultimately leading to diminished overall survival rates [3,4]. Moreover, the financial implications linked to SSIs, including expenses related to emergency department visits, readmissions, and extended hospital stays, are significant. Estimates suggest that the cost of all SSIs in the United States contributes to an annual health care expenditure of $3.5 to 10 billion [5]. Broad spectrum prophylactic perioperative antibiotics have been proven to decrease the rates of infections [6,7]. However, the choice of prophylactic antibiotic has been under recent investigation in order to attempt to improve the frustratingly high rates of SSI and their downstream consequences.

COMMON ORGANISMS CAUSING INFECTION

When considering prophylactic preoperative antibiotics, it is essential to target specific organisms that are commonly associated with SSIs and other postoperative complications. The choice of antibiotics should be tailored to cover a broad spectrum of potential pathogens that might be encountered during the surgical procedure. In particular, Whipple procedures pose a unique risk of infection due to the possibility of bowel contents contaminating a sterile field, and also due to the high probability of prior bile duct instrumentation. Preoperative biliary ductal instrumentation is associated with increased rates of SSIs due to the introduction of bacteria to the previously sterile biliary system [8,9]. Oftentimes, the biliary system becomes contaminated with antibiotic-resistant bacteria which infers an increased postoperative morbidity and mortality risk.

Bacterial cultures from pancreatoduodenectomy are predominantly gram-negative bacteria, including *Escherichia coli, Klebsiella pneumoniae, Enterobacter cloacae, Klebsiella oxytoca, and Pseudomonas aeruginosa.* This is followed by gram-positive organisms such as *Enterococcus spp, Staphylococcus spp,* and *Streptococcus spp* [10,11]. Additionally, over 50% of SSIs are reported to be polymicrobial [10].

Enterococcus faecalis is an organism of interest because prior research has suggested that colonization of intestinal tissue with this bacteria may increase the risk of anastomotic leak [12]. The proposed mechanism behind this finding is that *E faecalis* is a collagenase-producing bacteria. As such, it is able to degrade collagen and activate tissue matrix metalloproteinase 9 (MMP9) in host intestinal tissues. Studies have demonstrated that by eradicating strains of *E faecalis* with increased collagen-degrading activity and increased ability to activate host MMP9, anastomotic leak rates decreased.

CHOICE OF PROPHYLACTIC PERIOPERATIVE ANTIBIOTIC

Current clinical guidelines recommend first- or second-generation cephalosporins as the choice prophylactic perioperative antibiotic for pancreatoduodenectomy [13]. The Surgical Care Improvement Project (SCIP), which was the outcome of the 2003 Centers for Medicare and Medicaid Services initiative to reduce preventable surgical complications, outlines measures related to perioperative prophylactic antibiotics, including (1) administration of antibiotics within 60 minutes of the initial incision; (2) selection of appropriate antibiotic therapy; and (3) discontinuation of antibiotic within 24 hours of finishing the surgery. For patients without a penicillin allergy, the recommended prophylactic antibiotics prior to gastrointestinal (GI) surgery, including pancreatoduodenectomy, include cefotetan, cefoxitin, cefazolin with metronidazole, or ampicillin-sulbactam [14].

Fong and colleagues [15] investigated the microbiology of post-pancreatoduodenectomy wound infection cultures and the effectiveness of institution-based perioperative antibiotic protocols. The investigators identified substantial variability across the 3 included institutions in intraoperative bile and wound cultures as well as antibiotic-resistance patterns. In this study, Institution A mainly administered cefoxitin for perioperative coverage, Institution B administered cefazolin and metronidazole, and Institution C used ampicillin/sulbactam. Institution A (cefazolin) predominantly grew Enterococcus and Enterobacter in their wound cultures. Of note, there are strains of *E faecalis* that are cephalosporin resistant, and Enterobacter is essentially not covered by cefoxitin. Institution B (cefazolin and metronidazole) predominantly cultured *Staphylococcus aureus* and *K pneumoniae*, which were resistant to cefazolin. Institution C (ampicillin-sulbactam) grew strains of *E faecalis* and *E coli* that were resistant to their choice prophylactic antibiotic. None of these institutions were administering effective prophylactic perioperative antibiotics. Moreover, this study suggests that the antibiotic regimen recommended by the SCIP for GI surgery, may be inadequate for pancreatoduodenectomy given the unique biliary and enteric intraoperative contamination associated with this surgery.

In April 2023, a multi-institutional registry-linked randomized clinical trial investigating the effect of broad-spectrum perioperative antimicrobial prophylaxis in pancreatoduodenectomy was published [16]. The study, which stratified patients for the presence of prior biliary instrumentation, randomized 778 patients with no history of penicillin allergy to either piperacillin-tazobactam or cefoxitin. The primary outcome was the development of postoperative SSI within 30 days. The study found that patients who received piperacillin-tazobactam had a 13% decrease in SSI (19.8% vs 32.8%). Additionally, patients given piperacillin-tazobactam had lower rates of clinically relevant postoperative pancreatic fistula (12.7% vs 19.0%) and postoperative sepsis (4.2% vs 7.5%). The results of this study support the use of broad-spectrum antibiotics as perioperative prophylaxis prior to pancreatoduodenectomy. For patients with no penicillin allergy, this study clearly shows that piperacillin-tazobactam is a very good choice for antibiotic prophylaxis in a patient undergoing a pancreatoduodenectomy. It is unclear what is a good broad-spectrum antibiotic for patients with an allergy to β-lactam antimicrobials. True Type I, IgE-mediated cross-allergic reactions between β-lactam antimicrobials (ie, penicillin, cephalosporins, and carbapenems) are uncommon. In fact, the overall cross-reactivity of patients with a penicillin allergy who have a reaction to a first-generation cephalosporin or a cephalosporin with a similar R1 side chain is approximately 1% [17]. Current clinical practice supports the use of cephalosporins in patients without a history of a documented or presumed IgE-mediated penicillin allergy reaction (eg, anaphylaxis, urticaria, bronchospasm) [13]. In patients with a documented β-lactam allergy, clindamycin/vancomycin with gentamicin is recommended as an alternative for surgical prophylaxis [18].

In this study, the use of piperacillin-tazobactam, in addition to decreasing the rates of SSI and sepsis, has the additional benefit of decreasing need for additional antibiotics, which therefore reduces risk of development of *Clostridium difficile* (0.3% in piperacillin-tazobactam group vs 3.5% in cefoxitin group). Furthermore, the rate of clinically relevant pancreatic fistulas was reduced. There are 2 proposed hypotheses for this: First, piperacillin-tazobactam antibiotic prophylaxis more appropriately covers *E faecalis* strains which are known collagenase-producing bacteria and have been associated with anastomotic breakdown and leaks. Second, it is possible that the use of broad-spectrum antibiotic prophylaxis reduced the clinical severity of the clinically relevant fistula, essentially converting it to a biochemical leak with a lower probability of diagnosis.

Prior to this landmark trial, no randomized controlled trial had been conducted in order to investigate perioperative prophylactic antibiotics in pancreatoduodenectomy [19]. This is starkly different from other abdominal surgical procedures, such as colectomy, which have an immense amount of data supporting the recommended surgical prophylaxis. Dozens of randomized controlled trials (RCTs) have been completed in the field of colorectal surgery in order to reduce rates of SSIs; these trials have investigated various prophylactic antibiotics with differing coverage patterns, timing and duration of prophylactic antibiotic coverage, and even routes of antibiotic administration [13,20]. Together with other studies aimed at optimizing the key contributors to postoperative infections, these trials have led to the development of bundles that are evidence-based tools for decreasing SSIs in colorectal surgery [21].

ROLE OF INTRAOPERATIVE BILE CULTURES AND POSTOPERATIVE ANTIBIOTICS

Current guidelines recommend obtaining intraoperative bile cultures, especially in the setting of a preoperative biliary system instrumentation [18]. The literature generally supports that there is typically concordance between intraoperative bile cultures and SSI and organ space infections [15]. By obtaining these intraoperative cultures, postoperative empiric antibiotics can oftentimes be more appropriately tailored if the cultures are positive and the patient develops signs of an infection. However, this is not a routinely accepted and implemented practice; there are some retrospective data that show intraoperative bile culture data do not reliably predict organisms contributing to postoperative SSI [22].

The postoperative use of antibiotics as prophylaxis for SSI is not currently recommended [18]. The 2019 Guidelines for Pancreatoduodenectomy Enhanced Recovery after Surgery (ERAS) cites 3 retrospective studies [23–25] that investigated the use of prolonged antibiotics until intraoperative bile culture data became available; 2 of these studies showed decreased SSI rates with the use of prolonged antibiotics. More recently, a dual-center cohort study was conducted in the Netherlands which compared organ/space infection rates in patients receiving perioperative (cefuroxime and metronidazole) versus prolonged antibiotic prophylaxis after pancreatoduodenectomy; in this study, "prolonged" was defined as 5 additional days of antibiotic administration [26]. This study showed that prolonged antibiotics decreased organ/space infections in patients with contaminated (ie, positive) intraoperative biliary cultures, but not in patients without. Although seemingly promising, there are several potential issues to consider before recommending prolonged antibiotic use. First, none of these studies utilized adequate prophylactic antibiotics (such as piperacillin-tazobactam) as the standard comparison. Second, the use of prolonged and potentially unnecessary antibiotics increases the risk of patients developing resistant bacteria, *C difficile* infections, and exposes them undue health care costs. Finally, none of these studies have provided reproducible methods for routinely implementing such practice patterns, or even reliably identifying patients who would benefit from additionally therapy. For these reasons, this remains an area of needed research in the field of pancreatoduodenectomy and postoperative prophylactic antibiotics are not currently recommended.

WHAT IS NEXT?

Antibiotic stewardship is paramount and surgical prophylaxis is an ideal application for evidence-based antibiotic administration. Recent data show that broader-spectrum antibiotics (piperacillin-tazobactam) should be utilized as perioperative prophylaxis in pancreatoduodenectomy, given its unique surgical risks and complexity in comparison to other GI procedures. However, additional work must be completed in order to identify protocols that allow for patient-specific antimicrobial targeting.

CLINICS CARE POINTS

- SSIs following pancreatoduodenectomy are typically polymicrobial and predominantly caused by gram-negative organisms, followed by gram-positive cocci.
- The use of piperacillin-tazobactam as perioperative surgical prophylaxis prior to pancreatoduodenectomy has been shown to decrease 30 day SSI rates, clinically relevant postoperative pancreatic fistula, postoperative sepsis, and *C difficile* infection.
- Intraoperative bile cultures should be obtained for all patients undergoing pancreatoduodenectomy, especially those with preoperative biliary instrumentation.
- Routine postoperative prophylactic antibiotics are not recommended.

Disclosure

The authors have nothing to disclose.

References

[1] Fernández-del Castillo C, Morales-Oyarvide V, McGrath D, et al. Evolution of the Whipple procedure at the Massachusetts General Hospital. Surgery 2012;152(3 Suppl 1):S56–63.

[2] Winter JM, Cameron JL, Campbell KA, et al. 1423 pancreaticoduodenectomies for pancreatic cancer: A single-institution experience. J Gastrointest Surg Off J Soc Surg Aliment Tract 2006;10(9):1199–210 [discussion: 1210-1211].

[3] Merkow RP, Bilimoria KY, Tomlinson JS, et al. Postoperative complications reduce adjuvant chemotherapy use in resectable pancreatic cancer. Ann Surg 2014;260(2):372–7.

[4] Lee GC, Fong ZV, Ferrone CR, et al. High performing whipple patients: factors associated with short length of stay after open pancreaticoduodenectomy. J Gastrointest Surg Off J Soc Surg Aliment Tract 2014;18(10):1760–9.

[5] Anderson DJ, Podgorny K, Berríos-Torres SI, et al. Strategies to Prevent Surgical Site Infections in Acute Care Hospitals: 2014 Update. Infect Control Hosp Epidemiol Off J Soc Hosp Epidemiol Am 2014;35(6):605–27.

[6] Mangram AJ, Horan TC, Pearson ML, et al. Guideline for Prevention of Surgical Site Infection, 1999. Centers for Disease Control and Prevention (CDC) Hospital Infection Control Practices Advisory Committee. Am J Infect Control 1999;27(2):97–132 [quiz: 133-134; discussion: 96].

[7] Berríos-Torres SI, Umscheid CA, Bratzler DW, et al. Centers for Disease Control and Prevention Guideline for the Prevention of Surgical Site Infection, 2017. JAMA Surg 2017;152(8): 784–91.

[8] Gavazzi F, Ridolfi C, Capretti G, et al. Role of preoperative biliary stents, bile contamination and antibiotic prophylaxis in surgical site infections after pancreaticoduodenectomy. BMC Gastroenterol 2016;16:43.

[9] Barreto SG, Singh MK, Sharma S, et al. Determinants of Surgical Site Infections Following Pancreatoduodenectomy. World J Surg 2015;39(10):2557–63.

[10] Feng W, Irfan A, Fleece M, et al. Understanding risk factors and microbial trends implicated in the development of Whipple-related surgical-site infections. Antimicrob Steward Healthc Epidemiol ASHE 2023;3(1):e36; https://doi.org/10.1017/ash.2022.377.

[11] Kondo K, Chijiiwa K, Ohuchida J, et al. Selection of prophylactic antibiotics according to the microorganisms isolated from surgical site infections (SSIs) in a previous series of surgeries reduces SSI incidence after pancreaticoduodenectomy. J Hepato-Biliary-Pancreat Sci 2013;20(3):286–93.

[12] Shogan BD, Belogortseva N, Luong PM, et al. Collagen degradation and MMP9 activation by Enterococcus faecalis contribute to intestinal anastomotic leak. Sci Transl Med 2015;7(286):286ra68.

[13] Bratzler DW, Dellinger EP, Olsen KM, et al. Clinical practice guidelines for antimicrobial prophylaxis in surgery. Am J Health Syst Pharm 2013;70(3):195–283.

[14] Donald GW, Sunjaya D, Lu X, et al. Perioperative antibiotics for surgical site infection in pancreaticoduodenectomy: Does the SCIP-approved regimen provide adequate coverage? Surgery 2013;154(2):190–6.

[15] Fong ZV, McMillan MT, Marchegiani G, et al. Discordance Between Perioperative Antibiotic Prophylaxis and Wound Infection Cultures in Patients Undergoing Pancreaticoduodenectomy. JAMA Surg 2016;151(5):432–9.

[16] D'Angelica MI, Ellis RJ, Liu JB, et al. Piperacillin-Tazobactam Compared With Cefoxitin as Antimicrobial Prophylaxis for Pancreatoduodenectomy: A Randomized Clinical Trial. JAMA 2023;329(18):1579–88.

[17] Campagna JD, Bond MC, Schabelman E, et al. The use of cephalosporins in penicillin-allergic patients: a literature review. J Emerg Med 2012;42(5):612–20.

[18] Melloul E, Lassen K, Roulin D, et al. Guidelines for Perioperative Care for Pancreatoduodenectomy: Enhanced Recovery After Surgery (ERAS) Recommendations 2019. World J Surg 2020;44(7):2056–84.
[19] Brajcich BC, Ko CY, Liu JB, et al. A NSQIP-based randomized clinical trial evaluating choice of prophylactic antibiotics for pancreaticoduodenectomy. J Surg Oncol 2021;123(6): 1387–94.
[20] Nelson RL, Gladman E, Barbateskovic M. Antimicrobial prophylaxis for colorectal surgery. Cochrane Database Syst Rev 2014;2014(5):CD001181; https://doi.org/10.1002/14651858.CD001181.pub4.
[21] Vu JV, Collins SD, Seese E, et al. Evidence that a Regional Surgical Collaborative Can Transform Care: Surgical Site Infection Prevention Practices for Colectomy in Michigan. J Am Coll Surg 2018;226(1):91–9.
[22] Sutton TL, O'Grady J, Martindale R, et al. Intraoperative Bile Culture in Pancreaticoduodenectomy: Teaching Old Dogma New Tricks. J Gastrointest Surg Off J Soc Surg Aliment Tract 2022;26(1):30–8.
[23] Fathi AH, Jackson T, Barati M, et al. Extended Perioperative Antibiotic Coverage in Conjunction with Intraoperative Bile Cultures Decreases Infectious Complications after Pancreaticoduodenectomy. HPB Surg World J Hepatic Pancreat Biliary Surg 2016;2016:3031749; https://doi.org/10.1155/2016/3031749.
[24] Sourrouille I, Gaujoux S, Lacave G, et al. Five days of postoperative antimicrobial therapy decreases infectious complications following pancreaticoduodenectomy in patients at risk for bile contamination. HPB 2013;15(6):473–80.
[25] Mohammed S, Evans C, VanBuren G, et al. Treatment of bacteriobilia decreases wound infection rates after pancreaticoduodenectomy. HPB 2014;16(6):592–8.
[26] Droogh DHM, Dam JL van, Groen JV, et al. Prolonged antibiotics after pancreatoduodenectomy reduce abdominal infections in patients with positive bile cultures: a dual-center cohort study. HPB 2023;25(9):1056–64.

Advances in Surgery 58 (2024) 87–106

ADVANCES IN SURGERY

Current Management of Diverticulitis

Richard Garfinkle, MD, MSc, PhD[a,b],
Marylise Boutros, MD, FRCSC[c,d,*]

[a]Division of Mayo Clinic Colon and Rectal Surgery, 200 First Street, SW, Rochester, MN 55905, USA; [b]Division of Colon and Rectal Surgery, Jewish General Hospital, Montreal, Quebec, Canada; [c]Department of Surgery, McGill University, Montreal, Quebec, Canada; [d]Department of Colorectal Surgery, Cleveland Clinic Florida, Ellen Leifer Shulman and Steven Shulman Digestive Disease Institute, 2950 Cleveland Clinic Boulevard, Weston, FL 33331, USA

Keywords

• Diverticulitis • Antibiotics • Emergency surgery • Elective surgery

Key points

- Acute left-sided diverticulitis is increasing in incidence, and the cost of care remains a major health care burden.
- In appropriately selected patients, uncomplicated diverticulitis may be managed as an outpatient treatment without antibiotics.
- There is an evolving role for resection and primary anastomosis, with or without diverting loop ileostomy, in the surgical management of perforated diverticulitis.
- Evidence supports elective surgery to improve the quality of life in patients with recurrent (3 or more episodes) diverticulitis or chronic abdominal symptoms related to diverticulitis.
- Surgical decision-making is more complex in immunosuppressed patients and more data are required to inform best practice.

INTRODUCTION

Sigmoid diverticulitis remains one of the greatest health care burdens facing general and colorectal surgeons across North America. In the United States alone, diverticulitis is responsible for close to 1 million outpatient visits, half a million emergency room visits, and over 200,000 hospital admissions

*Corresponding author. Ellen Leifer Shulman and Steven Shulman Digestive Disease Institute, 2950 Cleveland Clinic Boulevard, Weston, FL 33331. *E-mail address:* boutrom3@ccf.org

https://doi.org/10.1016/j.yasu.2024.04.017
0065-3411/24/

annually, at a cost of nearly US $9 billion [1]. It is also a very common cause for colectomy, second to only colorectal cancer [2]. It was previously estimated that 10% to 25% of individuals with diverticulosis of the colon would develop diverticulitis; with the current routine use of computed tomography (CT) scans for diagnosis, that number is likely closer to 4% to 5% [3]. However, the advancing age of the general population, combined with modern Western dietary habits, has maintained a high prevalence of diverticular disease, and the incidence of diverticulitis has been consistently rising over the last several decades [4,5].

Like many surgical pathologies of the gastrointestinal tract, the pathophysiology of diverticulitis had long been attributed to abnormalities in luminal pressure and obstruction [6]. Diverticula were thought to arise in high-pressure zones like the sigmoid colon, causing mucosa to bulge through the colonic wall in areas of muscular weakness. Obstruction or trauma of a diverticulum, most commonly from a hard piece of stool, would then result in local inflammation and infection with subsequent microperforation [7]. This long-standing, unproven theory formed the basis of several dietary recommendations for patients with diverticular disease, including fiber intake and the avoidance of nuts and seeds, the latter of which has been largely debunked [8]. Our modern understanding of the pathogenesis of diverticular disease is still evolving, but likely involves a complex interaction between systemic inflammation, genetic factors, and the gut microbiome [9]. Accordingly, several lifestyle (eg, obesity, physical inactivity, and smoking) and medical (eg, nonsteroidal anti-inflammatory use, immunosuppression, and connective tissue disorders) factors have been associated with disease incidence [9]. Additional studies have demonstrated an association between family history and diverticulitis [10,11], and more recently, a polygenic risk score was developed and validated for the incidence and severity of disease [12]. A better understanding of these factors over the coming years will allow for more precise counseling and clinical decision-making.

DIAGNOSIS AND CLASSIFICATION

A diagnosis of diverticulitis is made based on history, physical examination, and imaging. Left lower quadrant or lower abdominal pain is the most common presentation of diverticulitis. Additionally, patients may have fever, nausea, and altered bowel habits. Importantly, rectal bleeding is not typical of acute diverticulitis, and if present, it may suggest an alternative diagnosis such as ischemic colitis. High-grade fevers with rebound tenderness are suggestive of more severe disease, and diffuse peritonitis, with or without hemodynamic change, is worrisome for free perforation. Pneumaturia and fecaluria are typical manifestations of colovesical fistula, while obstipation and abdominal distension are consistent with a diverticular stricture. Blood work offers complementary information but may be normal in up to 50% of mild episodes of diverticulitis. Elevations in C-reactive protein (CRP) level are also more helpful, and prognostic, compared to white blood cell count; a CRP greater than 150 mg/L may portend complicated disease [13,14].

Multidetector-CT is the principal imaging modality used to diagnose acute colonic diverticulitis. It has a sensitivity and specificity of close to 99% and allows for the appropriate staging of disease severity and complications [15]. Common findings of acute diverticulitis on CT scan include mural edema, fat stranding, and wall thickening involving a region of diverticula. More severe cases may show engorgement of the colonic mesentery, air bubbles adjacent to the colonic wall (indicating microperforation), or extensive inflammatory changes associated with fluid and hyperdense soft tissue, often referred to as a phlegmon. With perforated disease, distant pneumoperitoneum may be visible and abscess formation can occur. Hyperdense free fluid in the pelvis and paracolic gutters, as well as enhancement/thickening of the peritoneum, is suggestive of peritonitis. CT can also be suggestive of other disease complications; for example, the presence of tracts or air bubbles in adjacent organs may be indicative of fistulizing disease. In pregnant patients, MRI is a suitable alternative to CT scan; sensitivity and specificity range from 85% to 90% [16]. Ultrasound has been reported to be used for diagnosis as well; however, it is very operator-dependent and offers limited additional information.

Based on radiological, clinical, and operative findings, several classification schemes have been developed to stage diverticulitis severity (Table 1). In clinical practice, the most important and commonly used taxonomy differentiates uncomplicated from complicated diverticulitis, the latter of which is defined as the presence of an abscess, fistula, stricture, or free perforation with peritonitis. Cases of microperforation and phlegmon are considered uncomplicated disease. The other commonly used scheme is the Hinchey classification, which is an intraoperative classification system that categorizes perforated diverticulitis according to the type of abscess and peritonitis [17]. Importantly, Hinchey III (purulent) peritonitis should be differentiated from Hinchey IV (feculent) peritonitis, as it has potential treatment implications at the time of surgery.

Smoldering diverticulitis is an additional entity that warrants mention. It represents a form of chronic diverticulitis that is particularly resistant to treatment and often necessitates semiurgent surgery. Boostrom and colleagues defined smoldering diverticulitis as ongoing pain with evidence of persistent inflammation (clinical, radiologic, or biochemical), which fails to improve with antibiotics or returns soon after the cessation of antibiotics, and lasts at least 3 months [18]. Smoldering diverticulitis has been associated with both worse short-term and long-term outcomes [19].

UNCOMPLICATED DIVERTICULITIS

Historically, the management of uncomplicated diverticulitis revolved around 3 main pillars of treatment: antibiotics, bowel rest, and hospital admission. However, a modern understanding of disease pathophysiology, combined with current emphasis on early enteral feeding and fast-tracking patients through their recovery and hospital discharge, has challenged the notion that any 1 of the 3 is absolutely necessary for each case.

Table 1
Classification schemes used to stage diverticulitis severity

Name	Type	Classification Scheme
Hinchey	Operative	I: Pericolic abscess II: Pelvic, abdominal, retroperitoneal abscess III: Purulent peritonitis IV: Feculent peritonitis
Modified Hinchey	Radiologic	0: Mild diverticulitis Ia: Pericolic phlegmon Ib: Pericolic or mesocolic abscess II: Distant pelvic, abdominal, retroperitoneal abscess III: Purulent peritonitis IV: Feculent peritonitis
Ambrosseti	Radiologic	*Moderate*: Localized sigmoid wall thickening (<5 mm), pericolic fat stranding *Severe*: Abscess, extraluminal air, extraluminal contrast
Hansen-Stock	Radiologic/clinical	Diverticulosis 0: Diverticulosis Uncomplicated diverticulitis I: Uncomplicated diverticulitis Complicated diverticulitis IIa: Phlegmon, peridiverticulitis IIb: Abscess, sealed perforation IIc: Free perforation III: Chronic/recurrent diverticulitis
WSES	Radiologic	Uncomplicated diverticulitis 0: Thickening of the colonic wall, increased density of pericolic fat Complicated Ia: Pericolic air, pericolic fluid without abscess (within 5 cm from inflamed bowel) Ib: Abscess ≤4 cm IIa: Abscess >4 cm IIb: Distant air (>5 cm from bowel) III: Diffuse fluid without distant free air (no hole in colon) IV: Diffuse fluid with distant free air (persistent hole in colon)
Kruis	Radiologic/clinical	Diverticulosis 0: Asymptomatic diverticulosis Uncomplicated diverticulitis Ia: Diverticulitis without peridiverticulitis Ib: Diverticulitis with phlegmonous peridiverticulitis Complicated diverticulitis IIa: Microabscess IIb: Macroabscess IIc1: Purulent peritonitis IIc2: Feculent peritonitis Chronic diverticular disease IIIa: Symptomatic uncomplicated diverticular disease IIIb: Relapsing diverticulitis without complications IIIc: Relapsing diverticulitis with complications Diverticular bleeding

Abbreviation: WSES, World Society of Emergency Surgery.

The use of antibiotics for diverticulitis dates back to many years and is intimately linked to the notion that diverticulitis is an infectious entity resulting from microperforation of the colon [6]. Despite no trial ever demonstrating superiority with antibiotics, it became dogma to manage these patients with antibiotic therapy, perhaps out of fear that the disease would progress to a more complicated state with no treatment. However, antibiotics have a cost of their own, including adverse effects and drug resistance, the latter of which is increasingly being recognized a worldwide problem [20]. Recognizing that diverticulitis may, in fact, represent an inflammatory colonic disease in its early stages [21], researchers across Europe began challenging the use of routine antibiotic therapy for uncomplicated disease. Several small observational studies demonstrated no increased risk in complications or need for emergency surgery with antibiotic omission [22–24], and European guidelines on diverticulitis began supporting nonantibiotic therapy in immunocompetent patients. This was followed by 4 high-quality, multicenter randomized controlled trials (Table 2), all of which had a similar conclusion [25–28]. Long-term follow-up of these trials also confirmed no difference in recurrence rates or elective surgery [29,30]. With the accumulation of high-level evidence supporting antibiotic omission, several North American medical and surgical societies, including the American Society of Colon and Rectal Surgeons (ASCRS), the Society of American Gastrointestinal and Endoscopic Surgeons (SAGES), and the American Gastroenterological Association, all released updated clinical practice parameters supporting nonantibiotic therapy in select cases [31–33]. However, the adoption of this practice has been notably slower in North America as compared to Europe. The lack of high-quality North American data, as well as fear regarding medicolegal ramifications, have been cited as reasons for caution [34]. It remains to be seen how, and if, this practice will be integrated into modern diverticulitis management.

Table 2
Randomized controlled trials evaluating antibiotics in acute uncomplicated diverticulitis

RCT	Country	n Abx(−) vs Abx(+)	1° outcome Abx(−) vs Abx(+)
Chabok et al, [25] (AVOD). Br J Surg 2012	Sweden/ Iceland	309 vs 314	Disease complications 1.9% vs 1.0% NS
Daniels et al, [26] (DIABOLO). Br J Surg 2017	Netherlands	262 vs 266	Time to recovery 14 vs 12 d NS
Jaung et al, [27] Clin Gastroenterol Hepatol 2021	New Zealand	94 vs 84	Length of hospital stay 45.8 vs 40.0 h NS
Mora-Lopez et al, [28] (DINAMO). Ann Surg 2022	Spain	242 vs 238	Hospital admission 3.3% vs 5.8% NS

Abbreviation: NS, not significant.

It is important to recognize that nonantibiotic therapy is not appropriate for all cases. In addition to immunosuppression, several higher risk subgroups of uncomplicated diverticulitis–such as those with microperforation or very elevated CRP levels–are best treated with antibiotics. Though there are small studies demonstrating safety of nonantibiotic therapy in these subsets [35,36], it is the authors' preference to prescribe antibiotics in such cases. Patients with small abscesses also made up 10% of the study population in the DIABOLO trial [26]; however, most would consider this as complicated disease requiring antibiotics. The evidence supporting any one specific antibiotic regimen for diverticulitis, as well as route of administration (intravenous vs oral), is not particularly strong. A Cochrane review in 2012 found no difference in outcomes between single and double compound antibiotic therapy nor in short versus long duration intravenous administration [37]. Antibiotics should provide broad coverage against gram negative and anaerobic bacteria and are typically given for a 7 day course; however, the patient's general health status and clinical picture may dictate duration. Pragmatically, patients who are not tolerating diet or who appear to need a more prolonged hospitalization should receive intravenous antibiotics until it is appropriate to transition to oral medication.

Bowel rest during the acute episode of uncomplicated diverticulitis was also once routinely implemented. While most practice parameters omitted any guidance regarding nutrition during the early phase, over 80% of surveyed physicians reported some form of bowel rest as part of their personal protocol [38], which included clear liquid diet. A prospective cohort study from the Netherlands demonstrated very low rates of adverse events among patients admitted with uncomplicated diverticulitis and an unrestricted diet [39]. Patients admitted with an unrestricted diet are also more likely to be discharged sooner [40]. Low-residue diet in the early period may contribute toward less stool bulk and could improve symptomatic recovery in an inflamed colon. However, this is not an evidence-based practice.

Finally, outpatient management of uncomplicated diverticulitis should be strongly considered in all patients. The DIVER trial was the first multicenter randomized controlled trial to demonstrate safety for outpatient management, reporting no differences in treatment failure requiring hospitalization or quality of life (QoL), but a 3 fold reduction in the overall health care cost per episode [41]. This practice is supported by North American evidence and guidelines as well [31,42]. Even among the most contemporary trials of nonantibiotic therapy, patients were managed as an outpatient [28]. A systematic review in 2019 failed to identify any factors associated with failure of outpatient management, including previous episodes of diverticulitis, comorbidities, or even microperforation [43]; however, the overall clinical picture may dictate the need for admission in individual cases.

COMPLICATED DIVERTICULITIS

The management of complicated diverticulitis varies according to the complication. Diverticular abscess is the most common presentation of complicated disease, implicating approximately 10% to 15% of all cases [9]. What was once uniformly managed with surgery, the contemporary management of diverticulitis with an abscess is mainly nonoperative. Several population-level studies have demonstrated marked reductions in rates of urgent surgery for complicated diverticulitis; likely explanations include improvements in cross-sectional imaging, improvements in antibiotics and other resuscitative measures, and advancements in percutaneous drainage procedures. Patients who are not septic and peritonitic should be started on antibiotic therapy and typically admitted to hospital for observation. The decision to pursue drainage for additional source control is largely dependent on abscess size and accessibility for the interventional radiologist. Small retrospective studies have reported low rates of treatment failure with antibiotics alone for abscesses less than 3 cm in size [44,45]. A multicenter European study on nonoperative management of diverticular abscess included 447 patients, three-quarters of whom were managed with antibiotics alone [46]. Median abscess size was smaller in the antibiotics alone group (3.6 cm vs 6.4 cm), which is likely a reflection of selection bias; however, only 5% of patients managed with antibiotics alone ultimately went on to require a drainage procedure in short-term follow-up, suggesting that we are, at least, able to appropriately select those patients who do not need upfront drainage. On regression analysis, abscess size (>3 cm), rather than drainage versus no drainage, was associated with treatment failure and need for emergency surgery. Both SAGES and ASCRS recommend considering drainage for abscesses greater than 4 cm and 3 cm in size [31,32], respectively, which is a reasonable approach. Ultimately, with or without drainage, approximately 20% of patients with diverticular abscess will not improve with conservative measures alone and will require an operation [47]. At that point, surgical resection, or laparoscopic abscess drainage alone, is indicated.

For patients with a diverticulitis-related fistula or stricture, surgery is typically warranted for symptom control and the prevention of associated complications (eg, recurrent urinary sepsis from a colovesical fistula). Management in the acute setting should focus on the treatment of any active diverticulitis with antibiotics and subsequent planning for surgical intervention. Stricturing disease also falls on a spectrum of disease severity; patients who present with mild constipation and altered bowel habits can be managed with an elective operation, while those presenting with acute large bowel obstruction need more urgent intervention. The use of self-expanding metallic stents (SEMS) in diverticular strictures has been evaluated; however, its role in benign colorectal obstructions is not well supported. A systematic review and pooled analysis of 122 patients with benign colorectal obstructions reported high rates of stent-related complications (perforation, reobstruction, and stent migration), particularly when stenting across diverticular obstructions [48]. One must also consider the risk of any colonic stricture harboring an underlying malignancy, which would remain untreated following stent insertion. Therefore, when SEMS is employed, it should only be used as a bridge to surgery, and resection with pathologic evaluation of the specimen should ultimately be performed.

Diverticulitis complicated by macroperforation of the colon and/or diffuse pneumoperitoneum is typically managed with emergency surgery. However, in select patients without peritonitis and who are hemodynamically stable, nonoperative management with close observation can be attempted [49,50]. Although ASCRS guidelines recommend an interval colectomy in such patients [31], there is a paucity of data evaluating this specific clinical scenario and long-term expectant management has been described [50]. It is the authors' practice to primarily observe these patients and to selectively offer surgery according to other patient and disease characteristics.

INTERVENTIONS AFTER AN EPISODE OF DIVERTICULITIS

Following an episode of diverticulitis, interventions are focused at confirming the diagnosis, preventing recurrent diverticulitis, and improving QoL. Colonoscopy has traditionally been recommended after every case of diverticulitis and is rooted in an era where diverticulitis was diagnosed on clinical grounds alone or with a double barium enema. With modern, thin-sliced CT scanners, the likelihood of an occult malignancy is considerably lower. An important distinction must be made between uncomplicated and complicated diverticulitis. A recent systematic review and meta-analysis reported a pooled estimate of 0.7% (95% confidence interval [CI] 0.3%–1.4%) for cancer detection among 1497 patients with uncomplicated diverticulitis, comparable to the reported cancer detection rate among asymptomatic patients undergoing screening colonoscopy. However, in patients with perforation and an abscess, the cancer detection rate was estimated at 10.8% (95% CI 5.2%–21.0%) [51]. As such, routine colonoscopy is recommended after the resolution of complicated diverticulitis [31,32]. Guidelines are less committal after an episode of uncomplicated disease, but given the relative safety of colonoscopy, it should be considered in every case. It is the authors' practice to perform colonoscopy if one has not been performed within the last 2 years. Other high-risk features for cancer that should trigger colonic evaluation include atypical symptoms (eg, bleeding), nonresolving disease despite appropriate therapy, and certain radiological features (eg, absence of diverticula, asymmetric wall thickening, "shouldering" phenomenon, and regional lymphadenopathy) [52].

Following an episode of diverticulitis, the risk of recurrence ranges from 15% to 30%, and largely depends on how recurrence is defined. Nonetheless, several factors have been consistently associated with disease recurrence (Table 3), including previous episodes of diverticulitis, young age, and complicated disease [53]. Unfortunately, there are few interventions outside of surgery with a proven effect on reducing the risk of recurrence. Several large randomized controlled trials demonstrated no impact of mesalamine, rifaximin, or probiotics on diverticulitis recurrence [54], and 2 systematic reviews reported no strong evidence for fiber intake [55,56]. There may be a limited role for medical therapy in reducing chronic abdominal symptoms attributed to symptomatic

Table 3
Factors associated with recurrent diverticulitis*

Variable	Strong association	Moderate association	Low/no association
Age*	☑	—	—
Previous episodes	☑	—	—
Abscess formation	☑	—	—
Sex	—	☑	—
Inflammatory extension on CT	—	☑	—
Diverticular number/ location	—	☑	—
Family history	—	☑	—
Body mass index	—	—	☑
Diverticula size	—	—	☑
Ethnicity	—	—	☑
Comorbidity level	—	—	☑

*At younger ages, male sex is associated with recurrent diverticulitis; after the fifth to sixth decade of life, female sex is associated with recurrence.

Hupfeld, L., Burcharth, J., Pommergaard, HC. et al. Risk factors for recurrence after acute colonic diverticulitis: a systematic review. Int J Colorectal Dis 32, 611–622 (2017). https://doi.org/10.1007/s00384-017-2766-z.

uncomplicated diverticular disease [57]; however, true diverticulitis recurrence is not prevented. Additional lifestyle modifications, such as tobacco cessation, weight loss, and physical activity, may reduce diverticulitis recurrence [58–61]. These associations have been linked to several physiologic processes, such as increased circulating inflammatory mediators, effects on gastrointestinal motor function and intraluminal pressure, and changes in gut hormone secretion and activation. Furthermore, there are numerous other health benefits from these lifestyle modifications.

EMERGENCY SURGERY FOR DIVERTICULITIS

Emergency surgery for diverticulitis is indicated in patients who present in sepsis with diffuse peritonitis or who deteriorate after a trial of nonoperative management. The operation of choice is largely dependent on the patient's physiologic status and intraoperative findings. For the longest time, the Hartmann's procedure (sigmoid colectomy, end colostomy, and closed-off rectal stump) was the gold standard operation in the emergency setting. It minimizes operative time, avoids the risk of anastomotic leak, and represents a safe option when operating in the middle of the night. However, the risk of postoperative pelvic sepsis is not completely eliminated–the risk of rectal stump blowout can approach 15% [62]–and the nonreversal rate following a Hartmann's colostomy is notoriously high, ranging from 30% to 50% [63]. Sigmoid resection with primary anastomosis (PRA), with or without a diverting loop ileostomy, has become a popular alternative. Four randomized controlled trials have compared Hartmann's procedure to PRA for perforated diverticulitis (Table 4) [64–67]. A recent meta-analysis reported no difference in postoperative morbidity or mortality with PRA but significantly improved stoma-free survival at 12 months and significantly less morbidity following stoma reversal (see Table 4) [68].

Although most surgical guidelines now endorse PRA as the preferred surgical option in the emergency setting [31,32], there are still occasions where a Hartmann's procedure is preferable. Ultimately, patient factors (eg, severely comorbid and immunosuppression) and disease factors (eg, hemodynamic instability, physiologic derangement, extreme frailty, and malnutrition) may preclude a safe anastomosis. Patients with Hinchey IV diverticulitis also made up less than one-quarter of the studied populations in each trial, leaving some doubt regarding the application of PRA in true feculent peritonitis. The suitability of the rectum for anastomosis is another consideration as it is often thickened and edematous after having been left bathing in infected fluid for days. Finally, elderly patients with poor preoperative bowel function may be best managed with an end colostomy.

In pure Hinchey III peritonitis with a sealed off colonic perforation, laparoscopic lavage without colon resection is a third option. Initially, there was great enthusiasm for this technique when results from the LOLA, SCANDIV, and DILALA trials were published demonstrating no difference in 90 day or 1 year morbidity and mortality [69–71]. Many systematic reviews and meta-analyses were conducted on this subject, and the main conclusions were that laparoscopic lavage resulted in less stomas at the cost of higher rates of early reintervention [72,73]. However, with the decline of the Hartmann's procedure in favor of PRA (and the associated improvement in stoma reversal), the benefits of laparoscopic lavage have become marginal. Other technical concerns with laparoscopic lavage arose as well. The technique was not standardized (eg, volume of saline irrigation, number and location of surgical drains, how to confirm a sealed perforation without manipulating overlying adhesions), and it became clear that performing a proper lavage laparoscopically

Table 4
Risk ratio in randomized controlled trials comparing resection with primary anastomosis to Hartmann's procedure in the emergency setting

Trial	Postoperative Morbidity	Postoperative Mortality	Stoma-free Survival at 12 mo	Postoperative Morbidity at Stoma Reversal
Binda et al. 2012	0.38 (0.12–1.24)	0.27 (0.03–2.18)	1.07 (0.77–1.48)	0.52 (0.06–4.64)
Oberkofler et al. 2012	1.09 (0.61–1.97)	0.70 (0.17–2.88)	1.55 (1.09–2.21)	0.08 (0.00–1.54)
Bridoux et al. 2017	1.04 (0.39–2.75)	1.04 (0.07–16.18)	1.48 (1.19–1.84)	0.34 (0.04–3.13)
Lambrichts et al. 2019	0.79 (0.36–1.74)	2.06 (0.39–10.87)	1.28 (1.06–1.55)	0.13 (0.02–0.97)
Acuna et al. 2019 (meta-analysis)	0.88 (0.59–1.32)	0.84 (0.34–2.08)	1.34 (1.16–1.54)	0.23 (0.07–0.70)

in a hostile abdomen was challenging for most surgeons. Additionally, the risk of recurrent diverticulitis (21% vs 4%) and unplanned operations (26% vs 12%) on long-term follow-up [74], as well as the nontrivial risk of colon cancer, have mitigated the excitement surrounding nonresectional therapy. Altogether, ASCRS currently recommends colectomy over laparoscopic lavage in cases of purulent peritonitis [31].

Emergency colectomy for perforated diverticulitis is typically performed by laparotomy. Limited evidence suggest that laparoscopic Hartmann's procedure or PRA can be safely performed but should be limited to selected cases in experienced centers [75]. Laparoscopy is better utilized in cases of Hinchey I/II diverticulitis requiring urgent surgery for failure of nonoperative management. While it is required to resect distally in the upper rectum for a PRA, it is preferable to simply remove the diseased segment of bowel for a Hartmann's procedure where the distal margin will be revised during colostomy takedown. The use of surgical drains is left to the discretion of the operating surgeon.

ELECTIVE SURGERY FOR DIVERTICULITIS

Historically, elective colectomy was recommended for young patients (aged <50 years), those with recurrent diverticulitis (2 or more episodes), and those with complicated diverticulitis. These recommendations were mostly motivated by the fear of future diverticulitis complications, as these patients were thought to have a more virulent disease course [76,77]. However, numerous studies have demonstrated this not to be the case; current belief is that most perforations occur during the first episode of diverticulitis, while recurrent episodes tend to be less severe [78,79]. Among 181,115 eligible patients using a New York state-wide database, Ho and colleagues reported a 2.4% rate of "poor outcome" (complicated recurrence, colostomy, or death) after a first episode of diverticulitis [80]. In fact, in a large cohort study of patients with 2 or more episodes of uncomplicated diverticulitis, the stoma rate at 1 year was higher among patients who underwent elective surgery as compared to those managed with continued observation (4.0% vs 1.6%, $P<0.001$) [81]. Altogether, these data suggest that fear for a future complicated episode requiring emergency surgery and a stoma should not be used as motivation for an elective operation.

The decision regarding elective surgery in diverticulitis should focus more on QoL and the patient's risk profile for surgery [31]. Previous studies have demonstrated a negative association between symptomatic diverticular disease and health-related QoL [82], and the incidence of chronic abdominal pain after conservative treatment has been estimated as high as 38% [83]. Not surprisingly, QoL has been linked to recurrent diverticulitis and number of episodes. A Markov model study reported equivalent quality-adjusted survival between expectant management and surgery after a third episode of diverticulitis, and favored surgery thereafter [84]. Two randomized controlled trials have compared elective surgery to expectant management in diverticulitis; the

DIRECT trial and LASER trial are summarized in Table 5 [85,86]. Both trials demonstrated improvements in QoL with surgery, finally providing surgeons with some guidance on how to manage this common scenario.

Even following an episode of diverticular abscess managed conservatively, the decision for elective surgery should still center on QoL. The most recent ASCRS practice parameters recommend that surgery should be "considered," which is a significant change from their 2014 previous recommendation that "advised" interval surgery [31]. While the risk of recurrent disease is higher following diverticulitis with an abscess, emergency surgery is still rare [87,88]. Furthermore, the risks of an elective operation for complicated (rather than uncomplicated) diverticulitis are higher, including the need for stomas and conversion to open surgery [89].

Elective surgery for diverticulitis should always include a colorectal anastomosis, as the risk of postoperative recurrent diverticulitis is 4 fold higher if distal sigmoid colon is left in situ [90]. The proximal transection margin should be in soft, pliable, healthy colon. While splenic flexure mobilization is not mandatory, it is often required for sufficient length after removing the entire sigmoid colon. Some studies have demonstrated a reduced leak rate with the preservation of the superior rectal artery while others have reported no difference [91,92]. Ureteric stents can be considered in difficult resections and may have some benefit in identifying ureteric injuries, but there is no evidence supporting their routine use in diverticular surgery [93].

IMMUNOSUPPRESSION

Immunosuppression, no matter what indication or form, complicates the management of diverticulitis. Most, if not all, diverticulitis outcomes are worse in the immunosuppressed, compared to the immunocompetent, population.

Table 5
Comparison of the DIRECT and LASER randomized controlled trials

	DIRECT 2017	LASER 2021
Country	Netherlands	Finland
Number of patients	n = 109 (53 surgery, 56 no surgery)	n = 72 (37 surgery, 35 no surgery)
Inclusion criteria	3 or more episodes (37%) Persistent symptoms (63%)	3 or more episodes (66%) Abscess (27%) Persistent symptoms (7%)
GIQoL at 6 mo	Surgery: 114.4 No surgery: 100.4 Mean difference: 14.2 (7.1–12.1)	Surgery: 114.9 No surgery: 101.9 Mean difference: 11.9 (3.7–20.2)
Anastomotic leak	15%	5%
Long-term outcomes	5 y: improved QoL with surgery 5 y: 46% cross-over to surgery due to ongoing abdominal complaints	1 y: improved QoL with surgery 2 y: similar QoL in both groups 2 y: Less recurrent diverticulitis (11% vs 61%) with surgery

Abbreviation: GIQoL, gastrointestinal quality of life index.

The incidence of disease is higher, as is the risk for perforated diverticulitis and the need for an ostomy during emergency surgery [94]. However, immunosuppressed patients are typically poor operative candidates. Thus, the decision to offer elective surgery for diverticulitis to an immunosuppressed patient is more complex.

Based on the existing evidence, there is probably a higher risk of recurrent diverticulitis among immunosuppressed patients [53]. Biondo and colleagues studied 107 immunosuppressed patients, and among 81 patients with an uncomplicated first episode, only 1 had a complicated recurrence, suggesting that the notion of "the first attack is the worst" still applies to immunosuppressed patients. However, among 26 patients with a complicated first episode of diverticulitis, 9 suffered a complicated recurrence, which carries with it an increased risk for emergency surgery and stoma formation [95]. The risk of major postoperative adverse events in elective diverticular surgery must also be considered. An American College of Surgeons National Surgical Quality Improvement Program (ACS-NSQIP) study reported a nearly 50% increased odds of major morbidity (odds ratio [OR] = 1.46, 95% CI 1.17–1.83) among immunosuppressed patients, and 29% received a stoma [96].

Currently, the ASCRS guidelines recommend an individualized decision to elective surgery in immunosuppressed patients, which differs from older guidelines that more strongly advocated for surgical intervention after a single episode [31]. However, following a single episode of diverticulitis complicated by an abscess, the threshold to offer elective surgery should be lower, weighing the risks of a well-planned elective resection compared to those of a complicated recurrence with possibly devastating consequences. A better understanding of the natural history of immunosuppressed patients with diverticulitis, as well as a delineation of outcomes by immunosuppression subtype, is needed, particularly as indications for immunosuppressive therapies continue to expand.

SUMMARY

Over the last several decades, our understanding of the pathophysiology and natural history of sigmoid diverticulitis has greatly improved. This knowledge has challenged many of the traditional principles in the management for diverticulitis, such as routine antibiotic administration in all cases, number-based recommendations for elective surgery, and the necessity for an end colostomy in emergency surgery. Currently, level-1 data and multiple society guidelines support nonantibiotic therapy for mild uncomplicated diverticulitis. In patients with a diverticular abscess, consideration should be given to percutaneous drainage, though most abscesses less than 3 to 4 cm in size can be treated with antibiotics alone. The decision to offer elective surgery following resolution of an abscess is no longer clear, and most patients will have a favorable long-term outcome with expectant management. In the surgical treatment of diverticulitis, the main controversies rest in the indications for elective resection and the intraoperative decision-making in emergency surgery. While several randomized controlled trials have been published on this topic, more high-level data are required to provide stronger recommendations for treatment.

CLINICS CARE POINTS

- Antibiotics should not be routinely prescribed in cases of mild uncomplicated diverticulitis, as recently supported by multiple North American guidelines.
- Small diverticular abscesses may be treated with antibiotics alone without percutaneous drainage.
- The risk of emergency surgery with a stoma should not be used as motivation when considering elective surgery for diverticulitis; rather, the decision should be driven by how diverticulitis impacts the patient's QoL.
- The Hartmann's procedure remains an important and useful operation for perforated diverticulitis; however, in appropriate cases, the preferred surgical option in the emergency setting is a PRA (with or without diverting loop ileostomy).

Disclosure

The authors have no relevant disclosures.

References

[1] Peery AF, Crockett SD, Murphy CC, et al. Burden and cost of gastrointestinal, liver, and pancreatic diseases in the United States: update 2021. Gastroenterology 2022;162:621–44.
[2] Morris AM, Regenbogen SE, Hardiman KM, et al. Sigmoid diverticulitis: a systematic review. JAMA 2014;311:287–97.
[3] Shahedi K, Fuller G, Bolus R, et al. Long-term risk of acute diverticulitis among patients with incidental diverticulosis found during colonoscopy. Clin Gastroenterol Hepatol 2013;11:1609–13.
[4] Bharucha AE, Parthasarathy G, Ditah I, et al. Temporal trends in the incidence and natural history of diverticulitis: a population-based study. Am J Gastroenterol 2015;110:1589–96.
[5] Wheat CL, Strate LL. Trends in hospitalization for diverticulitis and diverticular bleeding in the United States from 2000 to 2010. Clin Gastroenterol Hepatol 2016;14:96–103.
[6] Beer E. Some pathological and clinical aspects of acquired (false) diverticula of the intestine. Am J Med Sci 1904;128:135–45.
[7] Humes DJ, Spiller RC. Review article: the pathogenesis and management of acute colonic diverticulitis. Aliment Pharmacol Ther 2014;39:359–70.
[8] Strate LL, Liu YL, Syngal S, et al. Nut, corn, and popcorn consumption and the incidence of diverticular disease. JAMA 2008;300:907–14.
[9] Strate LL, Morris AM. Epidemiology, pathophysiology, and treatment of diverticulitis. Gastroenterology 2019;156:1282–98.
[10] Cohan JN, Horns JJ, Ramsay JM, et al. Diverticulitis familiality: a statewide case-control study. J Am Coll Surg 2023 July;5; https://doi.org/10.1097/XCS.0000000000000799:-Online ahead of print.
[11] Almalki T, Garfinkle R, Kmiotek E, et al. Family history is associated with recurrence diverticulitis after an episode of diverticulitis managed nonoperatively. Dis Colon Rectum 2020;63:944–54.
[12] De Roo AC, Chen Y, Du X, et al. Polygenic risk prediction in diverticulitis. Ann Surg 2022 July 25; https://doi.org/10.1097/XCS.0000000000005623 Online ahead of print.

[13] Gallo A, Ianiro G, Montalto M, et al. The role of biomarkers in diverticular disease. J Clin Gastroenterol 2016;50:S26–8.
[14] Mäkelä JT, Klintrup K, Takala H, et al. The role of C-reactive protein in prediction of the severity of acute diverticulitis in an emergency unit. Scand J Gastroenterol 2015;50: 536–41.
[15] Rotert H, Nöldge G, Encke J, et al. The value of CT for the diagnosis of acute diverticulitis. Radiologe 2003;43:51–8.
[16] Heverhagen JT, Sitter H, Zielke A, et al. Prospective evaluation of the value of magnetic resonance imaging in suspected acute sigmoid diverticulitis. Dis Colon Rectum 2008;51: 1810–5.
[17] Hinchey EJ, Schaal PG, Richards GK. Treatment of perforated diverticular disease of the colon. Adv Surg 1978;12:85–109.
[18] Boostrom SY, Wolff BG, Cima RR, et al. Uncomplicated diverticulitis, more complicated than we thought. J Gastrointest Surg 2012;16:1744–9.
[19] Alnaki A, Garfinkle R, Almalki T, et al. Long-term implications of persistent diverticulitis: a retrospective cohort study of 915 patients. Dis Colon Rectum 2021;64:1112–9.
[20] Huston JM, Zuckerbraun BS, Moore LJ, et al. Antibiotics versus no antibiotics for thre treatment of acute uncomplicated diverticulitis: review of the evidence and future directions. Surg Infect 2018;19:648–54.
[21] Floch MH. A hypothesis: is diverticulitis a type of inflammatory bowel disease? J Clin Gastroenterol 2006;40:S121–5.
[22] Hjern F, Josephson T, Altman D, et al. Conservative treatment of acute colonic diverticulitis: are antibiotics always mandatory? Scand J Gastroenterol 2007;42:41–7.
[23] de Korte N, Kuyvenhoven JP, van der Peet DL, et al. Mild colonic diverticulitis can be treated without antibiotics. A case-control study. Colorectal Dis 2012;14:325–30.
[24] Isacson D, Andreasson K, Nikberg M, et al. No antibiotics in acute uncomplicated diverticulitis: does it work? Scand J Gastroenterol 2014;49:1441–6.
[25] Chabok A, Pahlman L, Hjern F, et al, AVOD Study Group. Randomized clinical trial of antibiotics in acute uncomplicated diverticulitis. Br J Surg 2012;99:532–9.
[26] Daniels L, Unlu C, de Korte A, et al. Dutch Diverticular Disease (3D) Collaborative Study Group. Randomized clinical trial of observational versus antibiotic treatment for a first episode of CT-proven uncomplicated acute diverticulitis. Br J Surg 2017;104:52–61.
[27] Jaung R, Nisbet S, Gosselink MP, et al. Antibiotics do not reduce length of hospital stay for uncomplicated diverticulitis in a pragmatic double-blind randomized trial. Clin Gastroenterol Hepatol 2021;19:503–10.
[28] Mora-Lopez L, Ruiz-Edo N, Estrada-Ferrer O, et al. Efficacy and safety of nonantibiotic outpatient treatment in mild acute diverticulitis (DINAMO-study): a multicentre, randomised, open-label, noninferiority trial. Ann Surg 2021;274:e435–42.
[29] van Dijk ST, Daniels L, Unlu C, et al, Dutch Diverticular Disease (3D) Collaborative Study Group. Long-term effects of omitting antibiotics in uncomplicated acute diverticulitis. Am J Gastroenterol 2018;113:1045–52.
[30] Isacson D, Smedh K, Nikberg M, et al. Long-term follow-up of the AVOD randomized trial of antibiotic avoidance in uncomplicated diverticulitis. Br J Surg 2019;106:1542–8.
[31] Hall J, Hardiman K, Lee S, et al. The American Society of Colon and Rectal Surgeons Clinical Practice Guidelines for the treatment of left-sided colonic diverticulitis. Dis Colon Rectum 2020;63:728–47.
[32] Francis NK, Sylla P, Abou-Khalil M, et al. EAES and SAGES 2018 consensus conference on acute diverticulitis management: evidence-based recommendations for clinical practice. Surg Endosc 2019;33:2726–41.
[33] Peery AF, Shaukat A, Strate LL. AGA clinical practice update on medical management of colonic diverticulitis: expert review. Gastroenterology 2021;160:906–11.
[34] Garfinkle R, Sabboobeh S, Demian M, et al. on behalf of the MUD Collaborative. Patient and Physician Preferences for Antibiotics in Acute Uncomplicated Diverticulitis: A Delphi

Consensus Process to Generate Non-Inferiority Margins. Dis Colon Rectum 2021;64: 119–27.
[35] Mali JP, Mentula PJ, Leppaniemi AK, et al. Symptomatic treatment for uncomplicated acute diverticulitis: a prospective cohort study. Dis Colon Rectum 2016;59:529–34.
[36] Bolkenstein HE, van Dijk ST, Consten ECJ, et al. Conservative treatment in diverticulitis patients with pericolic extraluminal air and the role of antibiotic treatment. J Gastrointest Surg 2019;23:2269–76.
[37] Shabanzadeh DM, Wille-Jorgensen P. Antibiotics for uncomplicated diverticulitis. Cochrane Database Syst Rev 2012;11:CD009092.
[38] Korte N, Klarenbeek B, Kuyvenhoven J, et al. Management of diverticulitis: results of a survey among gastroenterologists and surgeons. Colorectal Dis 2011;13:411–7.
[39] Stam MAW, Draaisma WA, van de Wall BJM, et al. An unrestricted diet for uncomplicated diverticulitis is safe: results of a prospective diverticulitis diet study. Colorectal Dis 2017;19: 372–7.
[40] van de Wall BJM, Draaisma WA, van Iersel JJ, et al. Dietary restrictions for acute diverticulitis: evidence-based or expert opinion? Int J Colorectal Dis 2013;28:1287–93.
[41] Biondo S, Golda T, Kreisler E, et al. Outpatient versus hospitalization management for uncomplicated diverticulitis: a prospective, multicenter randomized clinical trial (DIVER trial). Ann Surg 2014;259:38–44.
[42] Sirany AME, Gaertner WB, Madoff RD, et al. Diverticulitis diagnosed in the emergency room: is it safe to discharge home? J Am Coll Surg 2017;225:21–5.
[43] Cirocchi R, Randolph JJ, Binda GA, et al. Is the outpatient management of acute diverticulitis safe and effective? A systematic review and meta-analysis. Tech Coloproctol 2019;23: 87–100.
[44] Siewert B, Tye G, Kruskal J, et al. Impact of CT-guided drainage in the treatment of diverticular abscesses: size matters. AJR Am J Roentgenol 2006;186:680–6.
[45] Etzioni DA, Chiu VY, Cannom RR, et al. Outpatient treatment of acute diverticulitis: rates and predictors of failure. Dis Colon Rectum 2010;53:861–5.
[46] Lambrichts DPV, Bolkenstein HE, van der Does DCHE, et al. Multicentre study of non-surgical management of diverticulitis with abscess formation. Br J Surg 2019;106:458–66.
[47] Gregersen R, Mortensen LQ, Burcharth J, et al. Treatment of patients with acute colonic diverticulitis complicated by abscess formation: a systematic review. Int J Surg 2016;35: 201–8.
[48] Currie A, Christmas C, Aldean H, et al. Systematic review of self-expanding stents in the management of benign colorectal obstruction. Colorectal Dis 2014;16:239–45.
[49] Dharmarajan S, Hunt SR, Birnbaum EH, et al. The efficacy of nonoperative management of acute complicated diverticulitis. Dis Colon Rectum 2011;54:663–71.
[50] Costi R, Cauchy F, Le Bian A, et al. Challenging a classic myth: pneumoperitoneum associated with acute diverticulitis is not an indication for open or laparoscopic emergency surgery in hemodynamically stable patients. A 10-year experience with nonoperative treatment. Surg Endosc 2012;26:2061–71.
[51] Sharma PV, Eglinton T, Hider P, et al. Systematic review and meta-analysis of the role of routine colonic evaluation after radiologically confirmed acute diverticulitis. Ann Surg 2014;259:263–72.
[52] Lips LMJ, Cremers PTJ, Pickhardt PJ, et al. Sigmoid cancer versus chronic diverticular disease: differentiating features at CT colonography. Radiology 2015;275:127–35.
[53] Hupfeld L, Burcharth J, Pommergaard HC, et al. Risk factors for recurrence after acute colonic diverticulitis: a systematic review. Int J Colorectal Dis 2017;32:611–22.
[54] Balk EM, Adam GP, Cao W, et al. Evaluation and management after acute left-sided diverticulitis: a systematic review. Ann Intern Med 2022;175:388–98.
[55] Maconi G, Barbara G, Bosetti C, et al. Treatment of diverticular disease of the colon and prevention of acute diverticulitis: a systematic review. Dis Colon Rectum 2011;54: 1326–38.

[56] Unlu C, Daniels L, Vrouenraets BC, et al. A systematic review of high-fibre dietary therapy in diverticular disease. Int J Colorectal Dis 2012;27:419–27.
[57] Picchio M, Elisei W, Brandimarte G, et al. Mesalazine for the treatment of symptomatic uncomplicated diverticular disease of the colon and for primary prevention of diverticulitis: a systematic review of randomized clinical trials. J Clin Gastroenterol 2016;50: S64–9.
[58] Hjern F, Wolk A, Hakansson N. Obesity, physical inactivity, and colonic diverticular disease requiring hospitalization in women: a prospective cohort study. Am J Gastroenterol 2012;107:296–302.
[59] Dobbins C, Defontgalland D, Duthie G, et al. The relationship of obesity to the complications of diverticular disease. Colorectal Dis 2006;8:37–40.
[60] Harvey J, Roberts PL, Schoetz DJ, et al. Do appendicitis and diverticulitis share a common pathological link? Dis Colon Rectum 2016;59:656–61.
[61] Usai P, Ibba I, Lai M, et al. Cigarette smoking and appendectomy: effect on clinical course of diverticulosis. Dig Liver Dis 2011;43:98–101.
[62] Secher J, Balachandran R, Iversen LH. Incidence and risk factors of blowout within 90 days after a primary Hartmann's procedure: a retrospective cohort study. Langenbeck's Arch Surg 2023;408:275.
[63] Turner MC, Talbott MD, Reed C, et al. Disparities in colostomy reversal after Hartmann's procedure for diverticulitis. Tech Coloproctol 2019;23:445–51.
[64] Binda GA, Karas JR, Serventi A, et al. Primary anastomosis vs. nonrestorative resection for perforated diverticulitis with peritonitis: a prematurely terminated randomized controlled trial. Colorectal Dis 2012;14:1403–10.
[65] Oberkofler CE, Rickenbacher A, Raptis DA, et al. A multicenter randomized clinical trial of primary anastomosis or Hartmann's procedure for perforated left colonic diverticulitis with purulent or fecal peritonitis. Ann Surg 2012;256:819–26.
[66] Bridoux V, Regimbeau JM, Ouaissi M, et al. Hartmann's procedure or primary anastomosis for generalized peritonitis due to perforated diverticulitis: a prospective multicenter randomized trial (DIVERTI). J Am Coll Surg 2017;225:798–805.
[67] Lambrichts DPV, Vennix S, Musters GD, et al. Hartmann's procedure versus sigmoidectomy with anastomosis for perforated diverticulitis with purulent or faecal peritonitis (LADIES): a multicentre, parallel-group, randomized, open-label, superiority trial. Lancet Gastroenterol Hepatol 2019;4:599–610.
[68] Acuna SA, Dossa F, Baxter NN. The end of the Hartmann's era for perforated diverticulitis. Lancet Gastroenterol Hepatol 2019;4:573–5.
[69] Vennix S, Musters GD, Mulder IM, et al. Laparoscopic peritoneal lavage or sigmoidectomy for perforated diverticulitis with purulent peritonitis: a multicentre, parallel-group, randomized, open-label try. Lancet 2015;26:1269–77.
[70] Schultz JK, Yaqub S, Wallon C, et al. Laparoscopic lavage vs. primary resection for acute perforated diverticulitis: the SCANDIV randomized clinical trial. JAMA 2015;314: 1364–75.
[71] Angenete E, Thornell A, Burcharth J, et al. Laparoscopic lavage is feasible and safe for the treatment of perforated diverticulitis with purulent peritonitis: the first results from the randomized controlled trial (DILALA). Ann Surg 2016;263:117–22.
[72] Penna M, Markar SR, Mackenzie H, et al. Laparoscopic lavage versus primary resection for acute perforated diverticulitis: review and meta-analysis. Ann Surg 2018;267: 252–8.
[73] Marshall JR, Buchwald PL, Gandhi J, et al. Laparoscopic lavage in the management of Hinchey grade III diverticulitis: a systematic review. Ann Surg 2017;265:670–6.
[74] Azhar N, Johanssen A, Sundstrom T, et al. Laparoscopic lavage vs. primary resection for acute perforated diverticulitis: long-term outcomes from the Scandinavian Diverticulitis (SCANDIV) randomized clinical trial. JAMA Surg 2021;156:121–7.

[75] Beyer-Berjot L, Maggiori L, Loiseau D, et al. Emergency surgery in acute diverticulitis: a systematic review. Dis Colon Rectum 2020;63:397–405.
[76] Wong WD, Wexner SD, Lowry A, et al. Practice parameters for the treatment of sigmoid diverticulitis – supporting documentation. The Standards Task Force. The American Society of Colon and Rectal Surgeons. Dis Colon Rectum 2000;43:290–7.
[77] Kohler L, Sauerland S, Neugebauer E. Diagnosis and treatment of diverticular disease: results of a consensus development conference. The Scientific Committee of the European Association for Endoscopic Surgery. Surg Endosc 1999;13:430–6.
[78] Chapman J, Davies M, Wolff B, et al. Complicated diverticulitis: is it time to rethink the rules? Ann Surg 2005;242:576–81.
[79] Ritz JP, Lehmann KS, Frericks B, et al. Outcome of patients with acute sigmoid diverticulitis: multivariate analysis of risk factors for free perforation. Surgery 2011;149: 606–13.
[80] Ho VP, Nash GM, Milson JW, et al. Identification of diverticulitis patients at high risk for recurrence and poor outcomes. J Trauma Acute Care Surg 2015;78:112–9.
[81] Thornblade LW, Simianu VV, Davidson GH, et al. Elective surgery for diverticulitis and the risk of recurrence and ostomy. Ann Surg 2021;273:1157–64.
[82] Bolster L, Papagrigoriadis S. Diverticular disease has an impact on quality of life – results of a preliminary study. Colorectal Dis 2003;5:320–3.
[83] Andeweg CS, Berg R, Staal JB, et al. Patient-reported outcomes after conservative or surgical management of recurrent or chronic complaints of diverticulitis: systematic review and meta-analysis. Clin Gastroenterol Hepatol 2016;14:183–90.
[84] Andeweg CS, Groenewoud J, van der Wilt GJ, et al. A Markov decision model to guide treatment of recurrent colonic diverticulitis. Clin Gastroenterol Hepatol 2016;14:87–95.
[85] van de Wall BJM, Stam MAW, Draaisma WA, et al. Surgery versus conservative management for recurrent and ongoing left-sided diverticulitis (DIRECT trial): an open-label, multicentre, randomised controlled trial. Lancet Gastroenterol Hepatol 2017;2:13–22.
[86] Santos A, Mentula P, Pinta T, et al. Comparing laparoscopic elective sigmoid resection with conservative treatment in improving quality of life of patients with diverticulitis: the laparoscopic elective sigmoid resection diverticulitis (LASER) randomized clinical trial. JAMA Surg 2021;156:129–36.
[87] von Strauss Und Torney M, Moffa G, Kaech M, et al. Risk of emergency surgery or death after initial nonoperative management of complicated diverticulitis in Scotland and Switzerland. JAMA Surg 2020;155:600–6.
[88] Aquina CT, Becerra AZ, Xu Z, et al. Population-based study of outcomes following an initial acute diverticular abscess. Br J Surg 2019;106:467–76.
[89] Mizrahi I, Abu-Gazala M, Fernandez LM, et al. Elective minimally invasive surgery for sigmoid diverticulitis: operative outcomes of patients with complicated versus uncomplicated disease. Colorectal Dis 2021;23:2948–54.
[90] Thaler K, Baig MK, Berho M, et al. Determinants of recurrence after sigmoid resection for uncomplicated diverticulitis. Dis Colon Rectum 2003;46:385–8.
[91] Borchert DH, Schachtebeck M, Schoepe J, et al. Observational study on preservation of the superior rectal artery in sigmoid resection for diverticular disease. Int J Surg 2015;21: 45–50.
[92] Cirocchi R, Trastulli S, Farinella E, et al. Is inferior mesenteric artery ligation during sigmoid colectomy for diverticular disease associated with increased anastomotic leakage? A meta-analysis of randomized and non-randomized clinical trials. Colorectal Dis 2012;14: e521–9.
[93] Croghan SM, Zaborowski A, Mohan HM, et al. The sentinel stent? A systematic review of the role of prophylactic ureteric stenting prior to colorectal resections. Int J Colorectal Dis 2019;34:1161–78.

[94] Hwang SS, Cannom RR, Abbas MA, et al. Diverticulitis in transplant patients and patients on chronic corticosteroid therapy: a systematic review. Dis Colon Rectum 2010;53:1699–707.
[95] Biondo S, Borao JL, Kreisler E, et al. Recurrence and virulence of colonic diverticulitis in immunocompromised patients. Am J Surg 2012;204:172–9.
[96] Al-Khamis A, Abou-Khalil J, Demian M, et al. Sigmoid colectomy for acute diverticulitis in immunosuppressed vs immunocompetent patients: outcomes from the ACS-NSQIP database. Dis Colon Rectum 2016;59:101–9.

Advances in Surgery 58 (2024) 107–119

ADVANCES IN SURGERY

Repair of Parastomal Hernias

Andrew M. Fleming, MD, Elizabeth H. Wood, MD*

Department of Surgery, The University of Tennessee Health Science Center, 910 Madison Avenue Room 329, Memphis, TN 38103, USA

Keywords

- Parastomal hernia • Parastomal hernia repair • Ostomy • Hernia
- Colorectal surgery

Key points

- Multiple surgical techniques have been developed for the repair of parastomal hernias; however, evidence is inconclusive with regards to the optimal technique.
- Ultimate choice for repair is at the discretion of the operating surgeon and should be individualized to the patient.
- Mesh-based repairs appear superior to suture-only repair and the use of prophylactic mesh at the time of ostomy creation warrants additional study.

INTRODUCTION

The written history of modern ostomy surgery dates back to the 1700s, when Alexis Littré envisioned the use of a diverting stoma for a recently deceased infant with imperforate anus [1]. The first recorded attempt at such a surgery was by a French surgeon named Pillore of Rouen, who performed a cecostomy for a patient with an obstructing rectal tumor, though this was associated with early mortality [1]. Following these attempts, Duret published a successful account of a diverting sigmoid colostomy for the treatment of imperforate anus in an infant, with the patient surviving to the age of 45 years [1].

Gastrointestinal diversion via stoma creation is now commonly employed for a variety of intra-abdominal pathologies, including trauma, inflammatory conditions such as diverticulitis, and malignancy [2–4]. Moreover, a recent white paper from the Wound, Ostomy, and Continence Nursing Certification Board estimates up to 1,000,000 people in the United States are currently living with an ostomy [5]. While this procedure can be a life-saving maneuver for

*Corresponding author. *E-mail address:* ewood24@uthsc.edu

https://doi.org/10.1016/j.yasu.2024.04.007

some patients, ileostomy and colostomy, regardless of indication, remain fraught with complications. Incidence of stoma-related morbidity reported in randomized controlled trials (RCTs) has ranged as high as 81.1% [6]. Perhaps unsurprisingly, among the most common complications after stoma creation is parastomal hernia (PSH).

PSH causes significant harm and psychological distress for patients living with stomas and an ongoing challenge for surgeons. Morbidity from PSH can range in severity from pouching issues and local skin excoriation to giant PSH with associate herniation of other intra-abdominal organs and/or complete obstruction [7,8]. Paramount to the successful management of these patients is an understanding of the pathophysiology, diagnosis, classification, and surgical management of PSH [9].

PATHOPHYSIOLOGY

The creation of a stoma is the creation of an open fascial defect. Studies with longer follow-up periods continue to reveal increasing rates of PSH after ostomy creation (>50%) [9]. Accordingly, the question of PSH is often not one of "if?" but "when?" Several risk factors have been identified that may predispose patients to PSH. Foremost among patient-related factors are increased patient age (≥65 years), increased body mass index (≥25 kg/m^2), and history of diabetes mellitus [10–12]. These variables are fairly intuitive and likely correlate with patient frailty, increased procedural complexity, and local wound complications [13–15]. Interestingly, numerous analyses report female biological sex as an independent risk factor for PSH [10–12]. The underlying drivers of this phenomenon are unclear, though sex disparities in the treatment and outcomes of ventral and incisional hernia repair have been previously described [16]. Finally, one scoping review noted that lack of preoperative stoma site marking and ostomy nurse specialist care prior to ostomy creation was associated with increased stoma-related morbidity, including PSH [17].

DIAGNOSIS AND CLASSIFICATION

The primary method of diagnosing PSH is physical examination [9]. Prior societal guidelines have recommended examination in both a supine and erect position during a Valsalva maneuver, noting a sensitivity of 66% to 100% and negative predictive value of 75% to 100% [9]. The purpose of examination is to elicit symptoms, such as obstruction or pain, as these may indicate operative repair. Also worth considering at this time is whether the ostomy can simply be reversed and intestinal continuity be re-established. While computed tomographic (CT) scans and/or ultrasound can be employed in cases of uncertainty, false positives may result [9]. However, as noted by previous studies, CT provides additional information unable to be obtained on examination, such as the precise size and contents of the abdominal wall defect, as well as the presence of concomitant incisional hernia (cIH). These factors will need to be accounted for when deciding on the necessity of operative repair and, if indicated, the approach to be employed.

At this time, 5 separate classification systems of PSH have been described (Table 1) [18–22]. These vary in methodology and details of classification, as seen in Table 1. Most recently, the European Hernia Society defined their classification of PSH, which takes into account size of hernia defect, presence or absence of cIH, as well as stage modifiers for primary (P) versus recurrent (R) PSH. Data regarding the ideal classification system remain "very low quality" and warrant further investigation as each modern system is validated [9].

SURGICAL MANAGEMENT

Unfortunately, outcomes of PSH repairs (PSHRs) remain poor, and these procedures are associated with their own attendant complications [23]. Inherent to these challenging repairs, regardless of technique, is the paradox of performing herniorrhaphy and deliberately leaving behind a fascial defect. The study of PSHR is nearly as difficult as the operation, with very few high-quality data surrounding the subject.

Table 1
Summary of Classification Systems for Parastomal hernias

Parastomal Hernia classification system Author(s) (Year)	Method of classification	Details of classification system
Rubin et al, [18] 1994	Intraoperative Findings	Type I—"True" PSH Ia—Interstitial Ib—Subcutaneous Type II—Intrastomal Hernia Type III—Subcutaneous stomal prolapse Type IV—Pseudohernia
Devlin [19], 1998	Intraoperative	Type I—Interstitial Hernia Type II—Subcutaneous Hernia Type III—Intrastomal hernia Type IV—Peristomal hernia (stoma prolapse)
Moreno-Matias et al, [20] 2009	Radiographic	Type 0—Peritoneum adjacent to stoma bowel wall, no hernia sac Type Ia—Hernia sac < 5 cm Type Ib—Hernia sac > 5 cm Type II—Hernia sac containing omentum Type III—Hernia sac containing intestinal loop
Gil and Szczepkowski [21], 2011	Clinical	Type I—Isolated, small PSH Type II—PSH w/cIH (minimal abdominal deformation) Type III—isolated, large PSH Type IV—Large PSH with cIH (significant abdominal deformation)
Śmietański et al, [22] 2014	Intraoperative	Type I—PSH ≤5 cm without cIH. Type II—PSH ≤5 cm with cIH. Type III—PSH >5 cm without cIH. Type IV—PSH >5 cm with cIH. P—Primary PSH R—Recurrent PSH

At this time, the European Hernia Society guidelines on prevention and treatment of PSHR that there is "very low quality" evidence regarding the following items: optimal PSH classification system, optimal diagnostic modality, the implementation of watchful waiting for non-incarcerated PSH, the use of an extraperitoneal versus transperitoneal route, the use of a lateral pararectus versus transrectus stoma site, the ideal size of facial aperture, the use of laparoscopic versus open repair in the elective setting, the optimal technique for open PSHR with mesh, the optimal technique for laparoscopic PSHR with mesh, and the specific mesh material used during PSHR [9].

Conversely, the following tenets of PSH management have been sufficient data to support strong societal recommendations.

1. The use of prophylactic, synthetic, non-absorbable mesh during construction of a permanent end colostomy in elective surgery reduces the incidence of PSH [9].
2. There is a high rate of recurrence following primary suture repair, and a low rate of infectious complications from PSHR with synthetic mesh. Therefore, it is recommended to avoid suture repair in the elective setting [9].

PSHR with mesh is associated with improved rates of PSH recurrence in both open and laparoscopic surgery [24–26]. However, mesh types are rarely standardized among studies comparing outcomes of PSHR, and thus data surrounding their comparative efficacy are limited [27].

Types of repairs

Primary Suture Repair

There are multiple described approaches for primary fascial repair of a PSH, but the overall technique includes reducing the hernia by dissecting free and excising the hernia sac and primarily repairing the fascial defect with interrupted sutures (Fig. 1A). The hernia can be accessed via a midline, peristomal, or parastomal approach. Benefits of this technique include avoidance of mesh in a potentially contaminated field while disadvantages are the high recurrence rates which can be upwards of 57.6% [28].

Onlay Repair

To decrease recurrence rates after primary suture repair, mesh-based repairs were developed. First described by Rosin and Bonardi in 1977, following primary suture repair of the PSH and resection of any redundant colon, a polypropylene mesh with a central opening to allow passage of the stoma was sutured to the adjacent anterior rectus sheath (Fig. 1B). A drain was placed in the dissected subcutaneous space [29]. Variations of this technique include creating a keyhole or cruciate opening in the mesh and the "stove pipe" technique where a second piece of mesh is wrapped around the stoma itself within the subcutaneous tissue to further reinforce the repair [30].

Sugarbaker Repair

In 1985, Sugarbaker described a method where the contents of the hernia sac were reduced intra-abdominally, and the fascial edges of the defect were clearly

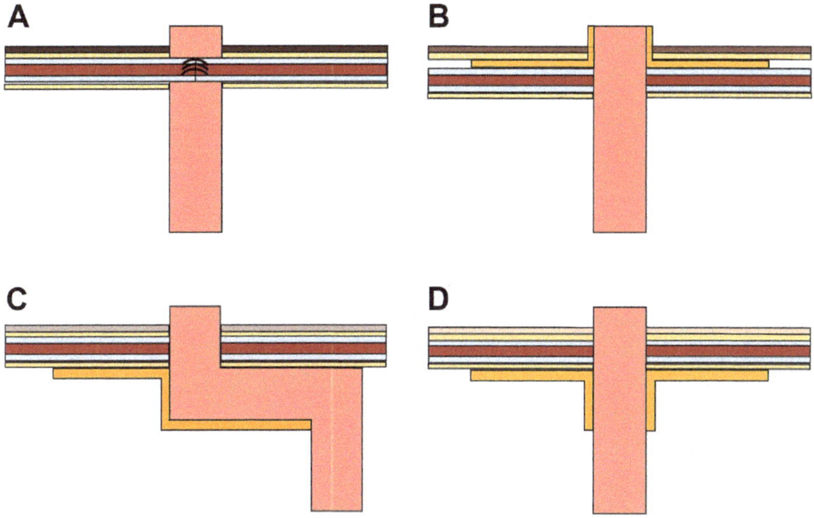

Fig. 1. Graphical representation of parastomal hernia repair techniques. (*A*) Primary suture repair of fascial defect. (*B*) Onlay of mesh over the anterior rectus sheath with "stove-pipe" modification. (*C*) Sugarbaker repair where intraperitoneal mesh is placed over lateralized bowel. (*D*) Keyhole repair where a slit or a cruciate incision is made in the intraperitoneal mesh.

delineated. Next, a prosthetic mesh was sutured to the defect except for a lateral portion where the colon entered the peritoneal cavity. The colon was then suture fixated to the lateral abdominal wall (Fig. 1C). In his initial series of 7 patients, no hernia recurrence was noted at 4 years follow up [31,32]. The Sugarbaker technique has also been modified for a minimally invasive approach. Typically, after entry is made into the abdomen, laparoscopic adhesiolysis is performed, the fascial defect is primarily closed with suture, and an underlay mesh is affixed to the abdominal wall using transfascial sutures or laparoscopic tackers. Many surgeons today ensure that there is at least an extra 4 to 5 cm of mesh around the fascial defect circumferentially. In the event there is an incisional hernia present, the mesh can be sized to incorporate these defects. Another advantage of Sugarbaker repairs is that the use of an underlay mesh avoids exposure of a prosthetic material to enteric contents [33,34].

Keyhole Repair

A second method for intraperitoneal mesh placement involves making a keyhole or cruciate incision within a mesh for the colon to pass through. To avoid taking down the ostomy, the mesh is split and subsequently sutured closed after encircling the bowel (Fig. 1D) [31–34]. Again, this technique can be applied with either an open or minimally invasive approach.

Sandwich Technique

A combination of the Sugarbaker and keyhole mesh repair was described laparoscopically by Berger and colleagues, Dubbed the "sandwich" technique, a keyhole mesh is first placed to reinforce the fascial defect. A second mesh is then placed so that the lateralized bowel is sitting between the two meshes. The second intraperitoneal mesh reinforces the cut slit in the keyhole mesh and allows coverage of any incisional hernias [35].

Pauli Parastomal Hernia Repair Technique

A novel approach was described by Pauli and colleagues in 2016, which couples a transverses abdominus release with a Sugarbaker repair. Entry into the abdomen is obtained via the midline, adhesiolysis is performed, and the hernia contents are reduced. An incision is made in the posterior rectus sheath 0.5 cm lateral to the linea alba spanning the entire length of the rectus. The retrorectal space is entered and dissected to the linea semilunaris taking care to spare the epigastric neurovascular bundle as it enters the rectus. The posterior rectus sheath is then incised 0.5 cm medial to the linea semilunaris to release the transversus abdominus muscle. The bowel proximal to the stoma is then brought through this defect which is then closed. This essentially lateralizes the bowel within the retromuscular space. Mesh is then placed into this space and affixed with transfascial sutures in the Sugarbaker manner. If needed, the mesh can be extended to cover any midline defects [36]. An initial case series of this retromuscular Sugarbaker repair reported an 11% recurrence rate at 13 month follow-up and 8% of patients experienced mesh complications requiring reoperation including bowel obstruction and mesh erosion into the stoma [37]. Owing to the technical difficulty of this operation and apparent morbidity, the Pauli technique has yet to be widely adopted. However, surgeons have described endoscopic and robotic modifications that may potentially improve patient outcomes [38,39].

Minimally Invasive Parastomal Hernia Repair

As minimally invasive surgery becomes more prevalent, many surgeons are approaching peristomal hernia repairs laparoscopically or robotically. By extrapolating the fundamentals of an open repair, surgeons can repair these hernias with decreased pain, discomfort, and length of stay. In 2020, Ayuso and colleagues published a series of 15 patients who underwent robot-assisted Sugarbaker repair of their peristomal hernias. With a mean follow up of 14 months, the authors reported a 6.7% recurrence rate with a mean length of stay was 4.2 days [40]. In a retrospective analysis using the American College of Surgeons National Surgical Quality Improvement Database comparing open to laparoscopic peristomal hernia repairs, the length of stay was significantly lower in the minimally invasive group (8.3 vs 4.12 days, $P < .001$). There were improved short-term outcomes in patients undergoing minimally invasive surgery regarding length of stay, risk of surgical-site infection, and overall morbidity [41].

Resiting

Historically, resiting the stoma was the recommended method of managing peristomal hernias as it was shown to have a lower recurrence rate than primary suture repair of the fascial defect [18]. It was then demonstrated that resiting the stoma alone continued to be associated with high hernia recurrence rates and practice patterns shifted to the use of mesh to reinforce the hernia [42]. In a study examining the trends of PSHR techniques, the proportion of patients undergoing stoma resiting decreased from 17% in 1998 to 7% in 2011. The authors attributed this to the increasing adoption of laparoscopic mesh-based repair techniques that carried lower complications and recurrence rates [43].

PREVENTION

The use of synthetic mesh at the time of ostomy formation has not yet been routinely adopted. However, 7 recent meta-analyses of 10 RCTs found moderate-level evidence demonstrating decreased odds of PSH formation and the need for surgical repair [44]. No evidence of increased morbidity was found in the same analysis [44]. These data are now reflected in societal guidelines, which, as mentioned earlier, recommend the use of prophylactic, synthetic, non-absorbable mesh during construction of a permanent end colostomy in elective surgery [9].

In 1958, Goligher noted that colostomies and ileostomies were prone to intra-abdominal adhesions and bowel obstructions [45]. He described tunneling the stoma extraperitoneal to avoid hernia formation. Modern case series report similar findings where extraperitoneal siting of the stoma at the index operation is associated with decreased PSH and intestinal obstruction rates [46]. These techniques have also been adapted for minimally invasive surgery with acceptable safety and feasibility [47]. A meta-analysis comparing extraperitoneal to intraperitoneal creation of stomas examined 7 studies comprising a total of 1071 patients and reported a lower rate of PSH in the extraperitoneal group. However, the studies were retrospective and observational in nature, and the length of follow up was largely unknown, making it difficult for the authors to recommend extraperitoneal siting for hernia prevention [11]. This, too, mirrors the recommendations of the European Hernia Society's guidelines on stoma prevention [9].

OUTCOMES

High-quality data surrounding PSHRs are sparse. In the elective setting, primary suture repair appears to be associated with high rates of recurrence and should be avoided [9]. In 2012, Hansson and colleagues reported a weighted pooled recurrence rate for patients undergoing primary suture repair of 69.4% (95% CI 59.7–78.3%) with a median follow-up time of 27 months [24]. In the same pooled analysis, onlay mesh repairs were associated with 17.2% recurrence (95% CI 11.9–23.4%; median follow-up 36 months), retromuscular repairs with 6.9% recurrence (95% CI 1.1–17.2%; median follow-up 12 months); open keyhole repairs with 7.2% recurrence (1.7–16.0%; median follow-up 28 months); open Sugarbaker repairs with 15% recurrence (n=1 study; median follow-up 42 months); laparoscopic keyhole repairs with

34.6% recurrence (95% CI 13.1–60.3%; median follow-up NR); laparoscopic Sugarbaker repairs with 11.6% recurrence (95% CI 6.4–18.0%; median follow-up NR); and laparoscopic sandwich repairs with 2.1% recurrence (n=1 study; median follow-up 20 months; Table 2).

These data, though dated, suggest that the keyhole repair is inferior to the Sugarbaker approach in the minimally invasive setting. Studies directly comparing outcomes of Sugarbaker versus Keyhole repairs are largely retrospective and observational in nature, making it difficult to exclude the possibility of significant selection bias [27,48–57] (Table 3). A more recent pooled analysis of 10 comparative studies comprising 347 Sugarbaker repairs and 246 keyhole repairs demonstrated decreased odds of PSH recurrence after the Sugarbaker repair (odds ratio 0.38; 95% CI 0.18–0.78; *P*=.008) [27]. However, this phenomenon disappeared upon subgroup analysis of more modern studies with larger patient cohorts and more robust statistical analysis [27]. The reasons for this finding are unclear but are potentially attributable to more rigorous research methodology. Rates of postoperative surgical-site infections and bowel obstructions were found to be similar between Sugarbaker and keyhole repairs in the same analysis, with the earlier data analyzed by Hansson and colleagues revealing no difference in rates of mesh infections or overall morbidity between mesh techniques [24].

These data signal that minimally invasive Sugarbaker approaches to PSHR are likely associated with the lowest rate of PSH recurrence with comparable morbidity to other mesh repairs. The remaining questions regarding data quality make the results of the upcoming RCT comparing retromuscular Sugarbaker to keyhole repairs all the more exciting [58]. Preliminary results report similar perioperative outcomes in both groups at 90 days [59]. Long-term results and data on hernia recurrence are hopefully forthcoming. Data comparing more modern modifications, such as sandwich repairs, 3-dimensional funnel meshes, and extraperitoneal approaches remain in early stages and warrant further analysis.

Table 2
Pooled summary data on PSH recurrence from the 2012 systematic review of PSHR outcomes by Hansson et al. [24]

Pooled recurrence rate data by Hansson et al.			
Repair technique	Number of Studies, n	Recurrence rate, % (95% CI)	Median follow-up, months
Primary suture	5	69.4% (59.7—78.3%)	27
Onlay	8	17.2% (11.9—23.4%)	36
Retromuscular	3	6.9% (1.1—17.2%)	12
Open keyhole	4	7.2% (1.7—16.0%)	28
Open Sugarbaker	1	15%	42
Laparoscopic keyhole	7	34.6% (13.1—60.3%)	NR
Laparoscopic Sugarbaker	6	11.6% (6.4—18.0%)	NR
Laparoscopic sandwich	1	2.1%	20

Table 3
Studies directly comparing recurrence rates after Sugarbaker to Keyhole Repairs

Author, year	Country	Study design	Number of patients		Indication for ostomy	Type of ostomy	Lap vs open repair	Mesh Composition	PSH Recurrence (%)	
			SB	KH					SB	KH
LeBlanc et al, [48] 2005	United States	Prospective	5	7	Not reported	Colostomy, Ileostomy, conduit	Lap	ePTFE	0	14
Muysoms [49], 2008	France	Retrospective	13	11	IBD, CA, other*	Colostomy, ileostomy	Lap	Composite, ePTFE	15	73
Craft et al, [50] 2008	United States	Retrospective	16	5	IBD, CA, other*	Colostomy, ileostomy, conduit	Lap	ePTFE	0	20
Pastor et al, [51] 2009	United States	Retrospective	7	3	IBD, CA, other*	Colostomy, ileostomy	Lap	ePTFE	29	67
Helgstrand et al, [52] 2013	Denmark	Prospective	56	57	IBD, CA, other*	Colostomy, ileostomy	Lap	Not reported	0	5
DeAsis et al, [53] 2015	United States	Prospective	25	18	Not reported	Colostomy, ileostomy	Lap	ePTFE	16	61
Kohler et al, [54] 2015	Austria	Retrospective	4	22	CA, other*	Colostomy, ileostomy, conduit	Lap	Composite	50	45
Oma et al, [55] 2018	Denmark	Retrospective	69	10	IBD, CA, other*	Colostomy, ileostomy	Lap, open	Composite	9	10
Gameza et al, [56] 2020	Denmark	Prospective	61	74	IBD, CA, other*	Colostomy, ileostomy, conduit	Lap	Composite, ePTFE	10	7
Mäkäräinen-Uhlbäck et al, [57] 2021	Finland	Retrospective	91	39	IBD, CA, other*	Colostomy, ileostomy	Lap, open	Polypropylene, polyester, PVDF	22	36

Abbreviations: SB, sugarbaker repair; KH, keyhole repair; CA, cancer; ePTFE, expanded polytetrafluoroethylene; IBD, inflammatory bowel disease; PVDF, polyvinylidene fluoride.

*Other indications for ostomy include diverticular disease, traumatic injury, iatrogenic injury

DISCUSSION

PSHs are an inevitable consequence of ostomy creation and remain a difficult problem to manage. Recurrence after hernia repair has required the continued evolution of surgical techniques for definitive repair. Most studies examining the various methods of repair are retrospective and observational in design and additional prospective studies are needed in order to provide further evidence of efficacy. As such, many surgeons allow for individual patient factors as well as their own experience and comfort level in determining a plan for hernia repair. Patient characteristics including size of defect, comorbidities, previous repair, and the presence of additional incisional hernia are all taken into consideration at the time of surgical planning. The type of mesh used is also at the discretion of the surgeon as synthetic, biologic, and biosynthetic meshes have all been utilized with varying degrees of success.

SUMMARY

The repair of peristomal hernias is challenging with many different techniques described in the literature. With limited prospective studies comparing surgical outcomes of the various techniques, most surgeons utilize their clinical judgment to determine the optimal repair for their patient.

CLINICS CARE POINTS

- The use of prophylactic, non-absorbable mesh during construction of a permanent end colostomy in elective surgery reduces the incidence of PSH
- Primary suture repair of PSH should be avoided in the elective setting due to high recurrence rates.
- Regardless of repair method, recurrence after PSHR remains an issue that warrants continued study to optimize surgical techniques.

Disclosure

The authors have nothing to disclose.

References

[1] Cataldo PA. Intestinal stomas: 200 years of digging. Dis Colon Rectum 1999;42(2): 137–42 [in English].

[2] Manley NR, Sharpe JP, Lewis RH, et al. Analysis of over 2 decades of colon injuries identifies optimal method of diversion: Does an end justify the means? J Trauma Acute Care Surg 2019;86(2):214–9 [in English].

[3] AlSulaim HA, Garfinkle R, Marinescu D, et al. Is the Hartmann's procedure for diverticulitis obsolete? National trends in colectomy for diverticulitis in the emergency setting from 1993 to 2018. Surg Endosc 2023;37(10):7717–28 [in English].

[4] Xiao J, Shen Y, Yang X, et al. The same parastomal hernia repairs rate in the different approaches to colostomy. J Surg Oncol 2023;128(2):304–12 [in English].

[5] United Ostomy Associations of America. The Critical Need to Provide Ostomy Supplies Specific to Patient Need to Improve Health Outcomes [white paper], 2021. https://www.ostomy.org/wp-content/uploads/2021/09/AAH_Ostomy_White-Paper_20210827.pdf.

[6] Malik T, Lee MJ, Harikrishnan AB. The incidence of stoma related morbidity - a systematic review of randomised controlled trials. Ann R Coll Surg Engl 2018;100(7):501–8 [in English].
[7] Bodimeade C, Troller R. Parastomal hernia containing the stomach-a rare complication. J Surg Case Rep 2023;2023(6):rjad204 [in English].
[8] Capitano S, Boccia L. A giant parastomal hernia with partial herniation of the right kidney. Tech Coloproctol 2022;26(3):231–4 [in English].
[9] Antoniou SA, Agresta F, Garcia Alamino JM, et al. European Hernia Society guidelines on prevention and treatment of parastomal hernias. Hernia 2018;22(1):183–98 [in English].
[10] Liu L, Zheng L, Zhang M, et al. Incidence and risk factors for parastomal hernia with a permanent colostomy. J Surg Oncol 2022;126(3):535–43 [in English].
[11] Niu N, Du S, Yang D, et al. Risk factors for the development of a parastomal hernia in patients with enterostomy: a systematic review and meta-analysis. Int J Colorectal Dis 2022;37(3):507–19 [in English].
[12] Ghoreifi A, Allgood E, Whang G, et al. Risk factors and natural history of parastomal hernia after radical cystectomy and ileal conduit. BJU Int 2022;130(3):381–8 [in English].
[13] Khan M, Patnaik R, Lue M, et al. Modified Frailty Index Predicts Postoperative Complications Following Parastomal Hernia Repair. Am Surg 2023; https://doi.org/10.1177/00031348231198102 31348231198102. [in English].
[14] Khan MTA, Patnaik R, Hausman-Cohen L, et al. Obesity Stratification Predicts Short-Term Complications After Parastomal Hernia Repair. J Surg Res 2022;280:27–34 [in English].
[15] Park J, Rivard SJ, Maguire L, et al. Parastomal Hernia Rates and Exercise After Ostomy Surgery. Dis Colon Rectum 2023;66(6):823–30 [in English].
[16] Howard R, Ehlers A, Delaney L, et al. Sex disparities in the treatment and outcomes of ventral and incisional hernia repair. Surg Endosc 2023;37(4):3061–8 [in English].
[17] Zelga P, Kluska P, Zelga M, et al. Patient-Related Factors Associated With Stoma and Peristomal Complications Following Fecal Ostomy Surgery: A Scoping Review. J Wound Ostomy Continence Nurs 2021;48(5):415–30 [in English].
[18] Rubin MS, Schoetz DJ, Matthews JB. Parastomal hernia: is stoma relocation superior to fascial repair? Arch Surg 1994;129(4):413–9.
[19] Devlin HK, AN. Management of abdominal hernias. 2nd edition. London: Arnold; 1998.
[20] Moreno-Matias J, Serra-Aracil X, Darnell-Martin A, et al. The prevalence of parastomal hernia after formation of an end colostomy. A new clinico-radiological classification. Colorectal Dis 2009;11(2):173–7.
[21] Gil G, Szczepkowski M. A new classification of parastomal hernias–from the experience at Bielański Hospital in Warsaw. Pol Przegl Chir 2011;83(8):430–7.
[22] Śmietański M, Szczepkowski M, Alexandre J, et al. European Hernia Society classification of parastomal hernias. Hernia 2014;18:1–6.
[23] Rubin MS, Schoetz DJ Jr, Matthews JB. Parastomal hernia. Is stoma relocation superior to fascial repair? Arch Surg 1994;129(4):413–8 [discussion: 418–9]. [in English].
[24] Hansson BM, Slater NJ, van der Velden AS, et al. Surgical techniques for parastomal hernia repair: a systematic review of the literature. Annals of surgery 2012;255(4):685–95 [in English].
[25] Carne PW, Robertson GM, Frizelle FA. Parastomal hernia. Br J Surg 2003;90(7):784–93 [in English].
[26] Cheung MT, Chia NH, Chiu WY. Surgical treatment of parastomal hernia complicating sigmoid colostomies. Dis Colon Rectum 2001;44(2):266–70 [in English].
[27] Fleming AM, Phillips AL, Drake JA, et al. Sugarbaker Versus Keyhole Repair for Parastomal Hernia: a Systematic Review and Meta-analysis of Comparative Studies. J Gastrointest Surg 2023;27(3):573–84 [in English].
[28] Rendell VR, Pauli EM. Parastomal Hernia Repair. Surgical Clinics 2023;103(5):993–1010.
[29] Rosin JD, Bonardi RA. Paracolostomy hernia repair with Marlex mesh: a new technique. Dis Colon Rectum 1977;20(4):299–302.

[30] Steele SR, Lee P, Martin MJ, et al. Is parastomal hernia repair with polypropylene mesh safe? Am J Surg 2003;185(5):436–40.
[31] Stelzner S, Hellmich G, Ludwig K. Repair of paracolostomy hernias with a prosthetic mesh in the intraperitoneal onlay position: modified Sugarbaker technique. Dis Colon Rectum 2004;47(2):185–91 [in English].
[32] Hansson BM, Morales-Conde S, Mussack T, et al. The laparoscopic modified Sugarbaker technique is safe and has a low recurrence rate: a multicenter cohort study. Surg Endosc 2013;27(2):494–500 [in English].
[33] Sugarbaker PH. Peritoneal approach to prosthetic mesh repair of paraostomy hernias. Annals of surgery 1985;201(3):344–6 [in English].
[34] Hansson BM, de Hingh IH, Bleichrodt RP. Laparoscopic parastomal hernia repair is feasible and safe: early results of a prospective clinical study including 55 consecutive patients. Surg Endosc 2007;21(6):989–93 [in English].
[35] Berger D, Bientzle M. Laparoscopic repair of parastomal hernias: a single surgeon's experience in 66 patients. Dis Colon Rectum 2007;50:1668–73.
[36] Pauli EM, Juza RM, Winder JS. How I do it: novel parastomal herniorrhaphy utilizing transversus abdominis release. Hernia 2016;20:547–52.
[37] Tastaldi L, Haskins I, Perez A, et al. Single center experience with the modified retromuscular Sugarbaker technique for parastomal hernia repair. Hernia 2017;21:941–9.
[38] Lambrecht JR. Endoscopic preperitoneal parastomal hernia repair (ePauli repair): an observational study. Surg Endosc 2021;35:1903–7.
[39] Morrell DJ, Blatnik JA, Pauli EM. Robotic parastomal hernia repair: modified retromuscular Sugarbaker. Robotic Hernia Surgery: A Comprehensive Illustrated Guide 2020;237–58.
[40] Ayuso S, Shao J, Deerenberg E, et al. Robotic Sugarbaker parastomal hernia repair: technique and outcomes. Hernia 2021;25:809–15.
[41] Halabi WJ, Jafari MD, Carmichael JC, et al. Laparoscopic versus open repair of parastomal hernias: an ACS-NSQIP analysis of short-term outcomes. Surg Endosc 2013;27:4067–72.
[42] Israelsson LA. Preventing and treating parastomal hernia. World J Surg 2005;29:1086–9.
[43] Gavigan T, Rozario N, Matthews B, et al. Trends in parastomal hernia repair in the United States: a 14-y review. J Surg Res 2017;218:78–85.
[44] Patel SV, Zhang L, Chadi SA, et al. Prophylactic mesh to prevent parastomal hernia: a meta-analysis of randomized controlled studies. Tech Coloproctol 2017;21(1):5–13 [in English].
[45] Goligher J. Extraperitoneal colostomy or ileostomy. Br J Surg 1958;46(196):97–103.
[46] Londono-Schimmer E, Leong A, Phillips R. Life table analysis of stomal complications following colostomy. Dis Colon Rectum 1994;37:916–20.
[47] Hamada M, Nishioka Y, Nishimura T, et al. Laparoscopic permanent sigmoid stoma creation through the extraperitoneal route. Surg Laparosc Endosc Percutaneous Tech 2008;18(5):483–5.
[48] LeBlanc KA, Bellanger DE, Whitaker JM, et al. Laparoscopic parastomal hernia repair. Hernia 2005;9(2):140–4 [in English].
[49] Muysoms F. Laparoscopic repair of parastomal hernias with a modified Sugarbaker technique. Acta Chir Belg 2007;107(4):476–80 [in English].
[50] Craft RO, Huguet KL, McLemore EC, et al. Laparoscopic parastomal hernia repair. Hernia 2008;12(2):137–40 [in English].
[51] Pastor DM, Pauli EM, Koltun WA, et al. Parastomal hernia repair: a single center experience. Jsls 2009;13(2):170–5 [in English].
[52] Helgstrand F, Rosenberg J, Kehlet H, et al. Risk of morbidity, mortality, and recurrence after parastomal hernia repair: a nationwide study. Dis Colon Rectum 2013;56(11):1265–72 [in English].
[53] DeAsis FJ, Linn JG, Lapin B, et al. Modified laparoscopic Sugarbaker repair decreases recurrence rates of parastomal hernia. Surgery 2015;158(4):954–9 [discussion: 959–61]. [in English].

[54] Köhler G, Mayer F, Wundsam H, et al. Changes in the Surgical Management of Parastomal Hernias Over 15 Years: Results of 135 Cases. World J Surg 2015;39(11):2795–804 [in English].
[55] Oma E, Pilsgaard B, Jorgensen LN. Clinical outcomes after parastomal hernia repair with a polyester monofilament composite mesh: a cohort study of 79 consecutive patients. Hernia 2018;22(2):371–7 [in English].
[56] Gameza VA, Bell Lybecker M, Wara P. Laparoscopic Keyhole Versus Sugarbaker Repair in Parastomal Hernia: A Long-Term Case-Controlled Prospective Study of Consecutive Patients. J Laparoendosc Adv Surg Tech 2020;30(7):783–9 [in English].
[57] Mäkäräinen-Uhlbäck E, Vironen J, Falenius V, et al. Parastomal Hernia: A Retrospective Nationwide Cohort Study Comparing Different Techniques with Long-Term Follow-Up. World J Surg 2021;45(6):1742–9 [in English].
[58] Miller BT, Thomas JD, Tu C, et al. Comparing Sugarbaker versus keyhole mesh technique for open retromuscular parastomal hernia repair: study protocol for a registry-based randomized controlled trial. Trials 2022;23(1):1–9.
[59] Maskal SM, Thomas JD, Miller BT, et al. Open retromuscular keyhole compared with Sugarbaker mesh for parastomal hernia repair: Early results of a randomized clinical trial. Surgery 2023;175(3):813–21.

Advances in Surgery 58 (2024) 121–133

ADVANCES IN SURGERY

Surgery or Endovascular Therapy for Chronic Limb-Threatening Ischemia

Thomas W. Cheng, MD[a], Alik Farber, MD, MBA, DFSVS[b,*]

[a]Division of vascular and Endovascular Surgery, Dartmouth-Hitchcock Medical Center, 1 Medical Center Drive, Lebanon, NH 03766, USA; [b]Department of Surgery, Division of Vascular and Endovascular Surgery, Boston Medical Center, Boston University Chobanian & Avedisian School of Medicine, 85 East Concord Street, 3rd Floor, Boston, MA 02118, USA

Keywords

• Chronic limb-threatening ischemia • Gangrene • Tissue loss • Ischemia • Limb

Key points

- Chronic limb-threatening ischemia (CLTI) is defined as ischemic rest pain or tissue loss (eg, ulceration/gangrene) that has been present for greater than 2 weeks.
- Workup includes a careful history, physical examination focused on evaluation of pulses and wounds, lower extremity noninvasive vascular studies (eg, ankle–brachial indices, toe pressures), saphenous vein mapping, and imaging of the lower extremity arterial anatomy (eg, computed tomography, magnetic resonance, or subtraction angiography) if a revascularization intervention is planned.
- Best Endovascular versus Best Surgical Therapy in Patients with Critical Limb Ischemia trial demonstrated that open bypass surgery with adequate single-segment saphenous vein is superior to endovascular therapy in treating patients with CLTI and infrainguinal arterial occlusive disease who are candidates for both revascularization strategies.

INTRODUCTION

Chronic limb-threatening ischemia (CLTI), an end-stage presentation of lower extremity peripheral artery disease (PAD), presents with ischemic rest pain or tissue loss (ulceration or gangrene) that has been present for at least 2 weeks [1]. PAD affects greater than 200 million people globally, and CLTI has been

*Corresponding author. *E-mail address:* Alik.Farber@bmc.org

https://doi.org/10.1016/j.yasu.2024.04.008

estimated to affect up to 11% of those with PAD [2,3]. The prevalence of CLTI has been estimated to continuously rise given the aging world population and continuous upsloping trend in diabetes and smoking [4]. A recent study analyzing approximately 65 million Medicare patients from 2017 to 2018 found that 480,227 patients carried the diagnosis of CLTI which corresponded to an annual incidence of 0.33% [5]. Untreated patients with CLTI have a 22% major amputation rate and a 22% all-cause mortality at 1 year [6,7]. Timely revascularization is associated with a significant improvement in limb salvage and quality of life [8,9].

Guideline-directed medical therapy, limb-related therapy, and revascularization are used to treat patients with CLTI. While both surgical and endovascular revascularization are the standard-of-care treatment strategies for CLTI, there is currently a lack of consensus on which approach is optimal [10]. To date, 3 randomized controlled trials have compared the efficacy of open surgical revascularization to endovascular therapy in patients with CLTI. These include the Bypass versus Angioplasty in Severe Ischemia of the Leg (BASIL), Best Endovascular versus Best Surgical Therapy in Patients with Critical Limb Ischemia (BEST-CLI), and BASIL-2 trials [11–13].

WORKUP

Patients with CLTI should undergo a detailed history that includes onset of rest pain/tissue loss, history of trauma to the area, ambulatory status/distance (if applicable), and provoking/alleviating factors such as leg elevation or recumbency. If leg pain is alleviated by hip flexion, neurogenic etiologies such as spinal stenosis are likely and should undergo workup. Relevant medical history includes smoking status, diabetes, hypertension, hyperlipidemia, coronary artery disease, chronic kidney disease (CKD), end-stage kidney disease (ESKD), and chronic obstructive pulmonary disease. Vascular-specific history includes prior endovascular/surgical interventions and prior amputations (minor [defined as below ankle] or major [defined as above ankle]). Relevant medications include antiplatelet agents, anticoagulants, statins, and agents, such as steroids that may affect wound healing.

Physical examination involves evaluation of palpable pulses at the femoral, popliteal, dorsalis pedis, and posterior tibial locations. If pulses are absent, continuous-wave Doppler insonation is performed. Wound examination is completed to assess the location and extent of ulceration/gangrene (ie, toe, midfoot, heel, malleolus) and signs of systemic/local infection. The lower extremity is then evaluated using noninvasive testing (ie, ankle–brachial indices, toe pressures, pulse volume recordings, or transcutaneous oximetry) to confirm the presence and degree of ischemia. The foot is then classified according to the wound, ischemia, and foot infection (WIfI) classification that is similar to the TNM staging system for cancer [14]. If revascularization is planned, vein mapping and computed tomography angiography, magnetic resonance angiography, arterial duplex ultrasound, or diagnostic subtraction angiography is performed to evaluate arterial anatomy and guide intervention.

SURGICAL THERAPY, ENDOVASCULAR THERAPY, AND OUTCOMES

Lower extremity open surgical revascularization includes inflow bypass to the groin, such as aortofemoral or axillofemoral bypass and femoral endarterectomy or infrainguinal bypass. Because most patients with CLTI have infrainguinal arterial occlusive disease, infrainguinal bypass is a common surgical revascularization procedure [15]. Bypass is typically constructed from the common femoral, superficial femoral, deep femoral or popliteal arteries to targets at the level of the knee, calf, or foot. Single-segment great saphenous vein (SSGSV) as the bypass conduit has best outcomes [16]. When great saphenous vein (GSV) is unavailable/inadequate, alternative conduits such as alternative autogenous vein (arm vein, short saphenous vein), expanded polytetrafluoroethylene, and cryopreserved saphenous vein allografts can be utilized [17–19]. Adjunctive procedures such as endarterectomy, distal vein patch, vein cuff, and fistula can be used to optimize outcomes [20,21]. There is a myriad of techniques utilized in endovascular revascularization. These include "plain old" balloon angioplasty (POBA), drug-coated balloon angioplasty (DCB), cutting balloon angioplasty, bare metal stent (BMS), drug-eluting stent (DES), stent graft placement, lithotripsy, and atherectomy.

Regardless of technique, outcomes of intervention are critical. Standard outcome measures reported include primary patency (time without any reinterventions), primary-assisted patency (time to first reintervention but not for thrombosis/occlusion [eg, angioplasty, stenting, atherectomy]), and secondary patency (time to thrombosis/occlusion). Other outcomes reported include major amputation, survival, amputation-free survival (AFS), and major adverse limb event (MALE), defined as reintervention, major amputation, or death. Major adverse cardiovascular event (MACE) is a common safety endpoint defined as stroke, myocardial infarction, or death.

CURRENT RESEARCH

Bypass versus angioplasty in severe ischemia of the leg

The BASIL trial, based in the United Kingdom, randomized patients with severe limb ischemia and primarily femoropopliteal occlusive disease to surgery-first or angioplasty-first therapy [11]. The trial enrolled 452 patients from 1999 to 2004 with 228 randomized to surgery-first and 224 to angioplasty-first. Randomization was stratified by center and clinical presentation (rest pain vs tissue loss; ankle pressure of $\geq$50 vs <50 mm Hg). Primary endpoint was AFS of the index leg (defined as major amputation/death). Secondary outcomes included reinterventions, quality of life, hospital resource utilization, 30 day morbidity/mortality, and all-cause mortality.

Overall, the most common age group was 70 to 79 year, 59.5% were male, 36.2% were current smokers, and 42% had diabetes. Tissue loss was present in 74.3% of limbs. Prior intervention on the index limb was present in 21.4%, and 18.4% had a prior intervention on the contralateral limb. Baseline medical therapy included antiplatelet (57.7%), statin (33.6%), and warfarin (7.3%) use.

In the surgery-first cohort, most frequent infrainguinal bypass origin was the femoral artery (94%), and bypass targets were evenly distributed between above-knee popliteal artery, below-knee popliteal and tibial arteries. Autogenous saphenous vein was utilized in 75% of bypasses. In the angioplasty-first cohort, the superficial femoral artery was treated most (80%) followed by more distal vessels (62%). Technical success was 97% and 80% in the surgery-first and angioplasty-first groups, respectively.

The surgery-first cohort had a lower reintervention rate than the angioplasty-first cohort (18% vs 26%) in *intention-to-treat* analysis. In *as-treated* analysis, the reintervention rate between surgery-first and angioplasty-first was further augmented (17% vs 28%). The surgery-first cohort had a higher 30 day morbidity rate compared to angioplasty-first cohort (57% vs 41%), which was driven by infection, wounds, and cardiovascular events. The 30 day mortality rate was similar between groups (5% vs 3%).

The primary outcome of AFS was similar between the surgery-first and angioplasty-first arms, at 1 year (68% vs 71%) and 3 years (57% vs 52%), respectively. In post hoc analysis of outcomes after 2 years, the surgery-first group was associated with reduced likelihood of AFS (HR 0.37, 95% CI 0.17–0.77, $P = .008$) and all-cause mortality (HR 0.34, 95% CI 0.17–0.71, $P = .004$) compared to the angioplasty-first group. Clinical stratification groups (rest pain, tissue loss, ankle pressures), age, diabetes, and creatinine were associated with these outcomes. Quality-of-life metrics were similar between groups. The cost analysis demonstrated that surgery-first strategy had a 34% higher cost within the first year of intervention compared to angioplasty-first strategy.

In a subsequent publication with extended follow-up, an *as-treated* analysis was performed for AFS and overall survival [22]. Prosthetic grafts were utilized in 25% of cases. Vein bypass grafts had an improved AFS compared to prosthetic bypass, respectively (~47% vs ~17% at 5 years, $P = .003$). Survival was similar (~55% vs ~38% at 5 years, $P = .38$). Secondary bypass following failed index angioplasty had significantly lower AFS compared to first-time bypass (20% vs 40% at 5 years, $P = .006$). These data suggest that performing angioplasty as a first revascularization is not a "free shot" as a secondary bypass is not as durable as a primary bypass procedure.

BASIL was the first randomized controlled trial that compared open surgical bypass to endovascular techniques in patients with CLTI. Major criticisms include the use of AFS as a primary endpoint with its overemphasis of mortality events at the expense of underemphasis of limb-related outcomes. Angioplasty alone was not the standard-of-care endovascular intervention outside the United Kingdom.

BASIL-2 who require an infrapopliteal revascularization

The BASIL-2 trial was an open-label, pragmatic, multicenter, phase 3 trial randomized patients with CLTI to vein bypass or endovascular therapy as their index procedure [12]. The trial enrolled 345 patients from 2014 to 2020 at

39 UK centers, 1 Swedish center, and 1 Danish center. Importantly, only patients with infrapopliteal disease were eligible. There were 172 patients randomly assigned the bypass group and 173 patients to the endovascular treatment group. Minimization was utilized rather than stratification, which was based on age group (≤60, 61–70, 71–80, or >80 years), gender, type 2 diabetes only, CKD only, type 2 diabetes and CKD, ischemic rest pain only, tissue loss only, ischemic rest pain and tissue loss, prior index leg revascularization, and intention for hybrid procedure (combined open and endovascular revascularization). DCBs, BMSs, and DESs were permitted and utilized by operator's discretion; atherectomy was not permitted. Primary endpoint was AFS. Secondary outcomes included 30 day morbidity and mortality, reinterventions, wound healing, major amputation, MALE, MACE that included CLTI or major amputation of the nonindex leg, quality-of-life metrics, hemodynamic measures, and all-cause mortality.

Overall, the median age was 72.5 years, 81% of enrolled patients were male, 20.6% were current smokers, 44.3% ambulated independently, 68.7% had diabetes, and 34.2% had CKD stage III or worse. Tissue loss was present in 88.1% of patients with 20.6% having tissue loss only and 67.5% having tissue loss with ischemic rest pain. Prior intervention on the index and nonindex leg occurred in 35.1% and 28.1% of patients, respectively. Baseline medical therapy included antiplatelet (78%), statin (77.4%), and warfarin/other anticoagulation (27.8%) use.

In the vein bypass cohort, the most common bypass origins were the common femoral (26%), superficial femoral (33%), and below-knee popliteal (33%) arteries. Bypass targets involved the anterior tibial (24%), posterior tibial (42.4%), peroneal (14.4%), and dorsalis pedis (17.3%) arteries. Ipsilateral reversed GSV was the most utilized vein conduit (49%) followed by ipsilateral nonreversed GSV (34%). Arm vein was utilized in 4% of cases. Immediate technical success rate in the surgery arm was 96%.

In the endovascular cohort, treatment modalities included POBA (82%), DCB (13%), BMS (16%), and DES (13%). Most frequently intervened arterial segments were the anterior tibial (31.5%), posterior tibial (17%), and peroneal (14%) arteries. Single infrapopliteal artery interventions (65%) were most common, followed by double (33%) and then triple (2%) infrapopliteal arterial interventions. The immediate technical success rate was 86% and interventional radiologists (IRs) performed 84% of endovascular revascularization.

The primary outcome of AFS was 53% for the vein bypass cohort and 63% for the endovascular cohort (HR 1.35, 95% CI 1.02–1.8, $P = .037$). The median AFS time was 3.3 and 4.4 years for the vein bypass and endovascular groups, respectively. Thirty-day morbidity (46% vs 42%) and mortality (6% vs 3%) rates were similar. The reintervention rate was 29% in the vein bypass and 32% in the endovascular arms. Crossover intervention rates (defined as alternative revascularization strategy following initial revascularization therapy [ie, open to endovascular and vice versa]) were more frequent in the vein bypass than the endovascular cohort (27% vs 19%). Reinterventions by similar revascularization modality (ie, initial endovascular revascularization with further endovascular therapy) were lower for the vein bypass than the endovascular group (5% vs 19%). MALE, MACE, hemodynamic changes, relief of ischemic pain, or health-related quality of life were similar between cohorts. The overall mortality rate was 53% in the vein bypass cohort and 45% in the endovascular cohort (HR 1.37, 95% CI 1–1.87). Causes of death, most commonly cardiovascular and pulmonary-related, were similar between arms. BASIL-2 investigators concluded that patients with CLTI who require infrapopliteal revascularization should be considered for best endovascular-first treatment strategy.

Best endovascular versus best surgical therapy in patients with critical limb ischemia

The BEST-CLI trial was an international, multicenter, multispecialty, pragmatic, randomized, controlled trial that compared endovascular to open surgical therapy in patients with CLTI who were candidates for both strategies [13]. It was completed across 150 sites in the United States, Canada, New Zealand, Finland, and Italy. The trial had 2 cohorts where Cohort 1 included patients with adequate SSGSV while Cohort 2 included those without adequate SSGSV. Each cohort was stratified by clinical presentation (ischemic rest pain vs tissue loss) and anatomy (presence or absence of significant tibial occlusive disease). Patients were then randomized to endovascular or open surgical therapy with procedural details left at investigator's discretion. A total of 1830 patients were enrolled from 2014 to 2019 with 1434 patients in Cohort 1 (718 open surgical and 716 endovascular arms) and 396 patients in Cohort 2 (197 open surgical and 199 endovascular arms). Surgical bypass technique was determined by the operator, and any endovascular technique was permitted including POBA, BMS, DES, DCB, and atherectomy. The primary outcome was MALE/all-cause death, where MALE was defined as above-ankle amputation or major index limb revascularization (new bypass, interposition graft revision, thrombectomy, or thrombolysis). The secondary outcomes were MALE or 30 day mortality, major/minor reinterventions, AFS, hemodynamic failure, clinical failure, resolution of index CLTI, recurrent CLTI, MACE, healthcare-related quality-of-life measures, and cost.

Overall, in Cohort 1, the mean age was 66.9 years, 71.5% were male, 35.7% were current smokers, 53.8% ambulated independently, 71.8% had diabetes, and 10.6% had ESKD. Tissue loss was present in 79.7%. Significant infrapopliteal disease was present in 66.9%. A history of any prior infrainguinal intervention was 5.4%. Baseline medical therapy included aspirin (66.9%), clopidogrel (21.9%), statin (70.3%), warfarin (6.5%), and direct-acting oral anticoagulation (3.9%) use.

In Cohort 1, bypass origins were common/superficial femoral artery (75.7%) and popliteal artery (15.7%), and bypass targets were above-knee popliteal (15.3%), below-knee popliteal (24.7%), and tibial/pedal (51.4%) arteries. SSGSV was utilized in 84.6% of bypasses. POBA was performed in 19% of limbs, mostly in tibial arteries where it remains the standard of care. DES/DCB was used in 50.3% of limbs. Arterial segments treated endovascularly were the superficial femoral (67.1%), popliteal (53.1%), and tibial/pedal (51.4%) arteries. Technical success rates of the index procedure were 98.3% and 84.7% for surgical and endovascular groups, respectively. In the endovascular group, vascular surgeons performed 73.4% of cases followed by interventional cardiologists/radiologists (27.9%).

In Cohort 1, the primary outcome of MALE/death was 42.6% in the surgical arm and 57.4% in the endovascular arm (HR 0.68, 95% CI 0.59–0.79, $P < .001$). A major reintervention rate was 9.2% and 23.5% in the surgical and endovascular cohorts, respectively. A major amputation rate was 10.4% and 14.9% in the surgical and endovascular cohorts, respectively. Perioperative MACE was 3.9% and increased to 40.3% overall, which was similar between groups. The 30 day mortality was similar at 1.7% versus 1.3% for surgical and endovascular groups, respectively, and overall mortality was 33% versus 37.6%.

For Cohort 2, baseline characteristics were similar to Cohort 1 except for a slightly older population (68.6 vs 66.9 years), less diabetes (60.3% vs 71.8%), more coronary artery disease (51.6% vs 43.3%), and any prior index limb revascularization (10.4% vs 5.4%). In Cohort 2, tissue loss and significant infrapopliteal disease were present in 69.9% and 63.6% of cases, respectively. Baseline medical therapy in Cohort 2 included aspirin (71.1%), clopidogrel (24.6%), statin (77.9%), warfarin (7.9%), and direct-acting oral anticoagulation (5.6%) use.

In Cohort 2, bypass origins were common/superficial femoral (85.3%) and popliteal (8.4%) arteries, and targets were above-knee popliteal (23.2%), below-knee popliteal (24.7%), and tibial/pedal (45.8%) arteries. Prosthetic conduit was utilized in 55.3% of cases followed by alternative vein (21.1%). Vascular beds intervened endovascularly were the superficial femoral (65.6%), popliteal (57.4%), and tibial/pedal (43.1%) arteries. Technical success rates of the index procedure were 100% and 80.6% for the surgical and endovascular groups, respectively. In the endovascular arm, vascular surgeons performed 79% of cases followed by interventional cardiologists/radiologists (21.5%).

In Cohort 2, the primary outcome of MALE/death was 42.8% in the surgical arm and 47.7% in the endovascular arm (HR 0.79, 95% CI 0.58–1.06, $P = .12$). A major reintervention rate was 14.4% and 25.6% in the surgical and endovascular cohorts, respectively. A major amputation rate was 14.9% and 14.1% in the surgical and endovascular groups, respectively. Perioperative MACE was 3.3% and increased to 31.3% overall, but this was again similar between groups. The 30 day mortality was 2.6% and 0.5% for the surgical and endovascular groups, respectively, but the number of events was inadequate to evaluate for significance. Overall mortality rates were similar between surgical and endovascular arms, respectively, at 26.3% and 24.1%.

BEST-CLI investigators concluded that in CLTI, both surgical and endovascular revascularization procedures are effective and safe. Patients who are candidates for limb salvage should undergo an evaluation of surgical risk and conduit availability. Bypass with adequate saphenous vein should be considered as a first-line treatment option for suitable candidates with CLTI, as part of fully informed, shared decision-making. Level 1 evidence from BEST-CLI does not support an "endovascular-first" approach to *all* patients with CLTI or an "endovascular-only" approach. BEST-CLI supports a complementary role for open and endovascular revascularization strategies and highlights the need for expertise in both for optimal care of these patients.

Other published studies from BEST-CLI include perioperative complications and baseline health-related quality of life [23–25]. Perioperative MACE, nonserious adverse events, and serious adverse events were similar between surgical and endovascular arms for both Cohorts 1 and 2 [23]. MACE was 4.7% versus 3.13% for surgical and endovascular arms, respectively ($P = .12$), for Cohort 1 and 4.28% versus 1.05% for surgical and endovascular arms, respectively ($P = .15$), for Cohort 2. Risk-adjusted analysis for Cohorts 1 or 2 showed no difference in MACE. Acute renal failure was similar for Cohort 1 (3.6% surgical vs 2.5% endovascular arms) and Cohort 2 (4.2% vs 1.6%). Venous thromboembolism was also similar for Cohort 1 (0.9% vs 0.4%) and Cohort 2 (0.5% vs 0%). Overall, most common complications were related to infection, procedures, and cardiovascular. Factors associated with poor health-related quality of life were smoking history, nonindependent ambulation status, opioid use, and female sex [25]. Baseline mean health-related quality-of-life scores trended lower for patients in BEST-CLI compared to BASIL-1 (3.1±1.3 vs 2.9±1.1, P=.07), respectively, and PREVENT III (3.1±1.3 vs 2.8±1.1, P<.001). WIfI stage was associated with lower quality-of-life scores related to mental health rather than physical health [24]. Future reports from BEST-CLI will evaluate changes in quality-of-life measures postintervention.

Comparisons between best surgical therapy in patients with critical limb ischemia and bypass versus angioplasty in severe ischemia of the leg-2

The BEST-CLI and BASIL-2 trials are two recently completed randomized controlled trials in patients with CLTI. While BEST-CLI concluded that bypass with SSGSV outperformed endovascular therapy, BASIL 2 concluded that vein bypass was associated with lower AFS. Both trials demonstrated that mortality in CLTI patients is very high. In terms of primary outcomes, BEST-CLI used MALE or all-cause death, whereas BASIL-2 used AFS, which as previously mentioned, can overemphasize mortality events while underemphasizing limb-related outcomes. Different conclusions reached by these trials are partially related to differences in patient and procedural factors [26]. BEST-CLIs sample size is over 5 times that of BASIL-2. Median follow-up for BEST-CLI Cohort 1 was 2.7 years, 1.6 years for BEST-CLI Cohort 2, and 3.3 years for BASIL-2. The shorter follow-up for BEST-CLI Cohort 2 may contribute to a type II error. BASIL-2s follow-up was extended instead of increasing the sample size and, as such, this may preclude observation of limb events that commonly occur early after revascularization. There was a higher proportion of women in BEST-CLI compared to BASIL-2 (BEST-CLI Cohort 1: 28.5%, BEST-CLI Cohort 2: 28%, BASIL-2: 19%) and a lower proportion of patients of White race (BEST-CLI Cohort 1: 72.2%, BEST-CLI Cohort 2: 70.5%, BASIL-2: 91%). BEST-CLI patients were somewhat younger than those in BASIL-2 (72 vs 67 years) [26]. Comorbidities differed between the enrolled patient population for ESKD (BEST-CLI Cohort 1: 10.6%, BEST-CLI Cohort 2: 11.4%, BASIL-2: 4%) and prior lower extremity revascularization (BEST-CLI Cohort 1: 5.4%, BEST-CLI Cohort 2: 10.2%, BASIL-2: 35.1%). Diabetes was similar between the 2 trials at approximately 70%, and greater than 70% of patients were on an antiplatelet and/or statin therapy. Given different enrollment criteria, significant infrapopliteal disease was less common (BEST-CLI Cohort 1: 66.8%, BEST-CLI Cohort 2: 63.7%, BASIL-2: 100%). The prevalence of tissue loss was similar between trials.

Endovascular procedures in BEST-CLI were more commonly performed by surgeons while IRs completed them in BASIL 2. POBA alone was used in 19% of patients in BEST-CLI and was mostly limited to tibial arteries, while in BASIL 2, 82% of patients were treated using POBA alone. Drug elution was utilized in 50% of patients in BEST-CLI Cohort 1, but only in 13% of patients in BASIL-2. The technical success rate was similar between the 2 trials (85% for BEST-CLI vs 86% for BASIL-2).

The 30 day mortality after open surgical bypass was 1.7% for BEST-CLI Cohort 1 and 6% for BASIL-2. These postoperative mortality differences are staggering. The major amputation rates were significantly lower for BEST-CLI compared to BASIL-2 in both endovascular and open surgical arms (endovascular arm: 14.8% BEST-CLI Cohort 1, 18% BASIL-2; open surgical arm: 10.3% BEST-CLI Cohort 1, 20% BASIL-2). Mortality rates also differed with BEST-CLI having lower rates in endovascular and open arms (endovascular arm: 37.6% BEST-CLI Cohort 1 and 45% BASIL-2; open surgical arm: 33% BEST-CLI Cohort 1 and 53% BASIL-2).

In summary, BEST-CLI and BASIL-2 had significant differences in patient populations and interventions. While endovascular technical failure was similar, perioperative and overall death and major amputation rates were higher in BASIL-2. Outcomes of BASIL-2 appear to be driven primarily by mortality. One possibility for observed differences relates to differences between US and UK health care systems. More granular comparisons are needed to further delineate these results and leadership of both trials is currently planning a patient-level meta-analysis.

Other recent literature, guidelines, and research

The 2019 Global Vascular Guidelines remain the currently used guidelines for CLTI management [1]. Key objectives include establishment of a global definition for CLTI, description of a combination of noninvasive testing and wound classification (ie, WIfI) to diagnose and stage CLTI, prescription of optimal medical therapy, and creation of a global limb anatomic staging system (GLASS) for evidence-based revascularization. GLASS is a new anatomic classification system based on 2 concepts: target arterial path and limb-based patency. Angiographic findings are utilized to define a target arterial path for revascularization, whereas limb-based patency is the maintenance needed to provide in-line flow through the target arterial path. Research is ongoing to verify this new classification scheme and a meta-analysis has suggested that bypass is favored over endovascular therapy for advanced GLASS stages [27].

Recently, a European study compared long-term efficacy of infrainguinal revascularization (endovascular therapy vs surgical bypass) in patients with CLTI from 2015 to 2021 at 4 European vascular centers [28]. The key exclusion criteria were suprainguinal revascularization, prior ipsilateral infrainguinal revascularization, and no follow-up arteriogram/noninvasive testing. Primary outcome was AFS, and secondary outcome was wound healing within 6 months.

The study identified 793 patients, of which 236 were propensity score matched (236 bypasses and 236 endovascular procedures) [28]. Of the bypasses, 80.5% were autogenous vein bypass and 64% were infrapopliteal. Of the endovascular procedures, interventions were performed at the femoropopliteal (34.3%), femoropopliteal and infrapopliteal (42.8%), and infrapopliteal regions (22.9%). At 5 years, surgical bypass had a higher AFS compared to endovascular therapy (60.5% vs 35.3%, $P < .001$). Overall, a major amputation was 25.8% after bypass and 36% after endovascular therapy. These real-world results are similar to BEST-CLI results where bypass was found to be superior to endovascular therapy for major limb events/death. Overall mortality was also similar to BEST-CLI.

Other techniques have emerged to expand treatment options for patients with "no-option" CLTI defined as those requiring primary amputation rather than revascularization. One technique is a percutaneous deep vein arterialization that creates an arteriovenous fistula with stent grafts typically between the posterior tibial artery and vein. The PROMISE II trial recently completed, which is a single-arm, multicenter study that enrolled 105 patients with CLTI with the primary endpoint as AFS [29]. Another ongoing CLTI trial is BASIL-3 which compares 3 endovascular techniques, POBA ± BMS versus DCB ± BMS versus DES, in patients with femoropopliteal disease and similar outcome measures to that of BASIL-2 [30]. This trial has completed enrollment and is expected to be published in the spring of 2024.

SUMMARY

CLTI is a complex disease process that can be treated with open and endovascular revascularization procedures. Current level 1 evidence suggest that open surgical bypass with adequate vein is superior to endovascular intervention as first-line therapy for patients with CLTI and infrainguinal arterial occlusive disease who are candidates for both revasculaization strategies.

CLINICS CARE POINTS

- Endovascular and surgical revscularization are competing, standard of care revasculaization strategies for patients with CLTI.
- Patients with CLTI who are candidates for revascularization should undergo assessment of their operative risk and imaging of great saphenous vein.
- In patients with CLTI who are of acceptable surgical risk, who have adequate SSGSV and who have moderate to complex arterial anatomy infrainguinal bypass should be considered.
- In those who are of high surgical risk, do not have adequate SSGSV or have mild to moderate arterial disease endovascular therapy should be offered.

Disclosure

A. Farber was a national Principal Investigator for the BEST-CLI trial.

Funding

Funding to the BEST-CLI trial was provided by NHLBI/NIH U01HL107407, U01HL107352, and U01HL115662 (trial coordination and analysis) and, during the follow-up period (2019-2021), by the following sources: physician societies: Vascular InterVentional Advances (VIVA), Society for Vascular Surgery, New England Society for Vascular Surgery, Western Vascular Society, Eastern Vascular Society, Midwest Vascular Surgery Society, Southern Association of Vascular Surgeons, Canadian Society for Vascular Surgery, Society for Clinical Vascular Surgery, Society of Interventional Radiology, Vascular and Endovascular Surgery Society, and Society for Vascular Medicine; and industry sources: Janssen, Gore, Bard, Medtronic, Cook, Boston Scientific, Abbott, Cordis, and Cardiovascular Systems Inc.

References

[1] Conte MS, Bradbury AW, Kolh P, et al. Global vascular guidelines on the management of chronic limb-threatening ischemia. J Vasc Surg 2019;69(6s):3S–125S.e140.

[2] Fowkes FG, Rudan D, Rudan I, et al. Comparison of global estimates of prevalence and risk factors for peripheral artery disease in 2000 and 2010: a systematic review and analysis. Lancet 2013;382(9901):1329–40.

[3] Nehler MR, Duval S, Diao L, et al. Epidemiology of peripheral arterial disease and critical limb ischemia in an insured national population. J Vasc Surg 2014;60(3):686–695 e682.

[4] Duff S, Mafilios MS, Bhounsule P, et al. The burden of critical limb ischemia: a review of recent literature. Vasc Health Risk Manag 2019;15:187–208.

[5] Kwong M, Rajasekar G, Utter GH, et al. Updated estimates for the burden of chronic limb-threatening ischemia in the Medicare population. J Vasc Surg 2023;77(6):1760–75.

[6] Verwer MC, Wijnand JGJ, Teraa M, et al. Long term survival and limb salvage in patients with non-revascularisable chronic limb threatening ischaemia. Eur J Vasc Endovasc Surg 2021;62(2):225–32.

[7] Abu Dabrh AM, Steffen MW, Undavalli C, et al. The natural history of untreated severe or critical limb ischemia. J Vasc Surg 2015;62(6):1642–51.e1643.

[8] Mustapha JA, Katzen BT, Neville RF, et al. Determinants of long-term outcomes and costs in the management of critical limb ischemia: a population-based cohort study. J Am Heart Assoc 2018;7(16):e009724.
[9] Shan LL, Yang LS, Tew M, et al. Quality of life in chronic limb threatening ischaemia: systematic review and meta-analysis. Eur J Vasc Endovasc Surg 2022;64(6):666–83.
[10] Jones WS, Dolor RJ, Hasselblad V, et al. Comparative effectiveness of endovascular and surgical revascularization for patients with peripheral artery disease and critical limb ischemia: systematic review of revascularization in critical limb ischemia. Am Heart J 2014;167(4): 489–498 e487.
[11] Adam DJ, Beard JD, Cleveland T, et al. Bypass versus angioplasty in severe ischaemia of the leg (BASIL): multicentre, randomised controlled trial. Lancet 2005;366(9501):1925–34.
[12] Bradbury AW, Moakes CA, Popplewell M, et al. A vein bypass first versus a best endovascular treatment first revascularisation strategy for patients with chronic limb threatening ischaemia who required an infra-popliteal, with or without an additional more proximal infra-inguinal revascularisation procedure to restore limb perfusion (BASIL-2): an open-label, randomised, multicentre, phase 3 trial. Lancet 2023;401(10390):1798–809.
[13] Farber A, Menard MT, Conte MS, et al. Surgery or Endovascular Therapy for Chronic Limb-Threatening Ischemia. N Engl J Med 2022;387(25):2305–16.
[14] Mills JL, Sr, Conte MS, Armstrong DG, et al. The Society for Vascular Surgery Lower Extremity Threatened Limb Classification System: risk stratification based on wound, ischemia, and foot infection (WIfI). J Vasc Surg 2014;59(1):220–34, e221-222.
[15] Farber A, Eberhardt RT. The Current State of Critical Limb Ischemia: A Systematic Review. JAMA Surg 2016;151(11):1070–7.
[16] Pereira CE, Albers M, Romiti M, et al. Meta-analysis of femoropopliteal bypass grafts for lower extremity arterial insufficiency. J Vasc Surg 2006;44(3):510–7.
[17] Farber A, Major K, Wagner WH, et al. Cryopreserved saphenous vein allografts in infrainguinal revascularization: analysis of 240 grafts. J Vasc Surg 2003;38(1):15–21.
[18] Quiñones-Baldrich WJ, Prego AA, Ucelay-Gomez R, et al. Long-term results of infrainguinal revascularization with polytetrafluoroethylene: a ten-year experience. J Vasc Surg 1992;16(2):209–17.
[19] Chang BB, Darling RC 3rd, Bock DE, et al. The use of spliced vein bypasses for infrainguinal arterial reconstruction. J Vasc Surg 1995;21(3):403–10 [discussion 410-402].
[20] Aherne T, Kheirelseid E, O'Neill D, et al. The Use of Arteriovenous Fistulae as an Adjunct to Peripheral Arterial Bypass: A Systematic Review and Meta-analysis. Eur J Vasc Endovasc Surg 2016;51(5):707–17.
[21] Neville RF, Tempesta B, Sidway AN. Tibial bypass for limb salvage using polytetrafluoroethylene and a distal vein patch. J Vasc Surg 2001;33(2):266–71 [discussion 271-262].
[22] Bradbury AW, Adam DJ, Bell J, et al. Bypass versus Angioplasty in Severe Ischaemia of the Leg (BASIL) trial: Analysis of amputation free and overall survival by treatment received. J Vasc Surg 2010;51(5 Suppl):18s–31s.
[23] Siracuse JJ, Farber A, Menard MT, et al. Perioperative complications following open or endovascular revascularization for chronic limb-threatening ischemia in the BEST-CLI Trial. J Vasc Surg 2023;78(4):1012–20.e1012.
[24] Siracuse JJ, Rowe VL, Menard MT, et al. Relationship between WIfI stage and quality of life at revascularization in the BEST-CLI trial. J Vasc Surg 2023;77(4):1099–106.e1094.
[25] Powell RJ, Choudhry N, Conte M, et al. Factors associated with lower preoperative quality of life in patients with chronic limb-threatening ischemia in the BEST-CLI trial. J Vasc Surg 2022;76(6):1642–50.
[26] Conte MS, O'Banion LA. Apples and oranges? A comparison of BEST-CLI to BASIL-2. J Vasc Surg 2023;78(2):265–8.
[27] Shirasu T, Takagi H, Gregg A, et al. Predictability of the Global Limb Anatomic Staging System (GLASS) for Technical and Limb Related Outcomes: A Systematic Review and Meta-Analysis. Eur J Vasc Endovasc Surg 2022;64(1):32–40.

[28] Ricco JB, Roiger RJ, Schneider F, et al. Editor's choice - infra-inguinal endovascular revascularisation and bypass surgery for chronic limb threatening ischaemia: a retrospective european multicentre cohort study with propensity score matching. Eur J Vasc Endovasc Surg 2023;66(4):531–40.
[29] Shishehbor MH, Powell RJ, Montero-Baker MF, et al. Transcatheter Arterialization of Deep Veins in Chronic Limb-Threatening Ischemia. N Engl J Med 2023;388(13):1171–80.
[30] Hunt BD, Popplewell MA, Davies H, et al. BAlloon versus Stenting in severe Ischaemia of the Leg-3 (BASIL-3): study protocol for a randomised controlled trial. Trials 2017;18(1):224.

Advances in Surgery 58 (2024) 135–142

ADVANCES IN SURGERY

ELSEVIER
MOSBY

The Significance of Circulating Tumor Cells in Pancreatic Cancer

Joseph R. Habib, MD, Ammar A. Javed, MD, Christopher L. Wolfgang, MD, PhD*

Department of Surgery, New York University Langone Health, 550 First Avenue, New York, NY 10016, USA

Keywords

• Pancreatic cancer • Circulating tumor cells • Liquid biopsy • Biomarkers

Key points

- A local and systemic component of disease exist in pancreatic cancer, each requiring treatment for improved survival and potential cure.
- CA19-9 is currently the only available biomarker for pancreatic cancer, however it remains limited in its ability to guide management, and new biomarkers are urgently needed.
- Circulating tumor cells are a measure of systemic disease burden and tumor biology.
- The identification, enumeration, subtyping, and longitudinal assessment of circulating tumor cells serve as novel biomarkers to measure disease biology and has promising applications in multiple phases of care.

CIRCULATING TUMOR CELLS AND LIQUID BIOPSY

The earliest reference to circulating tumor cells (CTCs) dates back to 1869, when John Ashworth, an Australian pathologist, observed and described circulating cells that shared features with the primary tumor in the bloodstream of a deceased patient with metastatic disease. Since then, our understanding of CTCs has evolved considerably. CTCs are cells that are shed off of the primary tumor (or metastatic loci), into the blood circulation, disseminate, evade the immune system surviving biological and physical stressors, and are hypothesized to be the seeds of metastatic disease through extravasation into distant organs (Fig. 1) [1]. The life span of these circulating cells is estimated to be

*Corresponding author. *E-mail address:* Christopher.Wolfgang@nyulangone.org

https://doi.org/10.1016/j.yasu.2024.05.001
0065-3411/24/

Systemic spread of pancreatic cancer and potential role of circulating tumor cells as biomarkers

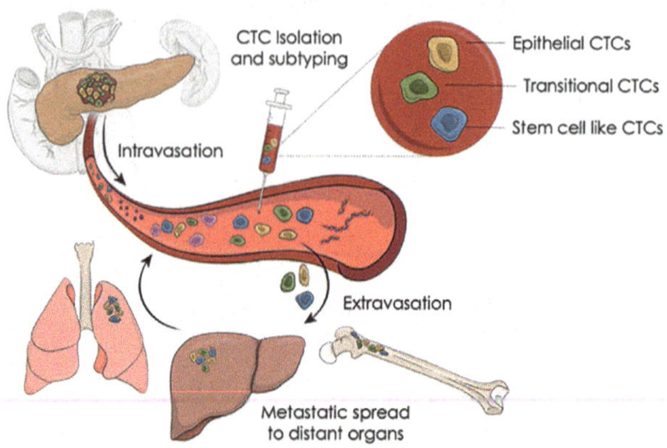

Fig. 1. Primary pancreatic cancer tumor shedding CTCs into blood via intravasation, dissemination, and extravasation leading to metastatic disease. Liquid biopsy is also illustrated displaying multiple CTC subtypes. (*Courtesy of* Kristen Dancel-Manning.)

in the matter of minutes to hours, and they have been noted to exist as clusters and form circulating tumor microemboli with even greater capacity for metastatic deposition [2]. More, they represent a heterogenous population of cells with variable molecular and functional features.

CTC extraction is performed via blood drawn for a liquid biopsy (see Fig. 1). As opposed to traditional tissue biopsies, often sampling primary tumor, which is ultimately resected, a liquid biopsy is less invasive, has lower risk, is cost-effective, and can be performed serially to sample and characterize the systemic component of disease in real-time both in the preoperative and postoperative setting. Furthermore, given the dynamic nature of cancer progression, cellular heterogeneity exists even within the primary tumor or metastatic deposit. Therefore, the degree of heterogeneity and tumor characteristics may vary overtime and is based on where the tissue sample is taken from. Thus, tissue biopsies have both spatial and temporal limitations. Serial CTC sampling via liquid biopsy can mitigate this concern. In support, studies have demonstrated the ability to measure this heterogeneity in CTCs documenting stemness features and an epithelial to mesenchymal cell type transition (see Fig. 1) [3]. Finally, these CTCs obtained via liquid biopsy can be isolated and enriched via a myriad of techniques for further analysis.

CIRCULATING TUMOR CELLS IN PANCREATIC CANCER

CTCs have been identified and isolated in all stages of pancreatic ductal adenocarcinoma (PDAC). Several subtypes of CTCs have been identified in PDAC with differing implications for survival [4]. Fig. 2, panel 1 (A–D) depicts an

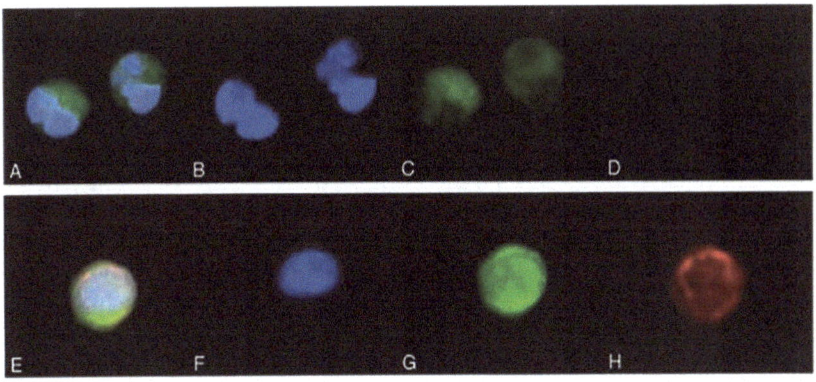

Fig. 2. CTCs expressing the nucleus marker 4′,6-diamidino-2-phenylindole (*blue*), epithelial marker CK (*green*), and mesenchymal marker vimentin (*red*). (*A–D*) display an epithelial CTC ($CK^+ V^-$) while (*E–H*) display a transitional CTC ($CK^+ V^+$).

epithelial CTC expressing cytokeratin (CK) using fluorescent techniques. Epithelial cell adhesion molecule is also commonly used as an epithelial cell marker. Moreover, an epithelial to mesenchymal transition (EMT) is a well-defined biological process where these epithelial tumor cells obtain mesenchymal properties enhancing invasiveness and resistance to apoptosis. Fig. 2 panel 2 (E–H) shows a CK-positive and vimentin-positive CTC called a transitional CTC. Vimentin is a type III intermediate filament expressed in mesenchymal cells. Importantly, these cells then have the ability to undergo a reverse EMT, or mesenchymal–epithelial transition, to induce new metastatic deposits in organs that are primed by forming a premetastatic niche, conducive to CTCs implantation [1].

CLINICAL APPLICATION OF CIRCULATING TUMOR CELLS AS A BIOMARKER

Early detection

Unlike colon and breast cancer, there is no good screening test for pancreatic cancer. Patients with pancreatic cancer remain asymptomatic until progression to late-stage disease which develops a mass effect leading to symptoms such as obstructive jaundice or abdominal pain. At presentation, it is estimated that only 20% of patients have resectable disease. Deploying CTCs for early cancer detection in high-risk populations would theoretically have impactful outcomes by detecting disease in less advanced stages while also increasing the number of patients with resectable disease. In fact, circulating epithelial cells have been implicated in precancerous lesions like intraductal papillary mucinous neoplasms (IPMNs) [5]. The presence of these circulating epithelial cells in the blood stream of patients with IPMNs was found to be associated with high-grade dysplasia, which is the optimal window for resection before progression to an invasive cancer. Potentially, the assessment of CTCs in high-risk cohorts could result in early detection of disease at a resectable stage.

Prognostication

There is mounting evidence supporting the use of CTCs as prognostic biomarkers in a variety of cancers including pancreatic cancer [6]. Currently, most of the robust prognostic factors such as nodal involvement, response to chemotherapy, and grade of differentiation can only be accurately evaluated after surgical resection and histopathologic evaluation. Again, these important prognostic factors are limited by time and space. Alternatively, CTCs can offer a window into the cancer biology both preoperatively and postoperatively and dynamically over various time points [4]. This becomes even more relevant in pancreatic cancer as our practice shifts further toward a neoadjuvant-first approach.

The simplest use of CTCs as a biomarker is the mere presence of CTCs and its subtypes in blood as a predictive indicator. A meta-analysis from 2014 concluded that patients with pancreatic cancer with the presence of CTCs had poorer progression-free survival and overall survival when compared to CTC-negative patients [7]. Furthermore, the presence of transitional CTCs has been shown to predict earlier systemic failure and recurrence [6]. The ratio of mesenchymal CTCs (CK negative, vimentin positive) to epithelial CTC has also been implicated in earlier recurrence.

Additionally, markers such as aldehyde dehydrogenase 1 have been shown to be an indicator for tumor initiating cell (TIC) expression in CTCs. TICs have stem cell like features with the capacity to initiate tumors and proliferate. CTCs expressing TIC phenotypes were independently associated with more cancer recurrence and worse disease-free survival [3]. In summary, the presence of any and an increased number of agressive CTC subtypes may be promising biomarkers for disease biology and patient prognostication.

Predicting treatment response

As the neoadjuvant approach becomes more common, one of the greatest challenges faced in the management of these patients is predicting treatment response in a timely manner. Currently, both multiagent therapies have shown to be effective, and in select patients, administration can result in complete pathologic response. However, assessment of treatment response is only possible 4 to 6 months later when the patients undergo surgical resection or progress to clinically overt metastatic disease in which case surgical resection is not possible. Tools for real-time noninvasive assessment of treatment response that could allow for early modification in treatment regimens are lacking.

In current practice, obtaining and trending serial carbohydrate antigen 19-9 (CA19-9) values and interval cross-sectional imaging evaluating response evaluation criteria in solid tumors (RECIST criteria) or changes in metastatic deposit sizes are the best ways to evaluate response to preoperative chemotherapy, inform cancer biology, and determine biologic and anatomy resectability. However, even when employing all these strategies, decision-making regarding the type of chemotherapy regimen, optimal number of chemotherapy cycles, or decision when to operate are imperfect [8]. CA19-9 is limited by its low specificity, and approximately 10% to 20% of patients are nonproducers. CEA (carcinoembryonic antigen) has also shown some promise when combined with CA19-9; however, their performance in predicting treatment response remains suboptimal. As far as the RECIST criteria is concerned, it is difficult to discern viable tumor from dead tissue, and therefore, this criterion fails to accurately predict treatment response [9]. Furthermore, it only assesses the primary tumor and may have limited implications in the assessment of systemic burden of disease. Dynamic CTC changes overtime may provide a promising adjunct for clinical utility. In fact, multiple studies have shown a reduction in CTC number after neoadjuvant chemotherapy is associated with pathologic treatment response to neoadjuvant chemotherapy [10]. Here, employing CTC dynamics as an additional aide may provide further insight into minimal residual disease not seen on imaging or estimated by CA19-9. Thus, CTCs offering insight into the degree of systemic disease may either inform oncologists when to switch chemotherapy regimens in cases or likelihood of poor response or help surgeons decide when to operate versus offer the patient additional cycles of chemotherapy.

Surgical decision-making

The debate between neoadjuvant chemotherapy and a surgery-first approach for patients with localized disease is ongoing. In the United States, neoadjuvant chemotherapy is given to most patients with resectable pancreatic cancer. Currently, CA19-9 is the best blood-based biomarker for PDAC and is often used as a surrogate for systemic disease. When within normal limits, it may encourage some surgeons to opt for a surgery-first approach. However, CA19-9 has multiple limitations as described earlier. Using CTCs, a more direct measure of systemic disease may provide enhanced foresight into optimal patient selection to identify the subset of patients who would more likely benefit from a surgery-first approach [4]. One could fathom that patients with a combination of low CA19-9 and undetectable/low CTC counts may be a good indicator of more localized disease, and hence, this patient may be more likely to benefit from upfront surgery. Evaluating CTC counts, subtypes, and dynamics may offer further assistance in optimizing patient preoperative selection for surgery or need for neoadjuvant chemotherapy.

Currently, cross-sectional imaging is the standard of care for determining preoperative presence of occult metastatic disease and anatomic resectability. A diagnostic laparoscopy is still often performed before pancreatectomy to ensure a lack of occult metastatic disease that would preclude surgery. In fact, the rate of aborted pancreatectomies for occult metastatic disease, most commonly found in the liver and peritoneum, is near 10% [11]. Notably, patients with occult abdominal metastatic disease have significantly more CTCs in circulation than those that successfully underwent pancreatectomy [12]. More, patients with aborted surgeries due to metastatic disease have comparable CTC counts to those with vascular involvement resulting in aborted pancreatectomy. Together, CTCs may play a potential role in predicting which patients are at a higher likelihood for aborted surgery and thus further inform likelihood of successful resection and potential need for additional neoadjuvant therapy.

Determining need for adjuvant therapy

The benefit of administering adjuvant chemotherapy in upfront surgery patients is well documented by the CONKO-001 randomized controlled trial. However, whether a patient requires additional chemotherapy after already receiving neoadjuvant chemotherapy still requires further research. Using the persistence of CTCs in the postoperative setting to determine adjuvant chemotherapy has been promising. In fact, a delay in the administration of adjuvant chemotherapy has been associated with poorer outcomes in patients with residual CTCs after resection [13]. Identification of these patients and prompt initiation of adjuvant therapy may be particularly beneficial and improve survival.

Surveillance for recurrence of disease

Postoperatively, the vast majority of patients unfortunately suffers from local and/or systemic recurrence of disease. Routine surveillance is currently performed by serial CA19-9 blood draws and cross-sectional imaging. The presence of CTCs in the postoperative setting, even after an R0 resection, is likely representative of minimal residual disease [4]. This has been implicated in disease recurrence in multiple studies. Even more important, dynamic changes and increase in CTCs in the postoperative setting have shown promise in predicting clinical disease recurrence before it is evident on imaging and prior to CA19-9-based prediction of recurrence. This may provide clinicians with an earlier window for intervention.

FUTURE DIRECTIONS AND LIMITATIONS

Despite considerable advancements in pancreas cancer research, there has been a minimal improvement in survival. This is largely a result of a lack of reliable biomarkers to guide diagnosis and therapy in all phases of care. The introduction of multianalyte tests and multiomic profiling (genomics, proteomics, metabolomics, transcriptomics, and so forth) are encouraging as we aim to improve our insight into this devastating disease and move to more personalized medicine [14,15].

CTCs serve as a direct representation of the systemic component of disease. On average, when treating this systemic component, patients are more likely to respond better to the more toxic FOLFIRINOX (Folinic acid, fluorouracil, irinotecan, and oxaliplatin) chemotherapy regimen compared to the relatively milder gemcitabine-based regimen. However, this is not the case for all patients. It has been documented that CTCs undergoing EMT can develop drug resistance with properties such as overexpression of ZEB-1 and vimentin that are associated with chemotherapy resistance. The prospective ability to sample the systemic component of disease by isolating CTCs, culturing them, and performing drug sensitivity profiling could have considerable implications both in the preoperative and postoperative setting.

However, the greatest limitation in widespread adoption of CTCs is the considerable variability in techniques and tools used for isolation, enumeration, and characterization. A streamlined approach is still needed. Nonetheless, harnessing CTCs has shown great promise in diagnostics, therapeutics, and prognostication in pancreatic cancer, and it provides an exciting avenue for future advancements.

SUMMARY

Current guidelines influencing the management of pancreatic cancer are fundamentally based on anatomic classifications. More recently, tumor biology and systemic disease is being recognized as an equally important consideration. As novel surgical techniques and modern multiagent chemotherapy increase surgical candidacy, it is imperative that we improve our understanding and treatment of systemic disease to meaningful improve outcomes and cure more patients.

CA19-9 remains the most widely used circulating biomarker for pancreatic cancer. However, additional biomarkers that can guide optimal management are urgently needed. CTCs particularly have shown great promise in multiple facets of care including in patient prognostication, ability to inform resection, predict treatment response, identify recurrence at an earlier timepoint than conventional imaging, and inform chemotherapy treatment decisions such as early initiation of adjuvant chemotherapy. Further studies are needed to validate these findings and streamline the integration of CTCs into the clinical care of patients with pancreatic cancer.

CLINICS CARE POINTS

- CA19-9 remains the most widely used circulating biomarker for pancreatic cancer; however, it remains limited in its ability to guide management.
- Additional biomarkers such as CTCs are urgently needed and have shown great promise in multiple facets of care including prognostication, surgical decision-making, postoperative therapy, and in surveillance.
- Further prospective studies are needed to validate these findings and streamline the integration of CTCs into the clinical the care of patients with pancreatic cancer.

Disclosure

The authors have nothing to disclose.

References

[1] Houg DS, Bijlsma MF. The hepatic pre-metastatic niche in pancreatic ductal adenocarcinoma. Mol Cancer 2018;17(1):95.

[2] Hasanain A, Blanco BA, Yu J, et al. The importance of circulating and disseminated tumor cells in pancreatic cancer. Surg Open Sci 2019;1(2):49–55.

[3] Poruk KE, Blackford AL, Weiss MJ, et al. Circulating tumor cells expressing markers of tumor-initiating cells predict poor survival and cancer recurrence in patients with pancreatic ductal adenocarcinoma. Clin Cancer Res 2017;23(11):2681–90.

[4] Gemenetzis G, Groot VP, Yu J, et al. Circulating tumor cells dynamics in pancreatic adenocarcinoma correlate with disease status: results of the prospective cluster study. Ann Surg 2018;268(3):408–20.
[5] Poruk KE, Valero V 3rd, He J, et al. Circulating epithelial cells in intraductal papillary mucinous neoplasms and cystic pancreatic lesions. Pancreas 2017;46(7):943–7.
[6] Javed AA, Ding D, Hasanain A, et al. Persistent circulating tumor cells at one year after oncologic resection predict late recurrence in pancreatic cancer. Ann Surg 2022;277(6): 859–65.
[7] Han L, Chen W, Zhao Q. Prognostic value of circulating tumor cells in patients with pancreatic cancer: a meta-analysis. Tumour Biol 2014;35(3):2473–80.
[8] Rompen IF, Habib JR, Sereni E, et al. The value of CA19-9 dynamics in decision making for treatment of locally advanced pancreatic cancer. Gland Surgery 2024;13(3):458–60.
[9] Perri G, Prakash L, Wang H, et al. Radiographic and serologic predictors of pathologic major response to preoperative therapy for pancreatic cancer. Ann Surg 2021;273(4): 806–13.
[10] Yu KH, Ricigliano M, Hidalgo M, et al. Pharmacogenomic modeling of circulating tumor and invasive cells for prediction of chemotherapy response and resistance in pancreatic cancer. Clin Cancer Res 2014;20(20):5281–9.
[11] Gemenetzis G, Groot VP, Blair AB, et al. Incidence and risk factors for abdominal occult metastatic disease in patients with pancreatic adenocarcinoma. J Surg Oncol 2018;118(8): 1277–84.
[12] Court CM, Ankeny JS, Sho S, et al. Circulating tumor cells predict occult metastatic disease and prognosis in pancreatic cancer. Ann Surg Oncol 2018;25(4):1000–8.
[13] Javed AA, Floortje van Oosten A, Habib JR, et al. A delay in adjuvant therapy is associated with worse prognosis only in patients with transitional circulating tumor cells following resection of pancreatic ductal adenocarcinoma. Ann Surg 2022;277(6):866–72.
[14] Kinny-Köster B, Habib JR, Wolfgang CL, et al. Favorable tumor biology in locally advanced pancreatic cancer-beyond CA19-9. Journal of Gastrointestinal Oncology 2021;12(5): 2484–94.
[15] Rompen IF, Habib JR, Wolfgang CL, et al. Anatomical and Biological Considerations to Determine Resectability in Pancreatic Cancer. Cancers (Basel) 2024;16(3):489.

Advances in Surgery 58 (2024) 143–160

ADVANCES IN SURGERY

Surgical Management of the Horrible Gallbladder

Andrew Barnes, MD, Brian Viscomi, MD,
Jessica Koller Gorham, MD, FACS, DABOM*

Department of General Surgery, Ochsner Medical Center, 1514 Jefferson Highway, New Orleans, LA 70121, USA

Keywords

• Cholecystectomy • Common bile duct • Cholecystitis • Cholangiography • Fluoroscopy • Intraoperative ultrasound • Transcystic exploration • Choledochoscopy

Key points

- Aberrant biliary anatomy is present in up to 40% of the population. Understanding normal and common variants of gallbladder, cystic duct, common bile duct, and hepatic artery anatomy reduces the risk of iatrogenic biliary or arterial injury.
- Complete dissection of the critical view of safety ensures accurate dissection of critical cystic structures prior to ligation during cholecystectomy.
- Risk factors for difficult cholecystectomy include history of prior surgery or instrumentation, pancreatitis, severe obesity, and moderate- or high-grade cholecystitis as defined by the Tokyo guidelines.
- Intraoperative adjuncts such as cholangiography, ultrasonography, choledochoscopy, and common bile duct exploration may be used to assist and identify critical structures and address choledocholithiasis.
- Bailout maneuvers, including cholecystostomy, subtotal cholecystectomy, conversion to open, and aborting the case, are appropriate when completing cholecystectomy is deemed unsafe by the surgeon.

INTRODUCTION

Cholecystectomy is one of the most commonly performed operations for a general surgeon, with up to 1 million cholecystectomies performed annually in the United States alone [1]. Despite the seemingly routine nature of this operation,

*Corresponding author. *E-mail address:* Jessica.kollergorham@ochsner.org

https://doi.org/10.1016/j.yasu.2024.04.009

however, general surgeons are equally familiar with the humbling, and often frustrating, challenge of a horrible gallbladder. These difficult cases often distort surgical anatomy, increasing the risk of technical errors and potentially disastrous complications. The pitfalls and frustrations associated with a difficult cholecystectomy can be mitigated, if not altogether avoided, with careful understanding and appreciation of the anatomy, pathophysiology, and surgical techniques, including that of standard laparoscopic approach and dissection of the critical view of safety (CVS), intraoperative adjuncts including imaging and available surgical tools, common bile duct (CBD) exploration, and bailout maneuvers.

Overview of biliary anatomy

Aberrant biliary anatomy is common and present in up to 40% of the population. Unanticipated abnormal anatomy is a potential source of iatrogenic injury and surgical complication and may compound surgical difficulty when faced with the difficult gallbladder [2–4]. Anatomic aberrance can be categorized into variations of the gallbladder, the extrahepatic biliary tree, and hepatobiliary vascular supply with variations in the latter two being the most common. Aberrant gallbladder anatomy is rare and includes complete agenesis, bilobed or duplicated gallbladder, and location to the left of the falciform ligament [2–4]. Within the extrahepatic biliary tree, the cystic duct travels between 0.5 and 4 cm to join the common hepatic duct (CHD) in the hepatoduodenal ligament to form the CBD [2]. The insertion site varies as the cystic duct can travel anteriorly, posteriorly, or descend inferiorly in relation to the CHD prior to its confluence or the cystic duct may insert into other portions of the extrahepatic biliary tree, most commonly into the right hepatic or right posterior sectoral duct in approximately 4% of the population [2–4]. The CBD is approximately 8 cm in length and extends inferiorly within the hepatoduodenal ligament toward the duodenum until it is enveloped by the pancreas and empties into the duodenum [2]. Within the hepatoduodenal ligament, the CBD rests in an anterolateral position relative to the portal vein and hepatic artery. The cystic artery provides the arterial supply to the gallbladder and originates from the right hepatic artery in approximately 80% of the population [2]. Alternative origins of the cystic artery include the proper hepatic and replaced right hepatic artery [2–4]. The right hepatic artery typically travels posteriorly to the CBD before giving rise to the cystic artery; however, in 20% of the population, an anterior course of the right hepatic is observed (Fig. 1) [4]. The spatial relationship between the CHD, cystic duct, and cystic artery was described by Calot in 1891 as the hepatocystic triangle. Contemporary definitions have replaced the cystic artery with the right lobe of the liver and serve as landmarks during dissection to establish the "Critical View of Safety" to be discussed later [2].

COMPLICATED CHOLELITHIASIS, EVALUATION, AND WORKUP

The underlying pathophysiology of most biliary disease results from an obstructive process impairing biliary clearance leading to increased pressure

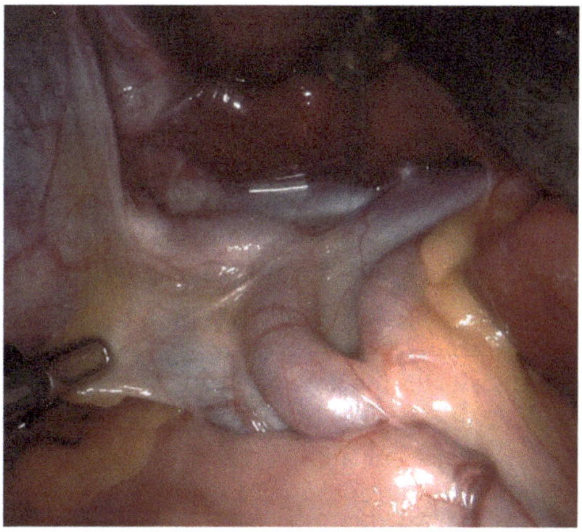

Fig. 1. Aberrant path and early takeoff of the right hepatic artery coursing anteriorly to the common bile and cystic duct.

and bacterial proliferation. The etiology of the obstruction includes benign and malignant causes; however, most commonly, it is the result of gallstones. While typically asymptomatic, obstructing stones result in a range of pathologic syndromes, collectively referred to as complicated cholelithiasis. Acute cholecystitis is the most common form of complicated cholelithiasis resulting from complete obstruction in the gallbladder neck or cystic duct. Obstruction progresses to inflammation manifesting with edema, pressure-induced gallbladder wall necrosis, and suppurative disease with sepsis. Untreated, perforation can occur resulting in biliary peritonitis, pericholecystic abscesses, or fistula formation. Chronic cholecystitis results from repeated episodes of mild cholecystitis and is characterized by mucosal atrophy and fibrosis. Choledocholithiasis refers to a stone within the biliary tree, and when obstructing may result in hepatic biliary inflammation and infection or acute cholangitis. Bacterial translocation may occur leading to systemic inflammatory response, sepsis, and end-organ dysfunction. Acute cholangitis is associated with a worse prognosis than acute cholecystitis with mortality rates of up to 10%. Other forms of complicated cholelithiasis include Mirizzi syndrome, gallstone pancreatitis, and gallstone ileus [5].

Symptoms associated with complicated cholelithiasis include abdominal pain localized to the right upper quadrant or epigastric region, fever, anorexia, nausea, and vomiting. Advanced cholecystitis or acute cholangitis may manifest with hemodynamic instability or other systemic symptoms. On physical examination, patients are commonly tender to palpation in the right upper quadrant. Occasionally, the gallbladder may be palpable in up to 25% of patients. Laboratory analysis can demonstrate leukocytosis, elevations in bilirubin and liver transaminases, but these may also be normal in many cases. Diagnostic imaging includes abdominal ultrasound, computerized tomography (CT), hepatobiliary scintigraphy hepatobiliary iminodiacetic acid (HIDA), and magnetic resonance cholangiopancreatography (MRCP). Abdominal ultrasound is widely considered to be the first line for evaluation of biliary disease. Ultrasonographic findings suggestive of cholecystitis include gallbladder wall thickening greater than 4 mm, pericholecystic fluid, cholelithiasis, or ultrasonographic Murphy's sign. Obstruction involving the biliary tree is suspected when the CBD is dilated to greater than 6 mm. In cases where ultrasound findings are inconclusive or the constellation of symptoms suggest an alternative diagnosis, CT scan, HIDA, and MRCP may be considered. HIDA scan can provide functional analysis of the gallbladder as it assesses the flow of bile through the biliary tree and gallbladder with time. The absence of contrast filling the gallbladder is consistent with cholecystitis. Its use is limited by expense and time; however, it does have higher sensitivity than ultrasonography with respect to cholecystitis and is considered to be the gold standard. CT is less sensitive than ultrasound for diagnosis of acute cholecystitis but outperforms ultrasound in diagnosing late complications of cholecystitis such as gangrenous and emphysematous cholecystitis and intraperitoneal abscess [6]. MRCP combines T1- and T2-weighted imaging to reconstruct the anatomy of the intraluminal biliary tree and surrounding soft tissues and is the best imaging modality to evaluate the biliary tree [3,7]. Table 1 [6,8] reviews the diagnostic criteria for acute cholecystitis according to the Tokyo guidelines.

SURGICAL ACCESS AND CRITICAL VIEW OF SAFETY

Surgical removal of the gallbladder is accomplished by open or minimally invasive techniques including laparoscopic and robotic approaches. In open cholecystectomy, access to the gallbladder is facilitated through a midline or subcostal incision. In minimally invasive surgery, 4 ports are generally used for dissection; however, 3 port, single port, and single-site techniques are also well described. The approach largely depends on surgeon's experience and preference as well as patient's habitus and prior surgical history [9,10].

Laparoscopic cholecystectomy was first performed in Germany by Muhe in 1985, and the technique quickly overtook open cholecystectomy in the early 90s [11,12]. Accompanying the rise in use of laparoscopic cholecystectomy was a rise in the incidence of biliary injuries. This complication is most attributed to misidentification and ligation of the CBD or an aberrant duct in lieu of the cystic duct. Methods to accurately identify the cystic structures were developed and first published as the "Critical View of Safety" in 1995. Derived from ductal identification in an open cholecystectomy, the CVS is achieved by ensuring only 2 structures enter the gallbladder prior to ligation of the cystic artery and duct. This is achieved by clearing the hepatocystic triangle of fat and fibrous tissue and separating the inferior gallbladder from the cystic plate; it is generally recommended to proceed until a third of the gallbladder is removed to ensure there is no doubt the only remaining attachments are the fibrous attachments between the gallbladder and cystic plate (Fig. 2A–D) [13,14].

Table 1
Diagnostic criteria for acute cholecystitis adapted from 2013 and 2018 Tokyo guidelines [6,8]

Diagnosis conferred by meeting criteria from all categories (only one imaging modality required)	
Category A: Findings localizing inflammation to gallbladder	Murphy's sign OR RUQ mass/pain/tenderness
Category B: Findings supporting activation of systemic inflammatory response	Fever OR elevated CRP OR leukocytosis
Category C: Imaging supporting acute cholecystitis[a]	Ultrasound Gallbladder wall thickening Pericholecystic fluid Acoustic shadowing secondary to cholelithiasis, debris, or gas Gallbladder distention CT/MRCP Gallbladder wall thickening and/or subserosa edema Pericholecystic fat stranding, fluid, or abscess Gallbladder distention Abnormal enhancement of gallbladder mucosa or of the surrounding liver Gas within the gallbladder HIDA Absence of radiotracer uptake in the gallbladder within 60 min of administration

Abbreviations: CRP, C-reactive protein; RUQ, right upper quadrant.
[a]Not all findings listed for any specific imaging modality must be met to meet criteria for category.

BILE DUCT INJURY

Bile duct injury (BDI) is the most feared complication following cholecystectomy due to its morbidity and difficulty of management. The constellation of BDI is complex and includes bile leak, bile duct stricture, partial/complete transection, thermal injury, and mechanical obstruction by surgical clips/suture. The morbidity of the BDI ranges widely depending on the nature and location of the injury. Some literature refers to "minor" and "major" BDI; however, these terms require a subjective interpretation. The Bismuth–Strasberg classification (Fig. 3) provides a more objective way to categorize BDI [15]:

The reported incidence of BDI in traditional open cholecystectomy was 0.1% to 0.2% [16]. Shorter length of stay, decreased postoperative pain, and reduction in overall morbidity lead the widespread adoption of the laparoscopic cholecystectomy [1]. However, the risk of BDI in laparoscopic cholecystectomy has been shown to be significantly higher than that of open procedures, ranging from 0.32% to 1.5% if all bile leaks are included [1,17]. Recent efforts in promoting safe cholecystectomy techniques have reduced BID rates to a plateau around 0.22% [17].

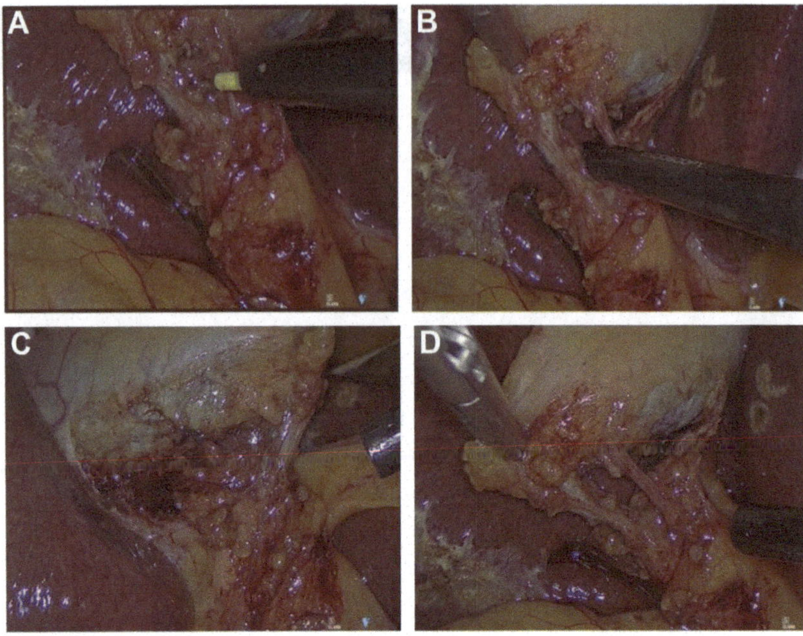

Fig. 2. Progressive clearance of the hepatocystic triangle utilizing cautery (*A*), blunt dissection (*B*), and contralateral exposure (*C*) to achieve the critical view of safety (*D*).

High-risk patients for difficult gallbladders

Although cholecystectomy is a common procedure for most general surgeons, each individual surgery requires vigilant consideration to identify and plan for the possibility of the "difficult gallbladder." Misidentification of the relevant biliary structures remains the primary cause of BDI attributed to 71% to 97% of all injuries [18]. Common variations in biliary anatomy including short cystic duct, parallel course of the cystic duct relative to the CBD, and aberrant right hepatic duct can distort the surgeon's assessment of a patient's anatomy [18]. History of prior biliary surgery or instrumentation, pancreatitis, and severe obesity can make surgery more technically challenging. Severity of cholecystitis, however, is the most significant factor resulting in BDI during cholecystectomy frequently cited as the most common cause for the difficult gallbladder. For Tokyo grade I cholecystitis (mild acute cholecystitis), there was no increased risk for BDI. For Tokyo grade II cholecystitis (moderate acute cholecystitis), the adjusted risk was more than doubled (odds ratio [OR] 2.41). Finally, for Tokyo grade III cholecystitis (severe cholecystitis), there was an 8 fold increase in the adjusted risk for BDI (OR 8.43) [19]. Systematic review and meta-analysis of over 41,000 patients in China who underwent laparoscopic cholecystectomy echoed these findings. Acute and subacute inflammation (OR 8.35) and thickening of the gallbladder wall greater than 4 mm (OR 3.18), both of which are correlated with the severity of biliary

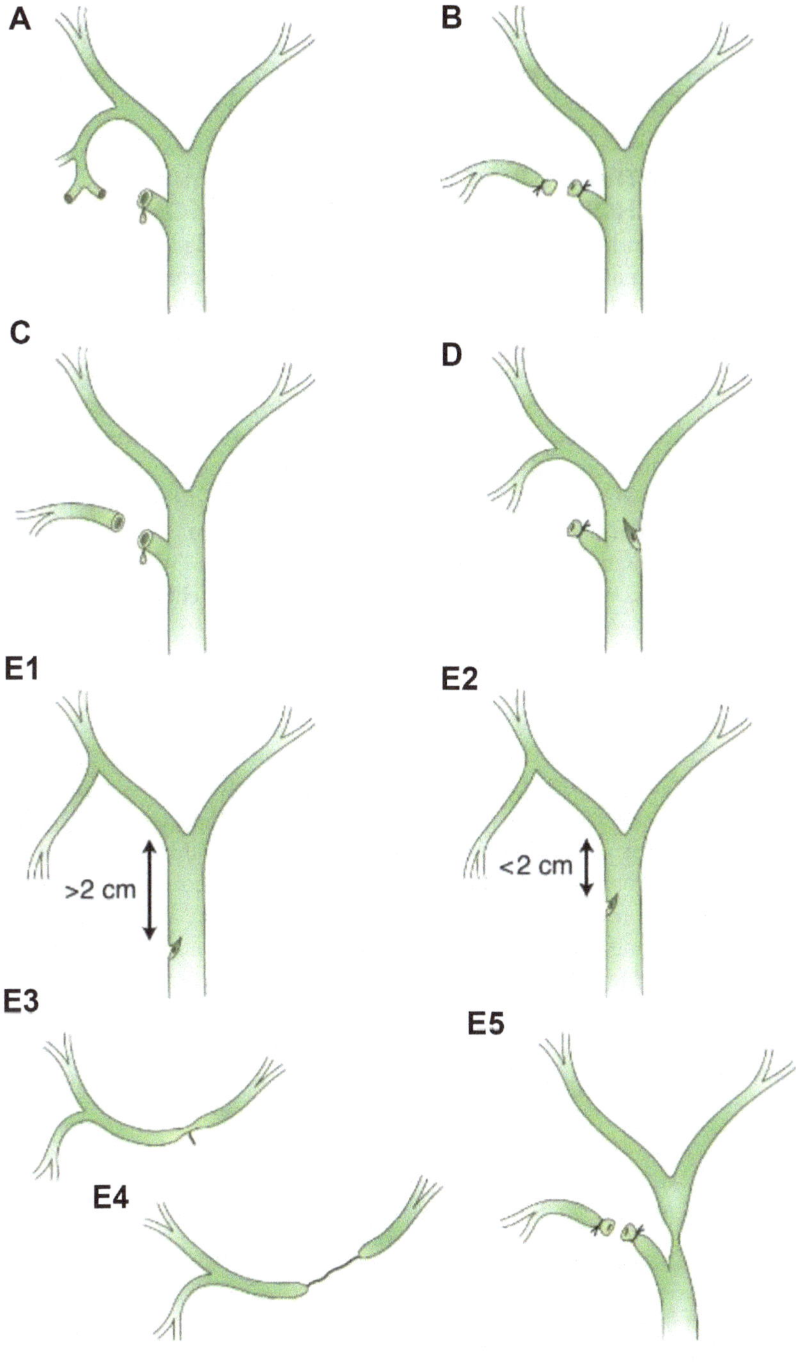
A
B
C
D
E1
>2 cm
E2
<2 cm
E3
E5
E4

disease, proved to be statistically significant risk factors for BDI. Other significant risk factors identified in this study include age over 40 years (OR 6.23), abnormal preoperative liver function (OR 2.01), and anatomic variations of the biliary tree (OR 11.82) [20].

INTRAOPERATIVE ADJUNCTS AND DECISION-MAKING INCLUDING CHOLANGIOGRAPHY AND ULTRASONOGRAPHY

Intraoperative findings associated with the difficult gallbladder can be categorized as inflammatory and noninflammatory. Inflammatory changes result from acute and/or chronic cholecystitis and can exacerbate surgical difficulty [6,21]. Adhesive disease, hepatomegaly, gallbladder distention, and substantial visceral fat can all add complexity and obscure visualization. Adhesiolysis utilizing blunt dissection may limit thermal injury to the colon and duodenum caused by electrocautery. Placement of additional ports may be required to improve visualization and retraction [21]. Needle decompression or toothed graspers can assist in managing an acutely inflamed or distended gallbladder [21]. Inflammation resulting in edema and loss of normal tissue planes can hinder the ability to achieve the CVS. Intraoperatively, adjuncts including imaging techniques, such as radiographic and fluorescence cholangiography and ultrasound can be used to better define biliary anatomy [6,21].

Cholangiography using radiographic contrast media to delineate biliary anatomy has been described since the 1930s. Developed as a mechanism to identify ductal injuries, intraoperative cholangiography (IOC) is a recommended modality for assessing biliary anatomy during difficult cases and facilitating the identification of intraductal stones. The degree to which IOC prevents injuries and the utility of routine use in cholecystectomy continues to be debated [14,21,22]. IOC is performed by injecting contrast material into the biliary system under fluoroscopy. Components of a successful cholangiogram include identification of the cystic and CBD, the left and right hepatic ducts, and contrast emptying into the duodenum. Contrast administration through specialized clamps (ie, Kumar clamp- Nashville Surgical Instruments) may facilitate injection of contrast into the gallbladder itself. Gallstones obstructing the cystic duct may prevent progression into the biliary tree with this technique. Alternatively, contrast may be injected through a cholangiocatheter placed

Fig. 3. Bismuth–Strasberg classification. (*A*) Bile leak from the cystic duct or small ducts of Luschka in the liver bed. (*B*) Injury to a sectoral duct (ie, aberrant right hepatic duct) with obstruction. (*C*) Injury to a sectoral duct with a subsequent bile leak. (*D*) Lateral injury to extrahepatic duct (ie, incomplete transection). (*E1*) Transection greater than 2 cm from the confluence. (*E2*) Transection less than 2 cm from the confluence. (*E3*) Transection at the confluence. (*E4*) Separation of the major ducts at the confluence. (*E5*) Complete occlusion of all bile ducts. (*From* Sabiston DC. Sabiston Textbook of Surgery: The Biological Basis of Modern Surgical Practice. Twenty-first ed. (Townsend CM, Beauchamp RD, Evers BM, Mattox KL, eds.). St. Louis, Missouri: Elsevier; 2022. Accessed November 14, 2023.)

directly or over a wire into the proximal cystic duct via ductotomy (Fig. 4) [21,22].

Near-infrared fluorescence cholangiography utilizing intravenous indocyanine green (ICG) is relatively new method for intraoperative biliary imaging (Fig. 5). Once in the bloodstream, hepatocytes absorb and excrete ICG into the bile allowing identification of biliary structures. The plasma half-life of ICG is relatively short; injection is recommended at least 30 minutes prior to surgery to ensure adequate uptake within the biliary system. Additional doses may be given intraoperatively to capture fluorescence during the vascular phase when arterial anatomy is unclear. A multicenter randomized controlled trial demonstrated cholangiography utilizing ICG reduced the time required to achieve the CVS without increasing postoperative complications when compared to cholecystectomy without cholangiography [23]. Compared to radiographic

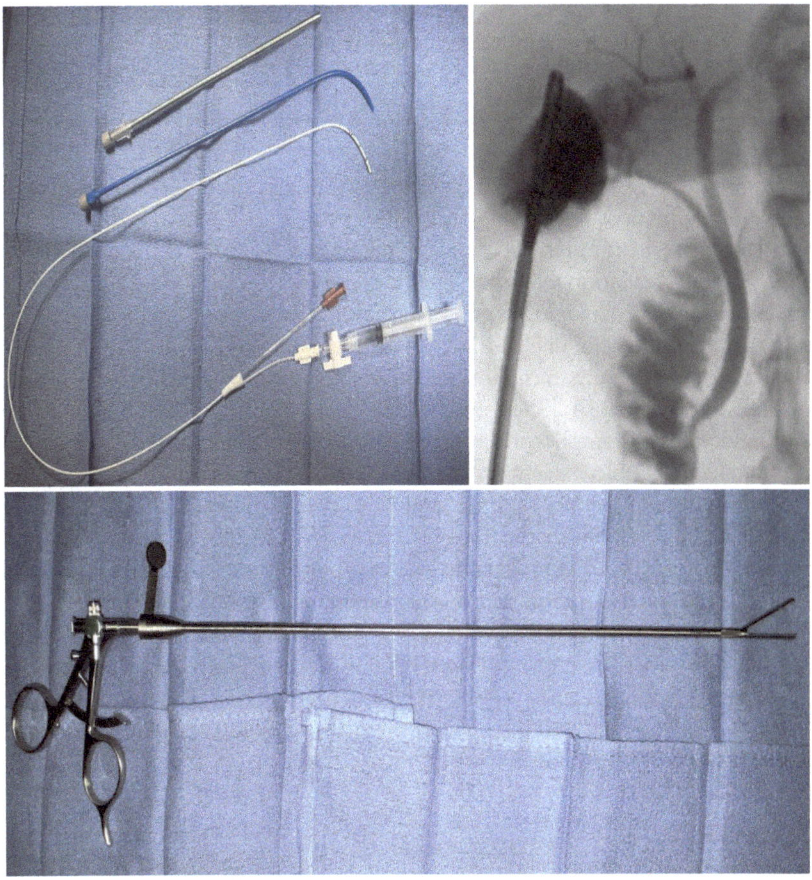

Fig. 4. Laparoscopic cholangiocatheter kit (*top left*). Normal cholangiogram with proximal filling of hepatic ducts and distal emptying into the duodenum (*top right*) utilizing Kumar clamp (*bottom*).

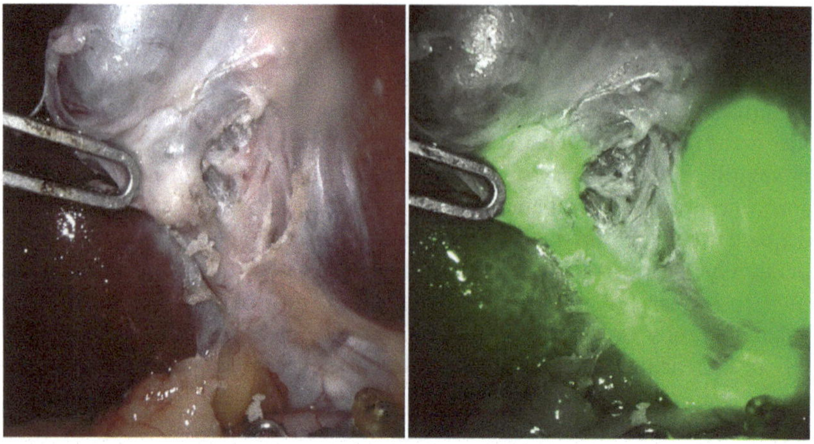

Fig. 5. Clearance of the hepatocystic triangle under plain light (*left*) and near-infrared fluorescence (*right*). Note the lack of fluorescence within the body of the gallbladder consistent with an obstructing stone at the neck.

cholangiography, ICGs ability to discern vascular anatomy may prove advantageous for difficult cholecystectomies; however, studies comparing rates of vascular injuries are limited [24]. ICG cholangiography obviates the need for ductotomy, avoids radiation exposure, and does not require additional equipment or staff as near-infrared imaging capture technology is ubiquitous in modern laparoscopic and robotic cameras [21,22,25]. Unfortunately, ICG fluorescence can be obscured by severe inflammation and distribution may limit its use in severe obesity. While a useful adjunct, studies have yet to demonstrate reduction in conversion or rates of complication rate with ICG cholangiography in both elective and nonelective cholecystectomy [23,25].

Laparoscopic ultrasound can be utilized to define biliary anatomy intraoperatively, facilitating safe dissection and the CVS. Intraoperative ultrasound is much less widely used compared to cholangiography, a discrepancy primarily attributed to lack of surgeon exposure and perceived difficulty [21,26]. A multifrequency ultrasound probe (Fig. 6) can be inserted through a 12 mm port in the epigastrium for image acquisition [21,26]. When placed transversely over the hepatoduodenal ligament, the typical anatomy is demonstrated in the "Mickey Mouse sign" with the anechoic appearing head, left, and right ear corresponding to the portal vein, CBD, and hepatic artery, respectively. Portal

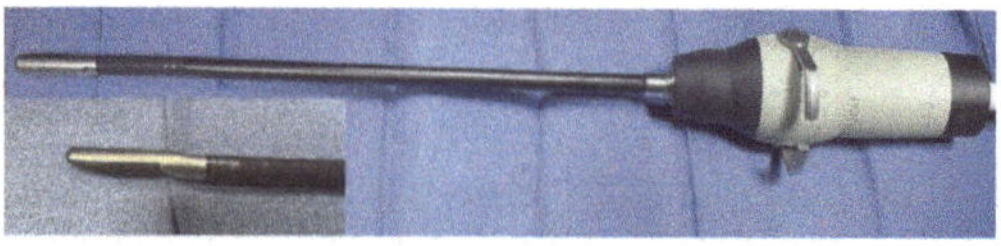

Fig. 6. BK Medical Laparoscopic ultrasound.

structures are imaged superiorly to the porta hepatis and inferiorly to the duodenum to identify relevant anatomy and variations [21]. Conceptually, the ability to visualize vascular structures is advantageous when compared to radiographic cholangiography and its ability to penetrate tissue edema and inflammation lends itself to improved visualization. Ultrasonography can be performed prior to dissection of biliary structures and does not involve radiation [21,26]. In a retrospective analysis of a single surgeon's use of ultrasound in 785 cholecystectomies, ultrasonography was able to identify relevant anatomy in 95% of cases and resulted in lower open conversion rates. In a subset of 125 patients, both traditional cholangiography and ultrasound were utilized. In these cases, ultrasound or cholangiography was typically successful when the other modality failed and was otherwise concordant in detection of choledocholithiasis. The use of laparoscopic ultrasound may be limited by the presence of intraluminal gas within the biliary tree or duodenum. Traditional cholangiography may outperform ultrasound in the ability to visualize the proximal hepatic ducts and associated anatomic variants [26].

TRANSCYSTIC AND DIRECT COMMON BILE DUCT EXPLORATION

Surgical exploration of the biliary tree is a treatment option for choledocholithiasis and was commonly performed following the widespread use of IOC by the 1980s. Though, in the modern era, endoscopic retrograde cholangiopancreatography (ERCP) is widely utilized for the management of choledocholithiasis, laparoscopic CBD exploration still plays a role. A Cochrane review and meta-analysis comparing single-stage laparoscopic cholecystectomy with laparoscopic CBD exploration versus 2 stage laparoscopic cholecystectomy plus ERCP group found no significant difference in overall mortality and morbidity rates between the two [27]. Indications for bile duct exploration include choledocholithiasis found during preoperative workup or intraoperative imaging, and patients whose anatomy would make traditional ERCP challenging (Roux-en-Y gastric bypass) [28].

Surgical approaches are generally categorized based on how access to the biliary tree is obtained, whereby an incision made either directly onto the CBD or indirect access via the cystic duct. Stones are identified through imaging modalities as described earlier (Fig. 7) or by direct visualization with a choledochoscope. Removal of stones is accomplished through a variety of methods including wire baskets, balloon catheters, irrigation, and manual advancement. Larger stones may be broken into more manageable sizes using lithotripsy [29]. Clearance of the CBD is achieved in greater than 85% of cases, and in modern series success rates exceed 95% [29–32]. For the transcystic approach, a clip or clamp is placed on the proximal cystic duct and a transverse ductotomy incision is made distally. If insertion of a choledochoscope is difficult, the cystic duct can be dilated with a balloon catheter, or if the duct is less than 5 mm, the incision can be extended perpendicularly along the cystic duct toward the confluence of the cystic and CBD forming a T-shape [30,32]. Successful

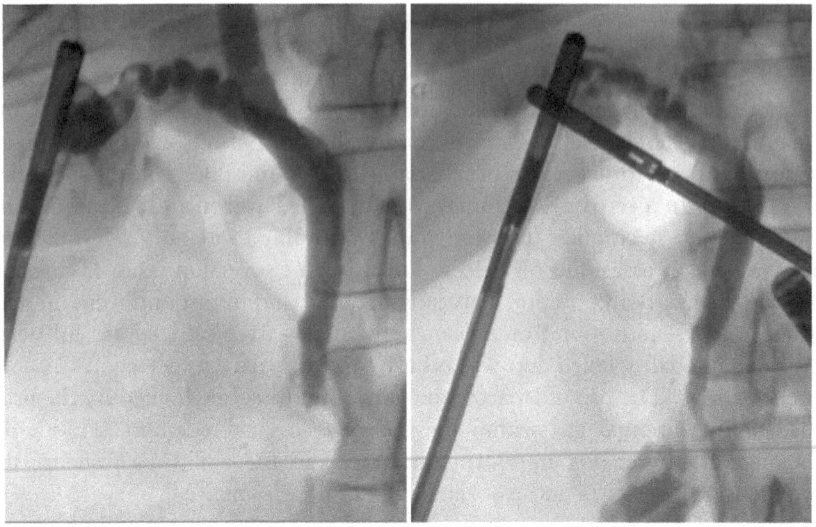

Fig. 7. Cholangiogram demonstrating obstructing stone (*left*) and resolution with contrast emptying into the duodenum (*right*).

cannulation of the cystic duct with the choledochoscope can be difficult and transductal approaches may be required when the duct is exceptionally small (<3 mm), is friable, or anatomic configuration prevents insertion [29,30,32]. The presence of large stones, greater than 1 cm, was historically a contraindication to the transcystic approach; however, this can be overcome with fragmentation utilizing lithotripsy [29,32]. Following removal of all stones, a completion cholangiogram is performed and the cystic duct stump is closed by suture ligation or clip placement [3–5,29,30]. The risk of complications from the transcystic approach is similar to those associated with cholecystectomy; however, compared to direct choledochotomy, the risk of bile duct leak and stricture is significantly less [29–31].

While the transcystic approach is often favored to avoid violating the CBD, choledochotomy remains a viable option. In patients with cystic duct diameter less than 4 mm, intrahepatic stones, and large stones that remain greater than 6 mm, choledochotomy is preferred. Choledochotomy should be avoided, however, in patients with a CBD diameter less than 7 mm to reduce the risk of stricture. When performing transcholedochal bile duct exploration, the anterior surface of the CBD is cleared for approximately 2 cm and a longitudinal choledochotomy is made sharply with endoscopic scissors. It is important to note that the blood supply to the CBD comes in laterally at the 3 and 9 o'clock position. Some advocate testing for bile using a 25 gauge needle prior to making the choledochotomy to avoid vascular injury at the porta hepatis. Once the choledochotomy is made, the stones may spontaneously spill out. An atraumatic grasper can also be used to remove additional stones through the incision as necessary. A choledochoscope can be inserted both distally (into the CBD) or proximally (into the common, left and right hepatic ducts) to facilitate wire basket retrieval of extrahepatic and intrahepatic stones [28]. Once the duct has been cleared, the choledochotomy is closed with a 4-0 or 5-0 absorbable suture. Many surgeons prefer to close over a T-tube, though meta-analysis shows a lower OR for complications when a T-tube is not utilized [33]. Direct choledochotomy and transcystic approaches are similar with respect to success in clearing the duct, conversion to open, and mortality rates; however, morbidity and complications (primarily bile leak and biliary stricture) are more common with direct choledochotomy techniques [29–31,34].

BAILOUT MANEUVERS

While laparoscopic cholecystectomy is a relatively low-risk, common procedure, the difficult gallbladder can be incredibly challenging for even the most experienced surgeon, leading to potential for devastating complications. Thus, it is important for each surgeon to be familiar with the various "bailout" maneuvers to address these challenging cases. Perhaps most importantly, the surgeon must recognize the potential for danger. In cases of severe cholecystitis with significant inflammation, perceived danger is readily apparent; however, there are situations where the risk of complications is not as easily appreciated. Awareness of "red flags" intraoperatively can help elucidate concern for missteps prior to making them. These red flags include an unusually large presumed cystic artery (may be hepatic artery), large pulsations behind the presumed cystic duct (may be the common hepatic or bile duct), failure of large clip to occlude the ductal lumen (may be the common hepatic or bile duct), and the presence of bile in the operative field in the setting of an intact gallbladder [35,36]. If these red flags are noted, it is important to pause, examine the anatomy, and reorient as necessary. It is recommended one ask another surgeon to weigh in (if available) during a difficult dissection or when there is concern for error. Injury to important vascular or biliary structures may be avoided in up to 18% of cases [35,37]. There are times when the degree of inflammation is such that no amount of careful dissection or second opinion will lead to identification of the critical view. In these cases, an understanding of bailout maneuvers is vital.

Common bailout strategies include (1) aborting the procedure, (2) fundus-first cholecystectomy, (3) subtotal cholecystectomy, and (4) conversion to open cholecystectomy.

Aborting the procedure

While this may be the best strategy in terms of avoiding injury, it does not address the underlying pathology; however, this may be necessary in cases where the degree of inflammation and adhesive disease is so great that the gallbladder cannot be safely visualized. If the decision is made to abort during a cholecystectomy for acute cholecystitis, the patient must be continued on antibiotics, and a percutaneous cholecystostomy tube should be considered [36]. If interval cholecystectomy is pursued after an aborted cholecystectomy, an extended interval (2–3 months) is advised [35,38].

Fundus-first cholecystectomy

When standard cholecystectomy technique cannot adequately demonstrate the CVS due to significant inflammation, proceeding cautiously with a fundus-first approach is reasonable. This technique involves dissecting the gallbladder from the liver bed using electrocautery from the fundus toward the neck. This is often used in conjunction with subtotal cholecystectomy which will be discussed further in this section. One must recognize the anatomic alterations of the cystic plate anatomy in the setting of severe inflammation and chronic cholecystitis. For example, the cystic plate can become contracted, thus shortening the distance between the end of the cystic plate and the right portal pedicle [35]. For this reason, it is important to stay right on the wall of the gallbladder during the dissection. Unfortunately, inflammation can also obscure and thicken the plane between the cystic plate and the gallbladder furthering this difficult dissection. In a retrospective cohort study of 772 patients with severe cholecystitis, Osawa and colleagues [39] found the fundus-down approach lowered the rate of subtotal cholecystectomy and reduced the length of stay compared to standard techniques. Converting from the fundus-down approach to a subtotal cholecystectomy is a safe alternative when the anatomy is obscured.

Subtotal cholecystectomy

This technique involves opening the gallbladder, aspirating its contents, removing as much of the gallbladder wall as feasible, and ablating the mucosa of the remnant gallbladder tissue, including the distal stump [35,40]. Subtotal cholecystectomy is further divided into "reconstituting" in which the gallbladder remnant is closed with suture (Fig. 8A, B) and "fenestrating" in which the remnant remains open with or without closure of the cystic duct [40]. If the cystic duct is closed, it is preferred to close internally with a purse string as exterior closure increases the risk of ligating the common hepatic or bile duct (see Fig. 2A–D [40]) [35,40]. As expected, there is an increased risk of bile leak with a fenestrating procedure when compared to a reconstituting procedure; however, these resolve spontaneously in most cases [40,41]. The reconstituting technique creates a remnant gallbladder, which increases the recurrence rate of biliary disease including remnant cholecystitis [41,42]. With this in mind, one could argue that a fenestrating approach may be more desirable; however, there are not sufficient data to suggest one technique over the other [14,40,42].

Conversion to open cholecystectomy

This technique begins with creating a right subcostal or upper midline incision. The gallbladder is then dissected from the surrounding structures either from the fundus down or from the hepatocystic triangle up. It is important to obtain the critical view prior to transecting structures even in the open approach. Subtotal cholecystectomy may be performed during an open

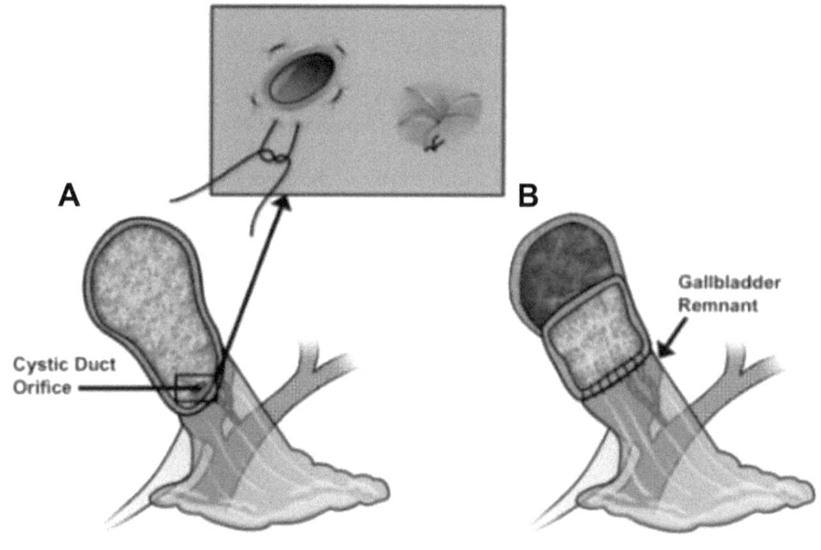

Fig. 8. Representation of "reconstituting" cholecystectomy with closure of the cystic duct orifice (*A*) and closure of the gallbladder remnant (*B*). (Seth J. Concors et al., Resection of gallbladder remnants after subtotal cholecystectomy: presentation and management, HPB, 20 (11), 2018, 1062-1066, https://doi.org/10.1016/j.hpb.2018.05.005.)

procedure as well. Although conversion to open has traditionally been the most common bailout maneuver, laparoscopic subtotal cholecystectomy should be considered prior to converting. A survey of experts in Japan, South Korea, and Taiwan showed that only 17.5% of responders felt that open conversion made surgery easier [14,43]. Additionally, a retrospective review of over 217,000 cholecystectomies from the National Surgical Quality Improvement Program (NSQIP) database showed a 100 fold increase in the rate of BDI following unplanned conversion to open cholecystectomy [35,44]. This is in part due to the selection bias of cases with severe inflammation and difficulty progressing through cholecystectomy prompting conversion to an open approach. However, it is worth noting that meta-analysis shows that while open conversion has lower rates of bile leak than that of laparoscopic subtotal cholecystectomy, the risk of BDI, reoperation, postoperative complications, and mortality is lower in laparoscopic subtotal cholecystectomy when compared to conversion to open [14,41,45].

CLINICS CARE POINTS

- Recognizing risk factors and clinical diagnosis of cholecystitis can prepare the surgeon for an encounter with the difficult gallbladder.
- When the critical view of safety can not be safely achieved, use of intraoperative adjuncts and bailout maneuvers can prevent iatrogenic biliary injury.

References

[1] Brunt LM, Deziel DJ, Telem DA, et al. Safe Cholecystectomy Multi-society Practice Guideline and State of the Art Consensus Conference on Prevention of Bile Duct Injury During Cholecystectomy. Ann Surg 2020;272(1):3–23.
[2] Crist DW, Gadacz TR. Laparoscopic anatomy of the biliary tree. Surg Clin North Am 1993;73(4):785–98.
[3] Abou-Khalil JE, Bertens KA. Embryology, Anatomy, and Imaging of the Biliary Tree. Surg Clin North Am 2019;99(2):163–74.
[4] Grimes N, Mark D, McKie L, et al. Anomalous biliary and vascular anatomy—Potential pitfalls during cholecystectomy. Clin Anat 2017;30(8):1103–6.
[5] Kimura Y, Takada T, Strasberg SM, et al. TG13 current terminology, etiology, and epidemiology of acute cholangitis and cholecystitis. J Hepato-Biliary-Pancreatic Sci 2013;20(1):8–23.
[6] Yokoe M, Hata J, Takada T, et al. Tokyo Guidelines 2018: diagnostic criteria and severity grading of acute cholecystitis (with videos). J Hepato-Biliary-Pancreatic Sci 2018;25(1):41–54.
[7] Hartwig W, Büchler MW. Acute cholecystitis: early versus delayed surgery. Adv Surg 2014;48:155–64.
[8] Yokoe M, Takada T, Strasberg SM, et al. TG13 diagnostic criteria and severity grading of acute cholecystitis (with videos). J Hepato-Biliary-Pancreatic Sci 2013;20(1):35–46.
[9] Haribhakti SP, Mistry JH. Techniques of laparoscopic cholecystectomy: Nomenclature and selection. J Minimal Access Surg 2015;11(2):113–8.
[10] Tao Z, Emuakhagbon VS, Pham T, et al. Outcomes of robotic and laparoscopic cholecystectomy for benign gallbladder disease in Veteran patients. J Robot Surg 2021;15(6):849–57.
[11] Reynolds W. The First Laparoscopic Cholecystectomy. J Soc Laparoendosc Surg 2001;5(1):89–94.
[12] Rutledge R, Fakhry SM, Baker CC, et al. The impact of laparoscopic cholecystectomy on the management and outcome of biliary tract disease in North Carolina: a statewide, population-based, time-series analysis. J Am Coll Surg 1996;183(1):31–45.
[13] Strasberg SM, Brunt LM. Rationale and use of the critical view of safety in laparoscopic cholecystectomy. J Am Coll Surg 2010;211(1):132–8.
[14] Wakabayashi G, Iwashita Y, Hibi T, et al. Tokyo Guidelines 2018: surgical management of acute cholecystitis: safe steps in laparoscopic cholecystectomy for acute cholecystitis (with videos). J Hepato-Biliary-Pancreatic Sci 2018;25(1):73–86.
[15] Berci G, Morgenstern L. An analysis of the problem of biliary injury during laparoscopic cholecystectomy. J Am Coll Surg 1995;180(5):638–9.
[16] Girard RM, Morin M. Open cholecystectomy: its morbidity and mortality as a reference standard. Can J Surg J Can Chir 1993;36(1):75–80.
[17] Pucher PH, Brunt LM, Davies N, et al. Outcome trends and safety measures after 30 years of laparoscopic cholecystectomy: a systematic review and pooled data analysis. Surg Endosc 2018;32(5):2175–83.
[18] Pesce A, Palmucci S, La Greca G, et al. Iatrogenic bile duct injury: impact and management challenges. Clin Exp Gastroenterol 2019;12:121–8.
[19] Törnqvist B, Waage A, Zheng Z, et al. Severity of Acute Cholecystitis and Risk of Iatrogenic Bile Duct Injury During Cholecystectomy, a Population-Based Case-Control Study. World J Surg 2016;40(5):1060–7.
[20] Yang S, Hu S, Gu X, et al. Analysis of risk factors for bile duct injury in laparoscopic cholecystectomy in China: A systematic review and meta-analysis. Medicine (Baltim) 2022;101(37):e30365; https://doi.org/10.1097/MD.0000000000030365.
[21] Asbun HJ, Shah MM, Ceppa EP, et al, editors. The SAGES manual of biliary surgery. Cham, Switzerland: Springer International Publishing; 2020; https://doi.org/10.1007/978-3-030-13276-7.
[22] Brunt LM. Should We Utilize Routine Cholangiography? Adv Surg 2022;56(1):37–48.

[23] van den Bos J, Schols RM, Boni L, et al. Near-infrared fluorescence cholangiography assisted laparoscopic cholecystectomy (FALCON): an international multicentre randomized controlled trial. Surg Endosc 2023;37(6):4574–84.
[24] Lim SH, Tan HTA, Shelat VG. Comparison of indocyanine green dye fluorescent cholangiography with intra-operative cholangiography in laparoscopic cholecystectomy: a meta-analysis. Surg Endosc 2021;35(4):1511–20.
[25] She WH, Cheung TT, Chan MY, et al. Routine use of ICG to enhance operative safety in emergency laparoscopic cholecystectomy: a randomized controlled trial. Surg Endosc 2022;36(6):4442–51.
[26] Deziel DJ. Laparoscopic Ultrasound for Bile Duct Imaging during Cholecystectomy: Clinical Impact in 785 Consecutive Cases. J Am Coll Surg 2022;234(5):849.
[27] Dasari BVM, Tan CJ, Gurusamy KS, et al. Surgical versus endoscopic treatment of bile duct stones. Cochrane Database Syst Rev 2013;2013(12):CD003327; https://doi.org/10.1002/14651858.CD003327.pub4.
[28] Clinical Spotlight Review: Laparoscopic Common Bile Duct Exploration - A SAGES Publication. SAGES. 2020. Available at: https://www.sages.org/publications/guidelines/clinical-spotlight-review-laparoscopic-common-bile-duct-exploration/. [Accessed 26 September 2023].
[29] Lyass S, Phillips EH. Laparoscopic transcystic duct common bile duct exploration. Surg Endosc Interv Tech 2006;20(2):S441–5.
[30] Huang J, Hu W, Liu J, et al. Laparoscopic Transcystic Common Bile Duct Exploration: 8-Year Experience at a Single Institution. J Gastrointest Surg 2023;27(3):555–64.
[31] Navaratne L, Martinez Isla A. Transductal versus transcystic laparoscopic common bile duct exploration: an institutional review of over four hundred cases. Surg Endosc 2021;35(1):437–48.
[32] Fang L, Wang J, Dai WC, et al. Laparoscopic transcystic common bile duct exploration: surgical indications and procedure strategies. Surg Endosc 2018;32(12):4742–8.
[33] Yin Z, Xu K, Sun J, et al. Is the end of the T-tube drainage era in laparoscopic choledochotomy for common bile duct stones is coming? A systematic review and meta-analysis. Ann Surg 2013;257(1):54–66.
[34] Hajibandeh S, Hajibandeh S, Sarma DR, et al. Laparoscopic Transcystic Versus Transductal Common Bile Duct Exploration: A Systematic Review and Meta-analysis. World J Surg 2019;43(8):1935–48.
[35] Gupta V, Jain G. Safe laparoscopic cholecystectomy: Adoption of universal culture of safety in cholecystectomy. World J Gastrointest Surg 2019;11(2):62–84.
[36] Stewart L. Perceptual errors leading to bile duct injury during laparoscopic cholecystectomy. In: Dixon E, Vollmer JrCM, May GR, editors. Management of benign biliary stenosis and injury: a comprehensive guide. Cham, Switzerland: Springer International Publishing; 2015. p. 165–86; https://doi.org/10.1007/978-3-319-22273-8_14.
[37] Iwashita Y, Hibi T, Ohyama T, et al. Delphi consensus on bile duct injuries during laparoscopic cholecystectomy: an evolutionary cul-de-sac or the birth pangs of a new technical framework? J Hepato-Biliary-Pancreatic Sci 2017;24(11):591–602.
[38] Borzellino G, Sauerland S, Minicozzi AM, et al. Laparoscopic cholecystectomy for severe acute cholecystitis. A meta-analysis of results. Surg Endosc 2008;22(1):8–15.
[39] Osawa T, Fukami Y, Komatsu S, et al. Impact of fundus-first laparoscopic cholecystectomy for severe cholecystitis. Surg Endosc 2023;37(8):6129–34.
[40] Strasberg SM, Pucci MJ, Brunt LM, et al. Subtotal Cholecystectomy-"Fenestrating" vs "Reconstituting" Subtypes and the Prevention of Bile Duct Injury: Definition of the Optimal Procedure in Difficult Operative Conditions. J Am Coll Surg 2016;222(1):89–96.
[41] Elshaer M, Gravante G, Thomas K, et al. Subtotal Cholecystectomy for "Difficult Gallbladders": Systematic Review and Meta-analysis. JAMA Surg 2015;150(2):159–68.
[42] van Dijk AH, Donkervoort SC, Lameris W, et al. Short- and Long-Term Outcomes after a Reconstituting and Fenestrating Subtotal Cholecystectomy. J Am Coll Surg 2017;225(3):371–9.

[43] Hibi T, Iwashita Y, Ohyama T, et al. The "right" way is not always popular: comparison of surgeons' perceptions during laparoscopic cholecystectomy for acute cholecystitis among experts from Japan, Korea and Taiwan. J Hepato-Biliary-Pancreatic Sci 2017;24(1):24–32.
[44] Mangieri CW, Hendren BP, Strode MA, et al. Bile duct injuries (BDI) in the advanced laparoscopic cholecystectomy era. Surg Endosc 2019;33(3):724–30.
[45] Henneman D, da Costa DW, Vrouenraets BC, et al. Laparoscopic partial cholecystectomy for the difficult gallbladder: a systematic review. Surg Endosc 2013;27(2):351–8.

Advances in Surgery 58 (2024) 161–189

ADVANCES IN SURGERY

What Is the Best Technique for Treating Carotid Disease?

Ahmed Abdelkarim, MD[a,b,c], Mohammed Hamouda, MD[a,b,c], Mahmoud B. Malas, MD, MHS, RPVI[a,b,c,*]

[a]Department of Surgery, Division of Vascular and Endovascular Surgery, UC San Diego, San Diego, CA, USA; [b]Center for Learning and Excellence in Vascular & Endovascular Research (CLEVER), UC San Diego, San Diego, CA, USA; [c]Altman Center for Clinical and Translational Research, 9452 Medical Center Drive - LL2W 502A, La Jolla, CA 92037, USA

Keywords

• Stroke • Carotid artery stenosis • Carotid artery revascularization • Endarterectomy • Stenting

Key points

- Carotid artery revascularization and aggressive medical management are recommended for symptomatic patients with greater than 50% and asymptomatic patients with greater than 70% carotid stenosis.
- Carotid endarterectomy (CEA) remains the gold standard technique for carotid revascularization with better outcomes, especially in the elderly and high-risk lesions (severe calcification and long lesions).
- Carotid artery stenting is favored for specific patients at high medical or anatomic risk, such as radiated neck, high-lesion, and restenosis.
- The current evidence suggests that transcarotid artery revascularization is both safe and effective, with comparable results to CEA and better results than transfemoral carotid artery stenting despite being performed in high-risk patients.
- Physicians should consider patient-specific risk and lesion-specific characteristics and involve patient in discussion about potential benefits, risks, and alternatives of each procedure.

INTRODUCTION

Stroke continues to be a common cause of morbidity and mortality in the United States, ranked as the first leading cause of disability and the fifth leading

*Corresponding author. Altman Center for Clinical and Translational Research, 9452 Medical Center Drive - LL2W 502A, La Jolla, CA 92037 *E-mail address:* mmalas@ucsd.edu

https://doi.org/10.1016/j.yasu.2024.04.010
0065-3411/24/

cause of death, killing approximately 140,000 Americans each year field [1], with ischemic strokes making almost 87% of all strokes [2]. The consequences of stroke have extended social and financial difficulties affecting both patients and the health care systems. It is estimated that the total cost of stroke in the United States between 2018 and 2019 was around $56.5 billion, and it is projected to reach $94.3 billion in 2035 [3].

It is estimated that carotid artery stenosis accounts for 8% of all ischemic strokes [4]. In a 2020 meta-analysis, the global prevalence of extracranial carotid stenosis greater than 50% was 1.8% in men and 1.2% in women and escalated with advanced age from 30 to 79 years [5]. Analysis of the Carotid Revascularization Endarterectomy Versus Stenting Trial (CREST) among 1-year survivors showed that stroke has adverse effects on a wide range of health-status domains exceeding that of myocardial infarction (MI) [6]. Owing to the debilitating effect of stroke and the massive burden on the health care system, carotid revascularization, whether through carotid endarterectomy (CEA) or carotid artery stenting (CAS), plays a crucial role in the realm of stroke prevention [7]. Symptomatic patients with prior stroke or transient ischemic attack (TIA) are at increased risk of recurrent cerebrovascular accidents. There is also an incremental relationship between the degree of carotid stenosis and the risk of recurrent stroke. However, this association is unclear in asymptomatic carotid patients [8–10].

CEA has been the gold standard for managing severe carotid artery stenosis for decades. However, in the past 3 decades, the introduction of minimally invasive transfemoral carotid artery stenting (TFCAS) presented an alternative to the open surgical approach. Nevertheless, major concerns have arisen due to the increased risk of periprocedural stroke after TFCAS. TransCarotid Artery Revascularization (TCAR) is a novel carotid revascularization technique developed to incorporate the benefits of a minimally invasive approach with the neuroprotection principles of CEA with common carotid artery clamping and adding an innovative flow reversal system [11]. As the management paradigm for carotid artery stenosis keeps evolving, it is crucial to investigate its indications and current management approaches.

INDICATIONS FOR CAROTID ARTERY REVASCULARIZATION

Intensive medical therapy must be offered to all patients with cerebrovascular diseases. Over the recent decades, there has been significant improvement in the best medical therapy for carotid artery stenosis patients, consisting of smoking cessation, hypertension and glycemic control, antiplatelet therapy, and lipid profile management [12–15]. Notably, statins have shown a substantial impact on the medical management of carotid atherosclerosis by stabilizing the atherosclerotic plaque and reducing stroke rate and all-cause mortality [16–18].

The indications and methods for carotid revascularization depend on the symptomatic status, degree of stenosis, and plaque morphology. The published guidelines of the American Heart Association (AHA) [12,13,19,20] and the Society for Vascular Surgery (SVS) [14,21,22] described in detail the indications and methods of revascularization for symptomatic and asymptomatic carotid artery stenosis patients.

SYMPTOMATIC PATIENTS

Symptomatic status is defined as experiencing an ipsilateral cerebrovascular accident (Stroke, TIA, Amaurosis fugax) within the past 6 months. In this group, there is a high risk of recurrent ipsilateral cerebrovascular accident, given the vulnerable nature of atherosclerotic plaque. This risk is directly proportional to the degree of carotid stenosis when adequate revascularization is not considered. The Effectiveness of CEA in symptomatic patients over medical therapy alone has been confirmed by 2 landmark clinical trials, the European Carotid Surgery Trial (ECST) and North American Symptomatic Carotid Endarterectomy Trial (NASCET) [23–26].

Based on societal guidelines, CEA is currently the standard management for symptomatic patients with greater than 50% stenosis. A minimally invasive CAS is recommended in patients with high-risk medical or anatomic factors for safe CEA (Table 1) [12,13,19,20] [14,21,22].

ASYMPTOMATIC CAROTID ARTERY STENOSIS

The evidence on the benefits of CEA over medical therapy alone in asymptomatic carotid stenosis patients is based on multiple clinical trials that took place in the mid-90s. The US Asymptomatic Carotid Atherosclerosis Study (ACAS) and the European Asymptomatic Carotid Surgery Trial (ACST) both found that CEA was more effective than medical treatment alone for stoke reduction in asymptomatic patients, resulting in a surge in the number of CEA procedures by expanding its indication to include asymptomatic patients with significant carotid stenosis [27–29].

Over the years, advances in medical therapy collectively led to a significant reduction in the yearly incidence of strokes, which are considered to be comparable to or even better than stroke rates achieved through carotid revascularization [30]. The cornerstone of medical therapy consists of antiplatelets, lipid-lowering agents, better blood pressure and glycemic control, and the significant decline in smoking rates in recent years. An ongoing CREST-2 randomized trial comparing both CEA and CAS to the best medical therapy (BMT) will further re-examine the outcomes of severe asymptomatic carotid artery stenosis.

In the meantime, based on the current societal recommendation, only asymptomatic patients with stenosis greater than 70% with standard surgical risk are considered for CEA. Asymptomatic patients with severe carotid stenosis who are at high surgical risk might be offered CAS as an alternative (Table 2) [12,13,19,20] [14,21,22].

TECHNICAL OPERATIVE DECISIONS IN CAROTID ENDARTERECTOMY

- Standard versus Eversion

Table 1
Societal guidelines for carotid endarterectomy and carotid artery stenting indication in neurologically symptomatic carotid stenosis

	American Heart Association [12,13,19,20]	Evidence	Society for Vascular Surgery [14,21,22]	Evidence
Carotid endarterectomy (CEA)	CEA is recommended for patients with (70%–90%) stenosis and estimated perioperative risk of morbidity and mortality below 6%.	Class I, LOE: A	CEA is preferred over carotid artery stenting (CAS) in low/standard risk patients with a >50% stenosis.	Grade 1, LOE: A
	CEA is recommended for patients with (50%–69%) stenosis based on patient-specific characteristics, such as age, sex, and comorbidities, if the estimated risk of perioperative morbidity and mortality is below 6%.	Class I, LOE: B		
	CEA should be selected over CAS in patients ≥70 y of age to reduce the periprocedural stroke rate.	Class IIa LOE B		

CAS	CAS is considered an alternative to CEA for patients with stenosis, which is >70% by noninvasive imaging or >50% by catheter-based imaging, who are at average or low risk of endovascular intervention complications and the expected combined stroke/death rate of procedure-related is <6%.	Class IIb, LOE: A	CAS is preferred over CEA in patients with >50% stenosis and hostile neck anatomy or lesions that extend proximal to the clavicle or distal to the C2 vertebral body.	Grade 2, LOE: B
	CAS is recommended for patients with >70% stenosis when CEA poses a high risk due to anatomic or medical factors, and the expected rate of procedure-associated stroke or mortality is below 6%.	Class IIa, LOE: C-LD	CAS is also preferred over CEA in symptomatic patients with >50% stenosis and severe uncorrectable CAD, congestive heart failure (CHF), or chronic obstructive pulmonary disease (COPD).	Grade 2, LOE: C
Both CAS &CEA	CAS or CEA procedures should be performed by operators with established periprocedural stroke and mortality rates of below 6%.	Class I LOE A		

Abbreviations: CAD, coronary artery disease; LOE, level of evidence.

Table 2
Societal guidelines for carotid endarterectomy and carotid artery stenting indication in neurologically asymptomatic carotid stenosis

	American Heart Association	Evidence	Society for Vascular Surgery [1,21,22]	Evidence
CEA	CEA is reasonable in asymptomatic patients who have >70% stenosis if the risk of perioperative stroke, myocardial infarction (MI), and death is low	Class IIa, LOE: A	For low surgical-risk patients with stenosis of >70% (documented by validated duplex ultrasound or CTA/ angiography), CEA with BMT is recommended over BMT alone.	GRADE 1, LOE: B
			For patients deemed high risk for CEA, BMT is recommended. CEA should only be considered for those patients when supported by evidence indicating that the risks of perioperative morbidity and mortality are below 3%	GRADE 1, LOE: B
CAS	Prophylactic CAS might be considered in highly selected patients (minimum 60% by angiography, 70% by validated Doppler ultrasound), but its effectiveness compared with BMT alone in this situation is not well-established	Class IIb, LOE: B	There is a lack of adequate data to endorse CAS as primary therapy for asymptomatic patients with (70% –99%) diameter stenosis. However, in highly selected patients, CAS can be deemed equivalent to CEA when conducted by skilled interventionists, assuming that the combined rate of stroke and death is below 3%.	GRADE 2, LOE: B
			For patients with a high risk for CEA, CAS should not be performed except as part of an ongoing clinical trial. Interventions in these patients should only be considered if the combined rate of stroke and death is below 3%.	GRADE 1, LOE: B

Abbreviations: CTA, computed tomography angiography.

CEA is classically described with the longitudinal arteriotomy extending from the common carotid to the internal carotid, exposing the plaque, which can be peeled off subsequently. Another technique is transecting the internal carotid artery (ICA) at its origin off the common carotid artery (CCA) and everting the former to peel off the plaque inside out (Fig. 1). Advantages of the eversion technique include shorter operative time and excluding the need for patch utilization. Nevertheless, outcomes of standard CEA with a patch and eversion CEA do not favor one technique over the other regarding stroke and death rates [31,32].

- General versus Regional Anesthesia

CEA can be done under general anesthesia (GA) as well as local/regional cervical block. A recent systematic review and meta-analysis showed no difference in stroke or death in either anesthesia type [33]. Similarly, a retrospective study by the authors' team on over 75,000 patients showed comparable stroke and death rates but significantly higher odds of MI, acute congestive heart failure (CHF), and longer hospital stays with GA compared to regional anesthesia (RA) [34]. However, the authors concluded that the adverse cardiac events after CEA are very low. Hence, the differences in outcomes may not be clinically

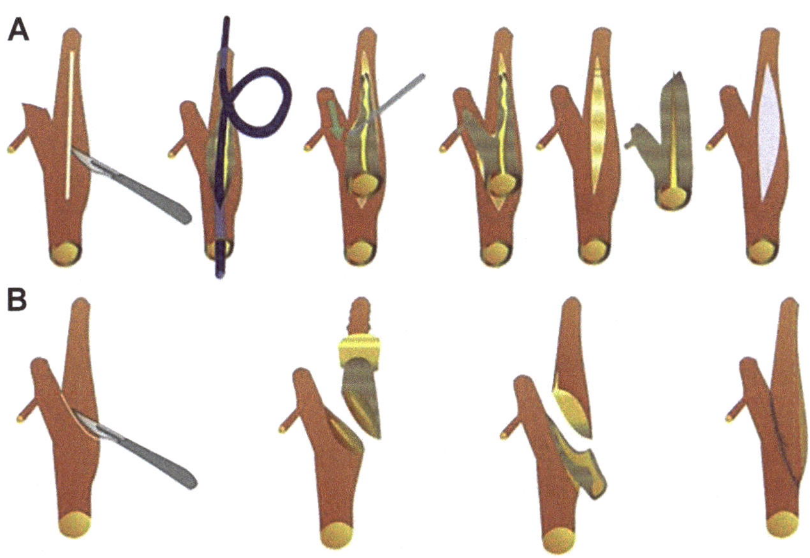

Fig. 1. Depicts the most frequently used techniques to perform carotid endarterectomy. (*A*) Displays the conventional open endarterectomy technique with patch closure. (*B*) Shows the eversion endarterectomy approach, which involves transecting the internal carotid artery at the bulb, followed by endarterectomy, then re-anastomosis. (*From*: Menezes FH, Pagliuso NP, Molinari GJDP. Modified Eversion Carotid Endarterectomy: A 14-Year Experience in a Tertiary Teaching University Hospital in Brazil (South America). *Ann Vasc Surg.* 2018;50:231 to 241. doi:10.1016/j.avsg.2017.12.009.).

relevant. Since the patient is awake during RA, close neuromonitoring and brain-function assessment is possible, which aids in decision-making regarding selective shunting after carotid cross-clamping [35].

- Shunting and Cerebral Monitoring

Surgeons perform CEA by routinely shunting all their cases, not shunting at all, or selectively shunting according to intraoperative monitoring (ie, selective shunting) [36]. Intraoperative cerebral monitoring can be performed by several methods, including transcranial Doppler, Electroencephalogram monitoring, carotid stump pressure, cervical block anesthesia, and cerebral oximetry [37]. Based on cerebral monitoring, deviations from normal cerebral perfusion after carotid cross-clamping alert the surgeon to utilize shunting selectively. In a retrospective study of over 28,000 patients, no difference in stroke or death was found in the routine, selective, or no-shunt utilization field [38]. Also, a metanalysis of 6 trials showed no difference in outcomes regarding the neuromonitoring method used during selective shunting Field [39]. However, in a large retrospective multi-institutional study by the authors' team, selective shunting under RA was associated with the highest stroke and mortality risk [40]. Shunting and cerebral monitoring decisions could be influenced by how the physician was trained and their preference/comfort in their regular practice [37].

- Patch versus No patch

Closing the CEA arteriotomy directly with continuous sutures is the classic technique described by Michael Debakey. However, over the years, CEA with patch angioplasty has consistently provided significantly better patency rates and has shown significantly more favorable outcomes when compared to CEA without patch utilization field [41,42]. The most recent SVS guidelines recommend routine patch angioplasty in all CEA cases [22]. Several patch materials are available today, and the most chosen one nowadays is Bovine pericardium. Other materials include Dacron, polytetrafluoroethylene (PTFE), and Autogenous Vein. Data in the literature show more promising outcomes with bovine pericardium compared to other patch materials [43].

DEVELOPMENT AND TECHNIQUE OF TRANSFEMORAL CAROTID ARTERY STENTING

CAS was introduced and developed as an option for carotid artery stenosis patients with medical and/or anatomic risk factors that put them at high surgical risk for CEA (Table 3) [44]. Almost 20 years ago, the food and drug administration (FDA) approved the utilization of the TFCAS procedure with a distal embolic protection device (EPD). Throughout the following years, notable advancements in TFCAS, including enhanced catheters, wires, sheaths, stents, and EPDs, significantly reduced stroke rates [45–47].

Placing a sheath in the CCA is necessary for CAS. Typically, this involves inserting a diagnostic catheter into the CCA and then advancing a glide wire

Table 3
High-risk factors for carotid endarterectomy

Anatomic factors	Medical factors
• Lesions above C2 • Lesions below the clavicle • Prior neck irradiation or surgery • Redo CEA • Contralateral occlusion • Contralateral cranial nerve injury/vocal cord injury • Severe tandem lesions • Cervical stoma (ex. Esophagostomy, Tracheostomy) • Carotid string sign up to middle cerebral artery (MCA) (*relative contraindication*) • Bilateral stenosis requiring treatment. • Cervical kyphosis or spinal immobility	• NYHA class III/IV • LVEF <30% • Abnormal stress test • unstable angina • Recent MI <6 wk. • Need for CABG • Severe lung disease • Uncontrolled HTN or DM • Liver failure • CKD

Abbreviations: CABG, coronary artery bypass graft; CEA, carotid endarterectomy; CKD chronic kidney disease; COPD, chronic obstructive pulmonary disease; DM, diabetes mellitus; HTN, hypertension; LVEF, left ventricular ejection fraction; NYHA, New York Heart Association; PT, prothrombin time.

into the external carotid artery (ECA). Subsequently, a wire exchange is performed to replace the glide wire with a stiff wire, which guides a 6 Fr Shuttle sheath. The senior author's techniques evolved to place a 125 cm Slip 6.5 F catheter configuration such as the JB1 and the VTK in the common carotid artery avoiding ECA selection and reducing the embolic risk. Under direct visualization, the shuttle introducer sheath is advanced until it reaches the desired position below the carotid bifurcation [48]. TFCAS should be performed under cerebral protection using a distal embolic protection (DEP) device placed in straight segment of the distal ICA.

In Type I aortic arch cases, typically angled catheters such as the angled taper Glidecath from Terumo Medical Corporation, a Berenstein catheter by Boston Scientific, or the JB1 catheter from Cook Medical tend to work effectively. However, when dealing with more complex aortic arch anatomy, such as Type II and Type III configurations (Fig. 2), reverse-curve catheters like the JB2 or the VTK catheter may be employed for better maneuverability (Fig. 3).

Stents used in TFCAS are either open-cell architecture or closed-cell architecture stents [49,50]. The struts for closed-cell stents are interconnected, whereas those in open-cell stents are not. Open-cell stents have a more flexible design allowing them to better conform to tortuous anatomy or complex lesions. On the contrary, closed-cell stents are less flexible but have the theoretic advantage of better plaque stabilization due to the smaller area between the struts. However, in the literature, a study by Schillinger and colleagues [51] comparing the 2 groups, there was no significant difference concerning the risk of stroke or mortality. A large national study by the authors' team showed a higher risk of stroke/death when closed cell stent deployed across the carotid bifurcation [52].

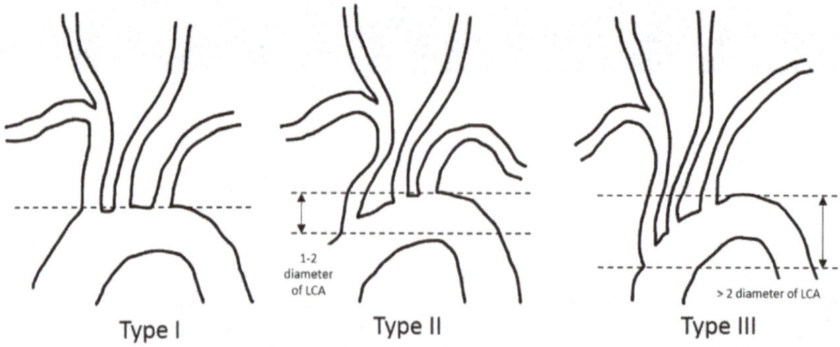

Fig. 2. Types of aortic arch. LCA, left carotid artery. (*From* Conway AM, Nguyen Tran NT, Qato K, et al. Complexity of Aortic Arch Anatomy Affects the Outcomes of Transcarotid Artery Revascularization vs Transfemoral Carotid Artery Stenting. *Ann Vasc Surg*. 2020;67:78–89. doi:10.1016/j.avsg.2020.04.016.).

Another option is a covered stent, where a recent study found that the MicroNet-covered stent significantly reduced periprocedural and postprocedural cerebral embolism. However, more research is needed in that regard [53].

LIMITATIONS OF TRANSFEMORAL CAROTID ARTERY STENTING

TFCAS popularity did not persist among vascular surgeons due to the increased stroke risk compared to CEA. Despite DEP, TFCAS still has to access the atherosclerotic aortic arch with difficult manipulation, especially in patients with arch type III and navigating through the carotid lesion before deploying the protection device (Fig. 4). Even after the protection device is employed, there is still a chance of embolization of small particles through the filter pores or around the device. Several randomized control trials (RCTs) were

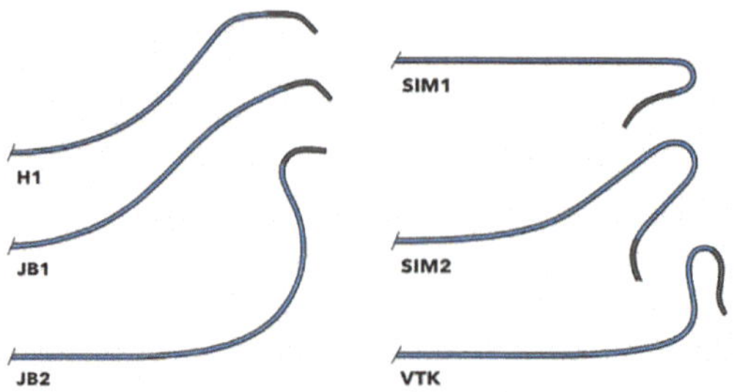

Fig. 3. Different types of catheters; reverse-curve catheters like JB2 or the VTK are preferred when dealing with more complex aortic arch anatomy, such as Type II and Type III. (*From* [Angioplasty-various-techniques-and-challenges in treatment of congenital and acquired vascular stenoses/ carotid angioplasty © 2012 by Parth Shah and Michael Dahn is licensed under CC BY 4.0]; with permission [48].)

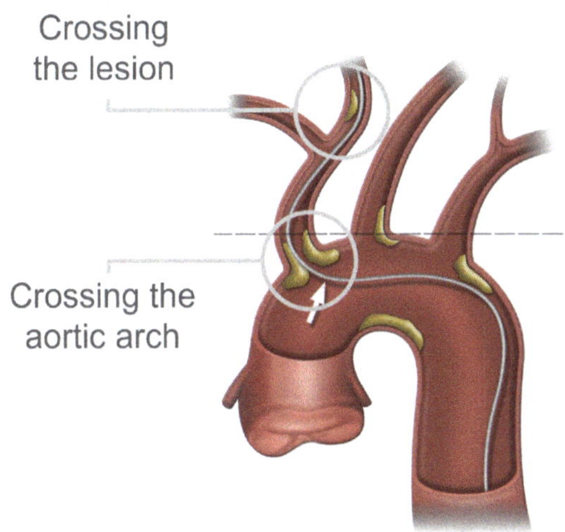

Fig. 4. Advancing a catheter through the aortic arch and crossing the carotid lesion before distal embolic protection establishment represent the basis of transfemoral carotid artery stenting anatomic limitations and increase the risk of periprocedural embolization. (*Courtesy of* Silk Road Medical, Inc.; Silk Road Medical, Inc. retains and reserves all rights, including copyrights.)

conducted to compare the results between CEA and TFCAS and showed that the latter was associated with lower MI but higher rates of perioperative stroke and death; however, long-term outcomes were comparable [6,46,54–57]. A recent meta-analysis by Vasavada and colleagues [58] showed similar results as CEA had lower odds of stroke and stroke/death compared to CAS. Therefore, CEA remains the preferred treatment for symptomatic and asymptomatic carotid artery stenosis. Moreover, in terms of long-term outcome, a recent analysis of the Vascular Quality Initiative (VQI)-linked to the Medicare database by our team found that CEA was associated with a lower rate of 10-year stroke (21% vs 27%; aHR, 0.6; 95% CI, 0.6–0.7; $P < .001$), death (58% vs 70%, aHR, 0.5; 95% CI, 0.4–0.5; $P < .001$), and stroke/death (65% vs 77%; HR, 0.5; 95% CI, 0.4–0.6; $P < .001$) compared to TFCAS [59].

Based on this combined evidence, multiple medical and anatomic risk factors have been defined by Medicare & Medicaid Services (CMS) to reconsider CAS reimbursement (Table 4, A). Despite rigorous patient selection, many studies on these risk factors have shown unexpected results. For instance, analysis on a matched cohort showed that the potential benefit for CAS in patients deemed High risk by CMS might be overrated. Contrarily, the benefits of CAS in standard-risk patients are overlooked [62].

DEVELOPMENT OF TRANSCAROTID ARTERY REVASCULARIZATION

Evidence keeps proving that in order to perform a safe CAS with minimal risk of perioperative embolization, it is imperative to avoid aortic arch manipulation

Table 4
Medicare decision summary for carotid artery stenting

A: Seventh Reconsideration [60]	B: Eighth Reconsideration[61]
CAS with embolic protection is recommended for the following patients: • High-risk and symptomatic carotid artery stenosis $\geq$70%. Coverage is limited to procedures performed using FDA-approved CAS systems and embolic protection devices. • High-risk and symptomatic carotid artery stenosis between 50% and 70%, in accordance with the Category B IDE clinical trials regulation or in accordance with the National Coverage Determination on CAS post-approval studies. • High-risk and symptomatic carotid artery stenosis $\geq$80%, in accordance with the Category B IDE clinical trials regulation or in accordance with the National Coverage Determination on CAS post-approval studies Significant comorbid conditions and anatomic risk factors contraindicating CEA: • Congestive heart failure class III/IV • Left ventricular ejection fraction <30% • Unstable angina • Contralateral carotid occlusion • Recent MI <6 wk • Previous CEA with recurrent stenosis • Previous radical neck dissection • Prior radiation treatment to the neck • Other conditions were used to determine patients at high risk for CEA in the prior carotid artery stenting trials and studies, such as ARCHER, CABERNET, SAPPHIRE, BEACH, and MAVERIC II.	CAS with embolic protection is recommended for the following patients: • Patients with symptomatic carotid artery stenosis $\geq$50%. • Patients with asymptomatic carotid artery stenosis $\geq$70%. This recent decision revises Medicare coverage for CAS by: • Expanding coverage to individuals previously only eligible for coverage in clinical trials. • Expanding coverage to standard surgical risk individuals by removing the limitation of coverage to only high surgical risk individuals. • Removing facility approval requirement. • Prior to furnishing CAS, a formal shared decision-making with the individual that includes: I. Discussion of all treatment options, including CEA, CAS, which includes transcarotid artery revascularization (TCAR), and optimal medical therapy. II. Explanation of risks and benefits for each option. III. Integration of clinical guidelines (eg, patient comorbidities and concomitant treatments). IV. Discussion and incorporation of beneficiary's personal preferences and priorities in choosing a treatment plan

Abbreviations: ARCHER, ACCULINK for revascularization of carotids in high-risk patients; BEACH, Boston Scientific EPI: a carotid stenting trial for high-risk surgical patients; CABERNET, carotid artery revascularization using the Boston Scientific FilterWire EX/EZ and the EndoTex NexStent; IDE, investigational device exemption; MAVERIC II, medtronic AVE self-expanding carotid stent system in the treatment of carotid stenosis; SAPPHIRE, stenting and angioplasty with protection in patients at high risk for endarterectomy.

and crossing the carotid lesion to place the EPD. In 2012, TCAR was introduced in the United States as a hybrid technique for high-risk patients combining CAS through direct surgical access of CCA with flow reversal technique to achieve optimal neuroprotection before any lesion manipulation (Silk Road Medical, Sunnyvale, CA) (Fig. 5) [63].

The safety and efficacy of ENROUTE (Silk Road Medical Inc., Sunnyvale, California) trans-carotid neuroprotection system (NPS) during TCAR procedures were assessed in 2 prospective single-arm multicenter clinical trials (Table 5). The Safety and Efficacy Study for Reverse Flow Used During Carotid Artery Stenting Procedure (ROADSTER 1) included patients at high-surgical-risk with ≥50% stenosis in symptomatic patients, and ≥70% stenosis in asymptomatic patients. In contrast to the 4.1% perioperative stroke rate among high-risk patients undergoing TFCAS in the CREST trial, in the ROADSTER1 trial, TCAR was associated with 1.4% 30-day stroke, indicating that the ENROUTE trans carotid NPS is both safe and efficient [64]. These promising results persisted at 1-year follow-up with stroke-free survival at 96% [65]. Following the remarkable success of ROADSTER 1, FDA approved TCAR for high-risk patients in 2015. After that, post-market analysis was conducted with the ROADSTER 2 trial, including a large multi-institutional cohort of high-risk CEA patients with symptomatic stenosis ≥50% and asymptomatic ≥80%. Similarly, early results from the ROADSTER 2 trial demonstrated excellent technical success alongside a low rate of perioperative stroke/death 2.3% and stroke/death/MI 3.2% [66].

OPERATIVE TECHNIQUE

TCAR can be performed under general or local anesthesia. A small incision is made in the triangle between the sternal and clavicular heads of the sternocleidomastoid muscle and superior border of the clavicle (Fig. 6). A longitudinal 2 cm

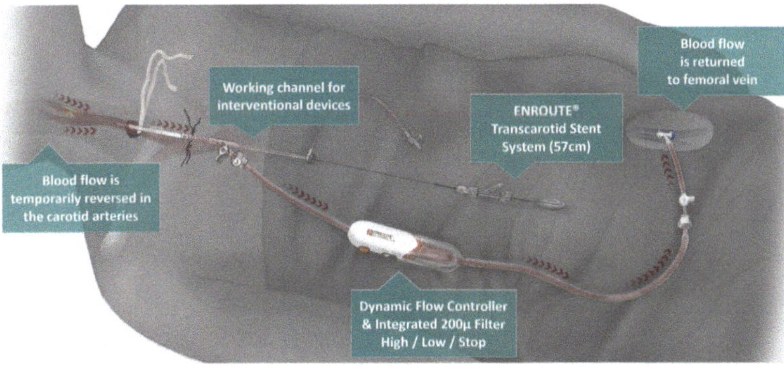

Fig. 5. Transcarotid artery revascularization procedure using the ENROUTE TransCarotid Neuroprotection & Stent System. Flow is reversed from trans carotid arterial sheath and filtered blood returned through percutaneous venous sheath. (*Courtesy of* Silk Road Medical, Inc.; Silk Road Medical, Inc. retains and reserves all rights, including copyrights.)

Table 5
Single-arm multicenter non-randomized control trial on transcarotid artery revascularization[a]

Study Name	Patients No.	Patients Characteristics	Outcomes
ROADSTER [64]	141	Asymptomatic stenosis >70% or symptomatic stenosis >50%	30-d all stroke = 1.4%; 30-d death = 1.4%; 30-d MI = 0.7%
ROADSTER I, 1-y follow-up [65]	165	Asymptomatic stenosis >70% or symptomatic stenosis >50%	1-y ipsilateral stroke = 0.6%, 1-y death = 4.2%
ROADSTER II [66]	692	Asymptomatic stenosis >80% or symptomatic stenosis >50%	30-d stroke = 1.9%. 30-d death = 0.4%. 30-d MI = 0.9%

Abbreviations: MI, myocardial infarction.
[a]Adapted from [What Is the Role of Transcarotid Artery Revascularization? [67]]; with permission.

incision is preferred (to allow access to a longer CCA segment). Meticulous dissection and circumferential control of the CCA is performed. Femoral vein access with ultrasound guidance is then obtained, followed by systemic heparinization, and a purse string suture is placed at the arterial access to facilitate puncture site closure at the end of the procedure. After that, arterial access is obtained with a micro needle and wire placed in distal CCA or ECA based on the lesion. The micro sheath is exchanged to the arterial 8 F sheath over a stiff wire. The arterial sheath is connected by the flow controller to the venous 8 F sheath. The CCA is then clamped proximal to the access site, initiating active flow reversal. Under fluoroscopy guidance, the lesion is crossed with 0.14-inch wire, and the

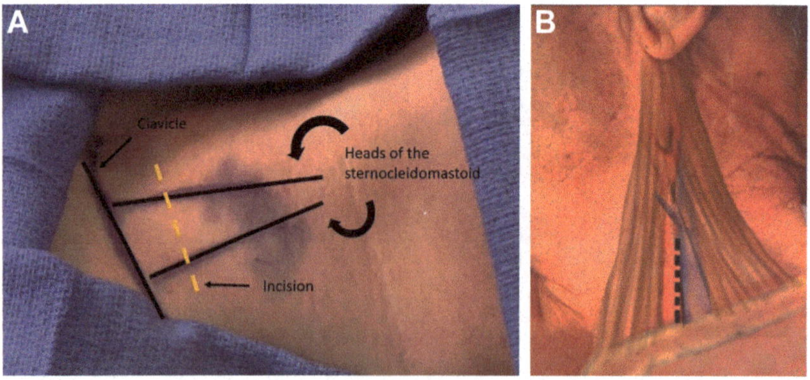

Fig. 6. The anatomic landmarks; (*A*) horizontal incision and (*B*) longitudinal incision for common carotid artery cut down during transcarotid artery revascularization. (*Courtesy of* Silk Road Medical, Inc.; Silk Road Medical, Inc. retains and reserves all rights, including copyrights.)

lesion is pre-dilated using a 2 to 4 mm × 15 to 20 mm balloon. Next, the ENROUTE self-expanding nitinol stent (7–10 mm × 30–40 mm) is deployed (Fig. 7). Blood flow to the CCA is then restored by removing the clamp and arterial sheath. The final steps of the procedure are the closure of the arterial access arteriotomy by tying the purse-string sutures, followed by the removal of the femoral vein sheath. Heparin is reversed, and closure of the neck incision in layers is performed with or without drain placement [63].

REAL WORLD OUTCOMES FOR TRANSCAROTID ARTERY REVASCULARIZATION

These promising early results led to the pervasive adoption of TCAR by vascular surgeons across the United States, superseding TFCAS (Fig. 8). In light of TCAR's increasing popularity and expansion, SVS launched the VQI TCAR Surveillance project (TSP) in 2016 in collaboration with the FDA and the CMS to evaluate the real-world safety and effectiveness of this new technique for carotid revascularization in comparison to the well-established CEA and TFCAS. Nearly 95% of all TCAR cases performed in North America were registered in this project [68].

In one of the earliest reports, and despite the fact that patients undergoing TCAR have significantly higher comorbidities than TFCAS, TFCAS showed double the odds of the composite outcome of stroke, TIA, and death (OR = 2.10; [95% CI: 1.08–4.08]; *P*=.03). This trend continued even after coarsened matching for potential confounders [69].

In another comparison between TCAR to TFCAS using larger matched cohorts, the risk of in-hospital stroke (1.3% vs. 2.4; *P*=.001), death (0.4% vs 1.0%; *P*<.01), and stroke/death (1.6% *v* 3.1%, RR, 0.51; 95% CI, 0. 37–0.72; *P*<.001) were significantly lower in TCAR; however, in-hospital MI rates were similar. At 1 year, TCAR was associated with a lower risk of ipsilateral stroke or death (5.1% vs 9.6%; hazard ratio, 0.52 [95% CI, 0.41–0.66]; *P*<.001) [70].

In another analysis by the authors' team, the authors compared TCAR and CEA and revealed that both procedures are comparable in terms of in-hospital

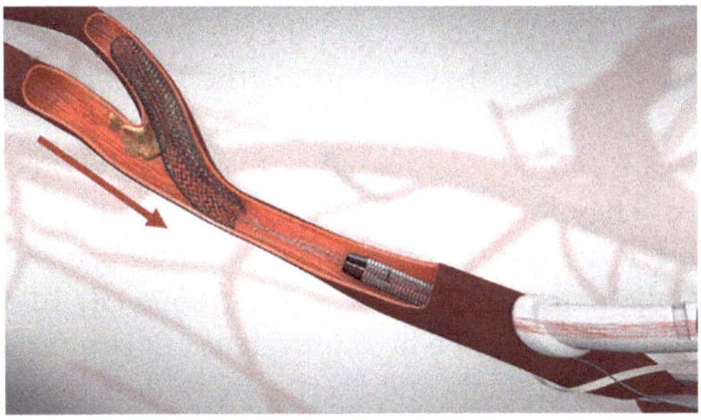

Fig. 7. Transcarotid access used to deploy the ENROUTE self-expanding nitinol stent; Red arrow parallel to the ICA showing reverse flow reversal. (*Courtesy of* Silk Road Medical, Inc.; Silk Road Medical, Inc. retains and reserves all rights, including copyrights.).

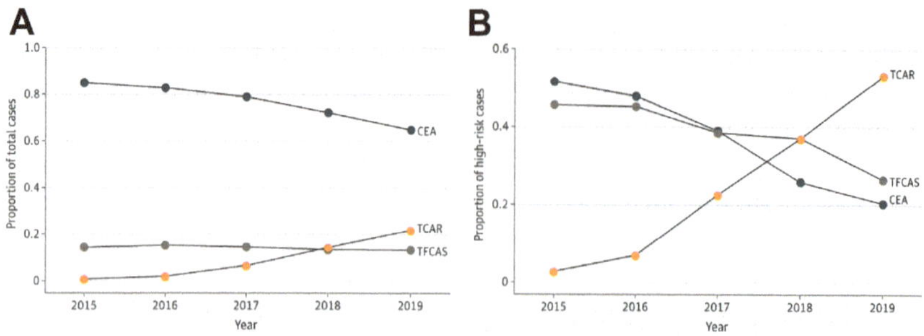

Fig. 8. Temporal Trends of different types of carotid revascularization procedures. (*A*): All carotid revascularizations. (*B*): Carotid revascularizations in high surgical risk patients. (*From* [Use of Transcarotid Artery Revascularization, Transfemoral Carotid Artery Stenting, and Carotid Endarterectomy in the US From 2015–2019]; with permission [44].)

stroke/death. Yet, TCAR exhibited a 47% and 86% reduction in the risk of in-hospital MI and cranial nerve injury (CNI), respectively, compared to CEA [71]. To build more robust evidence, the authors conducted a systematic review and meta-analysis to analyze data from 4012 patients from 2 nonrandomized studies, which confirmed that TCAR has a reduced risk of stroke (1.3% vs 2.6%, OR = 0.5, [95% CI: 0.36–0.74]) and death (0.8% vs 1.5%, OR = 0.5, [95% CI: 0.3, 0.8]) in comparison to TFCAS. Additionally, 4 other nonrandomized studies indicated that TCAR poses a similar risk of 30-day stroke, stroke/death, or combined stroke/death/MI, and lower risk of CNI (0.54% vs 1.84%, OR = 0.52, [95% CI: 0.36–0.74]) compared to CEA [72].

In another analysis by the authors' team, at 1-year follow-up, there was no difference in terms of ipsilateral stroke or death between TCAR and TFCAS as well as TCAR and CEA (6.1% vs 7.1%; HR, 0.85; 95% CI, 0.7–1.01; *P*=.07), although TCAR showed a lower risk of ipsilateral stroke or death compared to TFCAS only in asymptomatic patients (HR, 0.8; 95% CI, 0.6–0.98; *P*=.03) [73]. Based on these midterm results, it seems that the equivalent perioperative outcomes between TCAR and CEA appear to exist for up to 1 year, and TCAR's edge over TFCAS seems to be present mostly in the perioperative period, thus making it the best approach for high-risk patients.

The authors' team recently compared a 3-year mid-term survival between TCAR and CEA. They found that TCAR was associated with a minimal increase in death (HR = 1.16; 95% CI, 1.04–1.30; *P* = .008) that persisted only in symptomatic patients and (HR = 1.33; 95% CI, 1.08–1.63; *P* =.008) which could be contributed to the high prevalence of comorbid medical conditions in TCAR cohort that might still exert confounding bias even after matching [74]. Altogether, these results confirmed that CEA continues to be the preferred approach for standard-risk patients and ensures the safety and efficacy of TCAR as a minimally invasive option surpassing TFCAS to meet the needs of high medical or anatomic risk patients.

ANATOMIC LIMITATIONS OF TRANSCAROTID ARTERY REVASCULARIZATION

Silk Road Enroute Flow Reversal device listed certain anatomic requirements for device iinstructions for use (IFU) (Table 6). For a patient to be eligible for TCAR, the common carotid artery diameter needs to be more than or equal to 6 mm, with at least 5 cm distance from the clavicle to carotid bifurcation (Fig. 9). In a previous study on 224 carotid arteries, 72% were anatomically suitable for TCAR based on IFU. Short-distance clavicle to carotid bifurcation was the most common cause for not fulfilling TCAR IFU [75,76]. CCA could be sewn to prosthetic Dacron conduit to gain more distance to carotid bifurcation to insert arterial sheath safely. Nevertheless, it is considered outside the IFU and should be applied with high vigilance [77].

TIMING OF CAROTID REVASCULARIZATION IN SYMPTOMATIC PATIENTS

In symptomatic patients, carotid revascularization is recommended within 2 to 14 days after a neurologic event to ensure the best outcomes [21,78]. The authors' team performed two separate analyses using the VQI database on symptomatic patients and found the optimal timing for TCAR intervention within the same time period [79]. TFCAS was associated with higher odds of in-hospital stroke/death in all time periods compared to CEA; however, TCAR and CEA showed similar outcomes (aOR = 1.1 [95% CI: 0.7–1.7]; *P*=.66) [80].

DECISION-MAKING

Several patients' medical and anatomic factors put patients at high risk for each carotid revascularization approach: CEA, TFCAS, and TCAR (Tables 3 and 6; Table 7). Typically, patients with high surgical risk for CEA should be offered the minimally invasive CAS.

The following key factors should be evaluated when considering a patient for carotid revascularization to ensure proper patient selection.

Table 6
High-risk factors for transcarotid artery revascularization

Anatomic Factors	Medical Factors
• Severe ICA tortuosity • ICA diameter < 4 mm • CCA diameter < 6 mm • Clavicle to carotid bifurcation distance <5 cm • CCA depth from skin ≥4 cm • Heavily circumferential calcification • CCA Puncture site with moderate to severe plaque.	• Nickel allergy • Bleeding disorder • Contraindication to aspirin or P2Y12 inhibitors • Contraindication to anticoagulation • Severe CKD

Abbreviations: CCA, common carotid artery; CKD, chronic kidney disease; ICA, internal carotid artery.

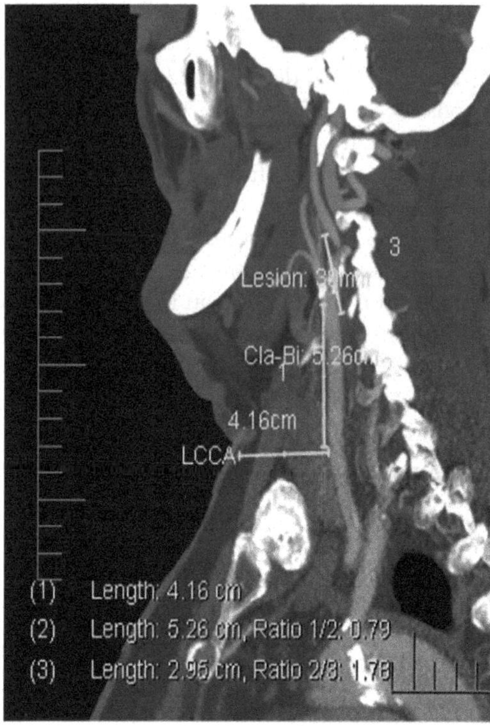

Fig. 9. Anatomic requirement for transcarotid artery revascularization (TCAR): healthy common carotid artery (CCA) of at least 6 mm in diameter, free of significant atherosclerosis and calcification, a landing zone of at least 5 cm from the clavicle to the carotid bifurcation to allow wire access and sheath support during advancement, the CCA should not be deeper than the actual length of the landing zone. (*From* Wu WW, Liang P, O'Donnell TFX, et al. Anatomic eligibility for transcarotid artery revascularization and transfemoral carotid artery stenting. *J Vasc Surg.* 2019;69(5):1452 to 1460. https://doi.org/10.1016/j.jvs.2018.11.051.)

PATIENT DEMOGRAPHICS AND MEDICAL COMORBIDITIES

Age

Advanced age tends to accelerate atherosclerotic plaque buildup in the aortic arch, leading to risky arch manipulation during CAS. Per AHA and SVS guidelines, in patients greater than 70, TFCAS tends to have worse outcomes compared to CEA. The authors previously found in a multicenter study that patient age affected the risk-adjusted efficacy of CAS, in contrast to the more consistent performance of CEA across different age groups [81].

On the other hand, TCAR emerges as a suitable minimally invasive alternative with favorable outcomes in older patients by evading harmful aortic arch manipulation [82–84]. In a retrospective study on octogenarians, TCAR showed a similar outcome to CEA but a significant reduction in the risk of in-hospital stroke/death compared with TFCAS (OR = 0.9 [95% CI: 0.5–0.1.7]; $P<.77$), (OR = 0.35 [95% CI: 0.2–0.6]; $P<.001$), respectively [85].

Table 7
High-risk factors for transfemoral carotid artery stenting

Anatomic factors	Medical factors
• High-risk aortic arch (Acute angulation, Type III arch) • Severely atherosclerotic aorta • Innominate vessel severe stenosis, occlusion • Left CCA severe stenosis, occlusion. • Severe ICA kinking • Unstable plaques • Carotid bifurcation fresh thrombus • Long (>10 mm) complex target lesion • Heavily circumferential calcification • Carotid string signs up to MCA (*relative contraindication*) • Poor access (Iliac artery occlusion or stenosis that impedes sheath placement).	• Advanced age (>70 y) • Symptomatic stenosis • Procedures within 14 d of neurologic deficit • Severe allergy to contrast media. • CKD

Abbreviations: CCA, common carotid artery; ICA, internal carotid artery; TFCAS, transfemoral carotid artery stenting.

Heart Disease

MI is considered to be the most common cause of perioperative and long-term death following CEA [86–88]. As a result, many surgeons recommend CAS instead of CEA for patients who have recent MI, unstable angina, or advanced CHF. Compared to TFCAS, TCAR is associated with a lower risk of perioperative complications and is viewed as an ideal option for these patients [69]. Even though recent MI is defined as a high-risk criterion for CEA, in a recent study by the authors' group, the authors showed that in patients with recent MI (<6 months), CEA is safer compared to TFCAS but similar to TCAR in terms of perioperative stroke/death/MI [89]. Moreover, in patients with symptomatic CHF, TFCAS was associated with the worst perioperative stroke/death/MI compared to CEA and TCAR, while TCAR was similar to CEA [90].

Renal Disease

The method of carotid revascularization should be chosen carefully for patients with chronic kidney disease [91]. These patients are at high risk of acute renal failure and ESRD following the intravenous contrast dye during CAS [92]. On the other hand, CEA poses a significant risk for patients on hemodialysis, especially for asymptomatic patients where the risks of CEA exceed the benefits [93]. TFCAS is associated with excessive perioperative death, stroke/death, and suboptimal long-term survival in hemodialysis patients [94]. Yet, a recent study by the authors' group found that in-hospital stroke or death following TCAR were similar between dialysis and non-dialysis patients, proving the safety TCAR offers for dialysis patients [95].

ANATOMIC CONSIDERATIONS

High Anatomic Risk Factors for Carotid Endarterectomy

Prior studies have shown conflicting results regarding CEA and TFCAS outcomes in patients with contralateral carotid occlusion (CCO) [96,97]. Based on an analysis of the VQI database in patients with CCO, the authors found that TCAR is associated with lower odds of in-hospital stroke or death in comparison to TFCAS. When comparing TCAR to CEA, the odds of in-hospital stroke or death were lower in TCAR only in asymptomatic patients [98].

A hostile neck, defined as a history of neck irradiation or any prior neck surgery, often has significant fibrotic scarring around the carotid artery. This poses a heightened anatomic risk for CEA, particularly increasing the risks for wound complications and CNI. The minimally invasive CAS tends to be the preferred method for these patients [99,100]. The authors' team analyzed the VQI database and found that among those patients, TFCAS has approximately four times higher risk of in-hospital death and technical failures when compared to TCAR (aOR = 3.8 [95% CI: 1.5–9.5]; P=.005), and (aOR = 3.7 [95% CI: 1.8–7.5]; P<.001), respectively [101]. A prior study also found that patients who undergo redo CEA for carotid stenosis are associated with almost 3-fold increase in the risk of stroke and double the risk of death [102]. However, the authors showed that TCAR was associated with a 59% reduction in stroke/death/MI compared to redoing CEA [103].

High Anatomic Risk Factors for Carotid Artery Stenting

Specific anatomic characteristics are considered high risk for any stenting procedure, whether TFCAS or TCAR, such as (1) severe tortuosity of ICA at the stenting site, (2) significant kinking of the ICA, and (3) extensive circumferential calcification of the ICA. Notably, if the ICA has a pronounced kinking at the EPD placement site, it is exclusively high-risk for TFCAS. Moreover, TCAR lacks TFCAS' contraindications of the high-risk aortic arch. More details about the specific anatomic criteria related to carotid artery access and sheath insertion that impede TCAR and TFCAS are summarized in Tables 6 and 7.

In the authors' analysis of national database, they found that among patients with calcification greater than 50% of carotid circumference, TCAR had more promising outcomes compared to TFCAS, specifically among those with heavy calcification in terms of stroke/death (OR = 0.50 [95% CI: 0.3–0.8]; P<.01) and stroke/death/MI (OR = 0.6 [95% CI: 0.4–0.9]; P<.01) [104]. Additionally, the authors found in another study that when lesion length extends beyond 25 mm, TCAR has reduced risk of stroke (aOR = 0.7 [95% CI: 0.5–0.9]; P<.01) and death (aOR = 0.3 [95% CI: 0.2–0.4]; P<.01) compared to TFCAS [105].

Even though TFCAS has shown worse outcomes than TCAR in every study, TCAR anatomic limitations could make TFCAS the only applicable option for a unique group of patients with a high risk for CEA and inadequate anatomy for TCAR [67]. In patients with a high risk for CEA and unsuitable anatomy for both TCAR and TFCAS, the decision to proceed with carotid revascularization and the specific approach should be tailored considering

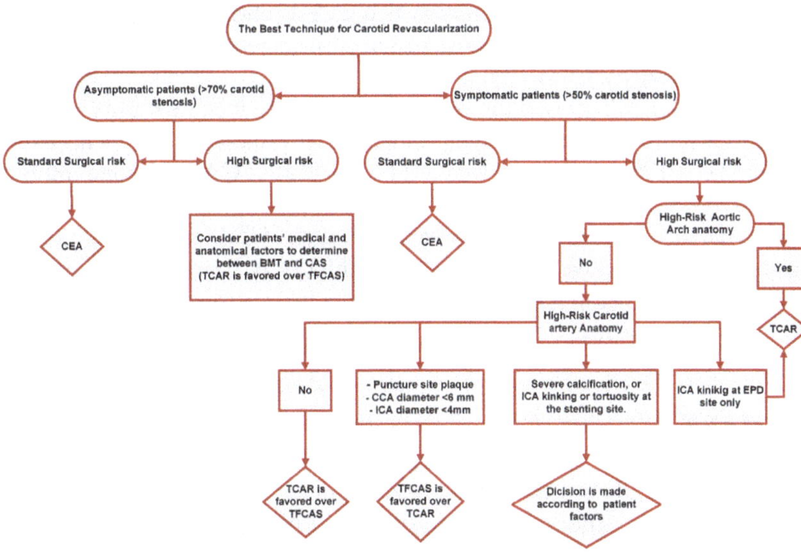

Fig. 10. Decision-making algorithm demonstrating the best technique for carotid artery revascularization. CEA, carotid endarterectomy; CAS, carotid artery stenting; TCAR, transcarotid artery revascularization; TFCAS, transfemoral carotid artery stenting; CCA, common carotid artery; ICA, internal carotid artery; EPD, embolic protection device.

several patient medical and lesion factors. In Fig. 10, the authors demonstrate a decision-making algorithm to determine the best technique for carotid revascularization.

TRANSCAROTID ARTERY REVASCULARIZATION AND STANDARD RISK PATIENTS BASED ON MEDICARE & MEDICAID SERVICES CRITERIA

TCAR was first approved for high-risk patients based on CMS definition [60]. Both ROADSTER 1 and 2 included only high-risk patients for CEA. It was considered an off-label use of TCAR in standard-risk patients and only approved for clinical trials under certain regulations. In April 2022, the FDA approved the expansion of TCAR indications to include standard-risk patients for CEA (P140026) [106]. Subsequently, a single-arm trial, ROADSTER 3 trial, was launched and started recruiting patients classified as standard risk by CMS. This trial will include symptomatic patients with greater than 50% stenosis or asymptomatic patients with greater than 60% stenosis by angiogram, aiming to enroll 400 patients [107].

CMS limitation of TFCAS reimbursement to high-risk patients was similarly applied to TCAR. However, these criteria were established in 2005 and included TCAR and TFCAS under the same category [60]. In a retrospective matched cohort study of prospectively collected data between 2016 and 2019, there was no significant difference between TCAR and CEA in the risk of 30-day stroke, death, or MI or 1-year stroke in patients who were considered standard surgical risk by CMS [108].

In Oct 2023, CMS revised the coverage for CAS to include standard-risk patients, both symptomatic and asymptomatic (see Table 4, B) [61]. This expansion did not differentiate between TFCAS and TCAR, despite multiple retrospective studies showing that periprocedural outcomes of TCAR were comparable to CEA, while TFCAS were inferior to CEA, even in high-risk patients. Furthermore, we should await CREST-2 trial results to determine whether medical therapy alone is better or equivalent to revascularization for asymptomatic patients.

SUMMARY

Carotid artery revascularization is recommended for symptomatic patients with greater than 50% stenosis and asymptomatic patients with greater than 70% stenosis. The choice between different carotid revascularization techniques has been debated in the last decade. While CEA stands as the gold standard technique for carotid revascularization, CAS is favored for specific patients at high surgical risk. The current evidence suggests that TCAR is both safe and effective, with comparable results to CEA and better results than TFCAS despite being performed in high-risk patients. Long-term outcomes of TCAR are not as extensively studied as those of CEA and TFCAS, and the evidence on the comparative outcomes between the 3 procedures is limited only to observational and retrospective studies. Even though sophisticated statistical analysis methods like propensity score matching (PSM) have been used, a well-designed RCT comparing CEA versus TCAR is crucial owing to the widespread adoption of this technique. Additionally, RCT will assess TCAR outcomes in standard-risk patients to further establish the role of TCAR in carotid artery stenosis management.

While asymptomatic patients with high-grade stenosis will benefit from carotid revascularization, asymptomatic patients with moderate stenosis should be offered medical management. While CREST-2 results will address if there is any advantage of both TFCAS and CEA over best medical management, unfortunately, this trial excluded TCAR, which leaves us to utilize VQI and Medicare-linked data, and we hope that the results from these real-world data will steer future conduction of more conclusive RCT.

While advancements in carotid revascularization have come a long way, uncertainties persist. Variability in individual anatomy can sometimes complicate the choice of technique, necessitating sufficient proficiency in all 3 approaches and tailored strategies to improve each patient's outcomes. Furthermore, it is essential to understand the patient's health care goals. While some patients prefer the minimally invasive options, others value the favorable long-term outcomes. Physicians should emphasize patient education with detailed discussion about potential benefits, risks, and alternatives.

CLINICS CARE POINTS

- Carotid revascularization is considered a vital intervention for stroke prevention. The choice of revascularization technique—whether CEA, TCAR, TFCAS—should be tailored to each patient's specific medical and anatomic profile to ensure the best possible clinical outcomes.
- CEA is recommended over CAS for low surgical risk patients with symptomatic carotid artery stenosis of greater than 50%.
- In asymptomatic patients with ≥70% carotid artery stenosis, assess the risk of CEA:
- For standard surgical risk patients, CEA is recommended.
- For high surgical risk patients, TCAR, TFCAS, or aggressive medical therapy may be recommended after considering multiple patient factors.
- Among carotid revascularization techniques, TFCAS has the highest morbidity and mortality rates. Yet, it could be the only revascularization technique available for patients with high surgical risk for CEA and unsuitable anatomy for TCAR.

DISCLAIMER STATEMENT

A. Abdelkarim has nothing to disclose. M. Hamouda has nothing to disclose. M.B. Malas was the principal investigator for ROADSTER 1 and ROADSTER 2 trial. He is a member of the steering committee of the Society for Vascular Surgery (SVS) Vascular Quality Initiative (VQI) Transcarotid Artery Revascularization (TCAR) Surveillance Project (TSP). He is also the national principal investigator for the ongoing RAODSTER 1 long-term follow-up trial. Educational grants to University of California San Diego were not used in this manuscript data.

References

[1] Yang Q, Tong X, Schieb L, et al. Vital Signs: Recent Trends in Stroke Death Rates — United States, 2000–2015. MMWR Morb Mortal Wkly Rep 2017;66:933–9.
[2] Virani SS, Alonso A, Benjamin EJ, et al. Heart Disease and Stroke Statistics—2020 Update: A Report From the American Heart Association. Circulation 2020;141(9):e139–596.
[3] Tsao CW, Aday AW, Almarzooq ZI, et al. Heart Disease and Stroke Statistics-2023 Update: A Report From the American Heart Association. Circulation 2023;147(8):e93–621.
[4] Flaherty ML, Kissela B, Khoury JC, et al. Carotid Artery Stenosis as a Cause of Stroke. Neuroepidemiology 2012;40(1):36–41.
[5] Song P, Fang Z, Wang H, et al. Global and regional prevalence, burden, and risk factors for carotid atherosclerosis: a systematic review, meta-analysis, and modelling study. Lancet Global Health 2020;8(5):e721–9.
[6] Brott TG, Hobson RW, Howard G, et al. Stenting versus Endarterectomy for Treatment of Carotid-Artery Stenosis. N Engl J Med 2010;363(1):11–23.
[7] Li B, Rizkallah P, Eisenberg N, et al. Symptom Status of Patients Undergoing Carotid Endarterectomy in Canada and United States. Ann Vasc Surg 2022;81:183–95.
[8] Conrad MF, Baloum V, Mukhopadhyay S, et al. Progression of asymptomatic carotid stenosis despite optimal medical therapy. J Vasc Surg 2013;58(1):128–35.e1.

[9] Conrad MF, Michalczyk MJ, Opalacz A, et al. The natural history of asymptomatic severe carotid artery stenosis. J Vasc Surg 2014;60(5):1218–26.
[10] Kakkos SK, Nicolaides AN, Charalambous I, et al. Predictors and clinical significance of progression or regression of asymptomatic carotid stenosis. J Vasc Surg 2014;59(4): 956–67.e1.
[11] Moacdieh MP, Khan MA, Layman P, et al. Innovation in the open and endovascular treatment of carotid artery stenosis. Semin Vasc Surg 2021;34(4):163–71.
[12] Kernan WN, Ovbiagele B, Black HR, et al. Guidelines for the Prevention of Stroke in Patients With Stroke and Transient Ischemic Attack: A Guideline for Healthcare Professionals From the American Heart Association/American Stroke Association. Stroke 2014;45(7): 2160–236.
[13] Powers WJ, Rabinstein AA, Ackerson T, et al. 2018 Guidelines for the Early Management of Patients With Acute Ischemic Stroke: A Guideline for Healthcare Professionals From the American Heart Association/American Stroke Association. Stroke 2018;49(3):e46–110.
[14] Ricotta JJ, AbuRahma A, Ascher E, et al, Society for Vascular Surgery. Updated Society for Vascular Surgery guidelines for management of extracranial carotid disease. J Vasc Surg 2011;54(3):e1–31.
[15] Patel RJ, Marmor R, Dakour H, et al. Dual Antiplatelet Therapy Is Associated with Increased Risk of Bleeding and Decreased Risk of Stroke Following Carotid Endarterectomy. Ann Vasc Surg 2023;88:191–8.
[16] Blauw GJ, Lagaay AM, Smelt AH, et al. Stroke, statins, and cholesterol. A meta-analysis of randomized, placebo-controlled, double-blind trials with HMG-CoA reductase inhibitors. Stroke 1997;28(5):946–50.
[17] van Dongen MME, Aarnio K, Martinez-Majander N, et al. Use of Statins After Ischemic Stroke in Young Adults and Its Association With Long-Term Outcome. Stroke 2019;50(12):3385–92.
[18] Anjorin AC, Marcaccio CL, Rastogi V, et al. Statin therapy is associated with improved perioperative outcomes and long-term mortality following carotid revascularization in the Vascular Quality Initiative. J Vasc Surg 2023;77(1):158–69.e8.
[19] Brott TG, Halperin JL, Abbara S, et al. 2011 ASA/ACCF/AHA/AANN/AANS/ACR/ASNR/CNS/SAIP/SCAI/SIR/SNIS/SVM/SVS guideline on the management of patients with extracranial carotid and vertebral artery disease: executive summary: a report of the American College of Cardiology Foundation/American Heart Association Task Force on Practice Guidelines, and the American Stroke Association, American Association of Neuroscience Nurses, American Association of Neurological Surgeons, American College of Radiology, American Society of Neuroradiology, Congress of Neurological Surgeons, Society of Atherosclerosis Imaging and Prevention, Society for Cardiovascular Angiography and Interventions, Society of Interventional Radiology, Society of NeuroInterventional Surgery, Society for Vascular Medicine, and Society for Vascular Surgery. Developed in collaboration with the American Academy of Neurology and Society of Cardiovascular Computed Tomography. Catheter Cardiovasc Interv Off J Soc Card Angiogr Interv 2013;81(1):E76–123.
[20] Kleindorfer DO, Towfighi A, Chaturvedi S, et al. 2021 Guideline for the Prevention of Stroke in Patients With Stroke and Transient Ischemic Attack: A Guideline From the American Heart Association/American Stroke Association. Stroke 2021;52(7):e364–467.
[21] AbuRahma AF, Avgerinos ED, Chang RW, et al. Society for Vascular Surgery clinical practice guidelines for management of extracranial cerebrovascular disease. J Vasc Surg 2022;75(1S):4S–22S.
[22] AbuRahma AF, Avgerinos ED, Chang RW, et al. The Society for Vascular Surgery implementation document for management of extracranial cerebrovascular disease. J Vasc Surg 2022;75(1, Supplement):26S–98S.
[23] Barnett HJM, Taylor DW, Eliasziw M, et al. Benefit of carotid endarterectomy in patients with symptomatic moderate or severe stenosis. N Engl J Med 1998;339(20):1415–25.

[24] North American Symptomatic Carotid Endarterectomy Trial Collaborators, Barnett HJM, Taylor DW, et al. Beneficial effect of carotid endarterectomy in symptomatic patients with high-grade carotid stenosis. N Engl J Med 1991;325(7):445–53.
[25] Rothwell PM, Gutnikov SA, Warlow CP, et al. Reanalysis of the final results of the European Carotid Surgery Trial. Stroke 2003;34(2):514–23.
[26] Warlow C. MRC European Carotid Surgery Trial: interim results for symptomatic patients with severe (70-99%) or with mild (0-29%) carotid stenosis. Lancet 1991;337(8752): 1235–43.
[27] Walker MD, Marler JR, Goldstein M, et al. Endarterectomy for Asymptomatic Carotid Artery Stenosis. JAMA 1995;273(18):1421–8.
[28] Halliday A, Mansfield A, Marro J, et al. Prevention of disabling and fatal strokes by successful carotid endarterectomy in patients without recent neurological symptoms: randomised controlled trial. Lancet Lond Engl 2004;363(9420):1491–502.
[29] Young B, Moore WS, Robertson JT, et al. An analysis of perioperative surgical mortality and morbidity in the asymptomatic carotid atherosclerosis study. Stroke 1996;27(12): 2216–24.
[30] Abbott AL. Regarding "Asymptomatic carotid artery stenosis—Medical therapy alone versus medical therapy plus carotid endarterectomy or stenting.". J Vasc Surg 2011;53(1):265.
[31] Dakour-Aridi H, Ou M, Locham S, et al. Outcomes following Eversion versus Conventional Endarterectomy in the Vascular Quality Initiative Database. Ann Vasc Surg 2020;65:1–9.
[32] Paraskevas KI, Robertson V, Saratzis AN, et al. Editor's Choice - An Updated Systematic Review and Meta-analysis of Outcomes Following Eversion vs. Conventional Carotid Endarterectomy in Randomised Controlled Trials and Observational Studies. Eur J Vasc Endovasc Surg Off J Eur Soc Vasc Surg 2018;55(4):465–73.
[33] Rerkasem A, Orrapin S, Howard DP, et al. Local versus general anaesthesia for carotid endarterectomy. Cochrane Database Syst Rev 2021;2021(10):CD000126; https://doi.org/10.1002/14651858.CD000126.pub5.
[34] Dakour Aridi H, Paracha N, Nejim B, et al. Anesthetic type and hospital outcomes after carotid endarterectomy from the Vascular Quality Initiative database. J Vasc Surg 2018;67(5):1419–28.
[35] Hye RJ, Voeks JH, Malas MB, et al. Anesthetic type and risk of myocardial infarction after carotid endarterectomy in the Carotid Revascularization Endarterectomy versus Stenting Trial (CREST). J Vasc Surg 2016;64(1):3–8.e1.
[36] Chuatrakoon B, Nantakool S, Rerkasem A, et al. Routine or selective carotid artery shunting for carotid endarterectomy (and different methods of monitoring in selective shunting). Cochrane Database Syst Rev 2022;6(6):CD000190.
[37] Aburahma AF, Mousa AY, Stone PA. Shunting during carotid endarterectomy. J Vasc Surg 2011;54(5):1502 10.
[38] Wiske C, Arhuidese I, Malas M, et al. Comparing the efficacy of shunting approaches and cerebral monitoring during carotid endarterectomy using a national database. J Vasc Surg 2018;68(2):416–25.
[39] Jahangiri FR, Liang M, Huckabey M, et al. Carotid Endarterectomy Surgeries: A Multimodality Intraoperative Neurophysiological Monitoring Approach. Cureus 2022;14(7):e26556.
[40] Dakour-Aridi H, Gaber MG, Khalid M, et al. Examination of the interaction between method of anesthesia and shunting with carotid endarterectomy. J Vasc Surg 2020;71(6):1964–71.
[41] Malas M, Glebova NO, Hughes SE, et al. Effect of patching on reducing restenosis in the carotid revascularization endarterectomy versus stenting trial. Stroke 2015;46(3): 757–61.
[42] AbuRahma AF, Robinson PA, Saiedy S, et al. Prospective randomized trial of carotid endarterectomy with primary closure and patch angioplasty with saphenous vein, jugular vein,

and polytetrafluoroethylene: long-term follow-up. J Vasc Surg 1998;27(2):222–32 [discussion: 233-234].
[43] Edenfield L, Blazick E, Eldrup-Jorgensen J, et al. Outcomes of carotid endarterectomy in the Vascular Quality Initiative based on patch type. J Vasc Surg 2020;71(4):1260–7.
[44] Stonko DP, Goldsborough E III, Kibrik P, et al. Use of Transcarotid Artery Revascularization, Transfemoral Carotid Artery Stenting, and Carotid Endarterectomy in the US From 2015 to 2019. JAMA Netw Open 2022;5(9):e2231944; https://doi.org/10.1001/jamanetworkopen.2022.31944.
[45] Naggara O, Touzé E, Beyssen B, et al. Anatomical and Technical Factors Associated With Stroke or Death During Carotid Angioplasty and Stenting. Stroke 2011;42(2):380–8.
[46] Mas JL, Chatellier G, Beyssen B, et al. Endarterectomy versus stenting in patients with symptomatic severe carotid stenosis. N Engl J Med 2006;355(16):1660–71.
[47] Cho YD, Kim SE, Lim JW, et al. Protected versus Unprotected Carotid Artery Stenting : Meta-Analysis of the Current Literature. J Korean Neurosurg Soc 2018;61(4):458–66.
[48] Shah P, Dahn M. Carotid Angioplasty. In: Forbes T, editor. Angioplasty, various techniques and challenges in treatment of congenital and acquired vascular stenoses. London, UK: IntechOpen; 2012; https://doi.org/10.5772/29253 Ch. 9.
[49] Nikas DN, Kompara G, Reimers B. Carotid stents: which is the best option? J Cardiovasc Surg 2011;52(6):779–93.
[50] Giri J, Kennedy KF, Weinberg I, et al. Comparative effectiveness of commonly used devices for carotid artery stenting: an NCDR Analysis (National Cardiovascular Data Registry). JACC Cardiovasc Interv 2014;7(2):171–7.
[51] Schillinger M, Gschwendtner M, Reimers B, et al. Does Carotid Stent Cell Design Matter? Stroke 2008;39(3):905–9.
[52] Faateh M, Dakour-Aridi H, Mathlouthi A, et al. Comparison of open- and closed-cell stent design outcomes after carotid artery stenting in the Vascular Quality Initiative. J Vasc Surg 2021;73(5):1639–48.
[53] JCM I Free Full-Text I Clinical Outcomes of Second- versus First-Generation Carotid Stents: A Systematic Review and Meta-Analysis. Available at: https://www.mdpi.com/2077-0383/11/16/4819. [Accessed 30 October 2023].
[54] Yadav JS, Wholey MH, Kuntz RE, et al. Protected carotid-artery stenting versus endarterectomy in high-risk patients. N Engl J Med 2004;351(15):1493–501.
[55] Rosenfield K, Matsumura JS, Chaturvedi S, et al. Randomized Trial of Stent versus Surgery for Asymptomatic Carotid Stenosis. N Engl J Med 2016;374(11):1011–20.
[56] International Carotid Stenting Study investigators, Ederle J, Dobson J, et al. Carotid artery stenting compared with endarterectomy in patients with symptomatic carotid stenosis (International Carotid Stenting Study): an interim analysis of a randomised controlled trial. Lancet 2010;375(9719):985–97.
[57] Brott TG, Howard G, Roubin GS, et al. Long-Term Results of Stenting versus Endarterectomy for Carotid-Artery Stenosis. N Engl J Med 2016;374(11):1021–31.
[58] Vasavada AM, Singh P, Firdaus A, et al. Carotid Endarterectomy Versus Stenting for the Treatment of Patients With Carotid Artery Stenosis: An Updated Systematic Review and Meta-Analysis. Cureus 2023;15(2):e35070; https://doi.org/10.7759/cureus.35070.
[59] Yei KS, Janssen C, Elsayed N, et al. Long-term outcomes of carotid endarterectomy vs transfemoral carotid stenting in a Medicare-matched database. J Vasc Surg 2023; https://doi.org/10.1016/j.jvs.2023.08.118.
[60] NCA - Carotid Artery Stenting (CAG-00085R) - Decision Memo. Available at: https://www.cms.gov/medicare-coverage-database/view/ncacal-decision-memo.aspx?proposed=N&NCAId=157. [Accessed 1 October 2023].
[61] NCA - Percutaneous Transluminal Angioplasty (PTA) of the Carotid Artery Concurrent with Stenting (CAG-00085R8). Available at: https://www.cms.gov/medicare-coverage-database/view/nca.aspx?ncaid=311&. Accessed October 30, 2023.

[62] Hicks CW, Nejim B, Locham S, et al. Association between Medicare high-risk criteria and outcomes after carotid revascularization procedures. J Vasc Surg 2018;67(6): 1752–61.e2.
[63] Malas MB, Leal J, Kashyap V, et al. Technical aspects of transcarotid artery revascularization using the ENROUTE transcarotid neuroprotection and stent system. J Vasc Surg 2017;65(3):916–20.
[64] Kwolek CJ, Jaff MR, Leal JI, et al. Results of the ROADSTER multicenter trial of transcarotid stenting with dynamic flow reversal. J Vasc Surg 2015;62(5):1227–34.e1.
[65] Malas MB, Leal Lorenzo JI, Nejim B, et al. Analysis of the ROADSTER pivotal and extended-access cohorts shows excellent 1-year durability of transcarotid stenting with dynamic flow reversal. J Vasc Surg 2019;69(6):1786–96.
[66] Kashyap VS, Schneider PA, Foteh M, et al. Early Outcomes in the ROADSTER 2 Study of Transcarotid Artery Revascularization in Patients With Significant Carotid Artery Disease. Stroke 2020;51(9):2620–9.
[67] Zarrintan S, Malas MB. What Is the Role of Transcarotid Artery Revascularization? Adv Surg 2023;57(1):115–40.
[68] Society for Vascular Surgery Patient Safety Organization. TransCarotid revascularization surveillance project of the society for vascular surgery vascular quality initiative. clinicaltrials.gov. 2021. Available at: https://clinicaltrials.gov/ct2/show/NCT02850588. [Accessed 19 August 2021].
[69] Malas MB, Dakour-Aridi H, Wang GJ, et al. Transcarotid artery revascularization versus transfemoral carotid artery stenting in the Society for Vascular Surgery Vascular Quality Initiative. J Vasc Surg 2019;69(1):92–103.e2.
[70] Schermerhorn ML, Liang P, Eldrup-Jorgensen J, et al. Association of Transcarotid Artery Revascularization vs Transfemoral Carotid Artery Stenting With Stroke or Death Among Patients With Carotid Artery Stenosis. JAMA 2019;322(23):2313.
[71] Malas MB, Dakour-Aridi H, Kashyap VS, et al. TransCarotid Revascularization with Dynamic Flow reversal versus Carotid Endarterectomy in the Vascular Quality Initiative Surveillance Project. Ann Surg 2020; https://doi.org/10.1097/SLA.0000000000004496.
[72] Naazie IN, Cui CL, Osaghae I, et al. A Systematic Review and Meta-Analysis of Transcarotid Artery Revascularization with Dynamic Flow Reversal Versus Transfemoral Carotid Artery Stenting and Carotid Endarterectomy. Ann Vasc Surg 2020;69:426–36.
[73] Malas MB, Elsayed N, Naazie I, et al. Propensity score-matched analysis of 1-year outcomes of transcarotid revascularization with dynamic flow reversal, carotid endarterectomy, and transfemoral carotid artery stenting. J Vasc Surg 2021; https://doi.org/10.1016/j.jvs.2021.07.242 S0741521421019868.
[74] Zarrintan S, Elsayed N, Patel RJ, et al. Propensity-Score Matched Analysis of Three Years Survival of Trans Carotid Artery Revascularization Versus Carotid Endarterectomy in the Vascular Quality Initiative Medicare-Linked Database. Ann Surg 2023;278(4):559–67.
[75] Wu WW, Liang P, O'Donnell TFX, et al. Anatomic eligibility for transcarotid artery revascularization and transfemoral carotid artery stenting. J Vasc Surg 2019;69(5):1452–60.
[76] Blears E, Patel S, Doyle M, et al. Predicting Transcarotid Artery Revascularization Adverse Outcomes by Imaging Characteristics. Ann Vasc Surg 2022;87:388–401.
[77] Liang P, Schermerhorn ML. Transcarotid Artery Revascularization: Is It Better than Carotid Endarterectomy? Adv Surg 2022;56(1):111–27.
[78] Cui CL, Yei KS, Ramachandran M, et al. In-hospital complications and long-term outcomes associated with timing of carotid endarterectomy. J Vasc Surg 2022;76(1):222–31.e1.
[79] Cui CL, Dakour-Aridi H, Eldrup-Jorgensen J, et al. Effects of timing on in-hospital and one-year outcomes after transcarotid artery revascularization. J Vasc Surg 2021;73(5): 1649–57.e1.
[80] Cui CL, Dakour-Aridi H, Lu JJ, et al. In-hospital Outcomes of Urgent, Early or Late Revascularization for Symptomatic Carotid Artery Stenosis. Stroke 2022;53(1):100–7.

[81] Nejim B, Alshwaily W, Dakour-Aridi H, et al. Age modifies the efficacy and safety of carotid artery revascularization procedures. J Vasc Surg 2019;69(5):1490–503.e3.
[82] Dias CG, Fajardo A, Martin GH, et al. Transcarotid Revascularization Results in Patients Over 70 Years of Age. Vasc Endovasc Surg 2023;57(2):114–8.
[83] Mehta A, Patel PB, Bajakian D, et al. Transcarotid artery revascularization versus carotid endarterectomy and transfemoral stenting in octogenarians. J Vasc Surg 2021;74(5):1602–8.
[84] Kibrik P, Stonko DP, Alsheekh A, et al. Association of carotid revascularization approach with perioperative outcomes based on symptom status and degree of stenosis among octogenarians. J Vasc Surg 2022;76(3):769–77.e2.
[85] Dakour-Aridi H, Kashyap VS, Wang GJ, et al. The impact of age on in-hospital outcomes after transcarotid artery revascularization, transfemoral carotid artery stenting, and carotid endarterectomy. J Vasc Surg 2020;72(3):931–42.e2.
[86] Jácome F, Nóbrega L, Pereira-Neves A, et al. Revised cardiac score index is a predictor of long-term outcomes after carotid endarterectomy. VASA Z Gefasskrankheiten 2022;51(2):93–8.
[87] Vernooij LM, van Klei WA, Moons KG, et al. The comparative and added prognostic value of biomarkers to the Revised Cardiac Risk Index for preoperative prediction of major adverse cardiac events and all-cause mortality in patients who undergo noncardiac surgery. Cochrane Database Syst Rev 2021;12(12):CD013139; https://doi.org/10.1002/14651858.CD013139.pub2.
[88] Squizzato F, Antonello M, Taglialavoro J, et al. Clinical Impact of Routine Cardiology Consultation Prior to Elective Carotid Endarterectomy in Neurologically Asymptomatic Patients. Eur J Vasc Endovasc Surg Off J Eur Soc Vasc Surg 2020;59(4):536–44.
[89] Straus S, Moghaddam M, Zarrintan S, et al. Modality-Specific Outcomes of Patients Undergoing Carotid Revascularization in the Setting of Recent Myocardial Infarction. J Vasc Surg 2023; https://doi.org/10.1016/j.jvs.2023.09.024.
[90] Moghaddam M, Zarrintan S, Willie-Permor D, et al. Transcarotid Artery Revascularization Is the Safest Carotid Artery Revascularization Option for Patients With Symptomatic Congestive Heart Failure. J Vasc Surg 2023;77(6):e109; https://doi.org/10.1016/j.jvs.2023.03.174.
[91] Patel AR, Dombrovskiy VY, Vogel TR. A contemporary evaluation of carotid endarterectomy outcomes in patients with chronic kidney disease in the United States. Vascular 2017;25(5):459–65.
[92] Pucciarelli A, Arcari A, Popusoi G, et al. Incidence and predictors of acute kidney injury in patients undergoing proximal protected carotid artery stenting. EuroIntervention J Eur Collab Work Group Interv Cardiol Eur Soc Cardiol 2018;14(3):e360–6.
[93] Cooper M, Arhuidese IJ, Obeid T, et al. Perioperative and Long-term Outcomes After Carotid Endarterectomy in Hemodialysis Patients. JAMA Surg 2016;151(10):947.
[94] Arhuidese IJ, Obeid T, Hicks CW, et al. Outcomes after carotid artery stenting in hemodialysis patients. J Vasc Surg 2016;63(6):1511–6.
[95] Elsayed N, Vasudevan RS, Zarrintan S, et al. TransCarotid Artery Revascularization Can Be Safely Performed in Patients Undergoing Dialysis. Ann Vasc Surg 2023;92:57–64.
[96] Kokkinidis DG, Chaitidis N, Giannopoulos S, et al. Presence of Contralateral Carotid Occlusion Is Associated With Increased Periprocedural Stroke Risk Following CEA but Not CAS: A Meta-analysis and Meta-regression Analysis of 43 Studies and 96,658 Patients. J Endovasc Ther Off J Int Soc Endovasc Spec 2020;27(2):334–44.
[97] Nejim B, Dakour Aridi H, Locham S, et al. Carotid artery revascularization in patients with contralateral carotid artery occlusion: Stent or endarterectomy? J Vasc Surg 2017;66(6):1735–48.e1.
[98] Dakour-Aridi H, Elsayed N, Malas M. Outcomes of Carotid Revascularization in Patients with Contralateral Carotid Artery Occlusion. J Am Coll Surg 2021;232(5):699–708.e1.

[99] Batarseh P, Parides M, Carnevale M, et al. Perioperative outcomes of carotid endarterectomy and transfemoral and transcervical carotid artery stenting in radiation-induced carotid lesions. J Vasc Surg 2022;75(3):915–20.
[100] Kang J, Woo SY, Yang SS, et al. Treatment results of carotid endarterectomy and carotid artery stenting for patients with radiation-induced carotid stenosis. Ann Surg Treat Res 2022;103(2):112–8.
[101] Khan MA, Abdelkarim A, Elsayed N, et al. Evaluating postoperative outcomes in patients with hostile neck anatomy undergoing transcarotid artery revascularization versus transfemoral carotid artery stenting. J Vasc Surg 2023;77(1):191–200.
[102] Arhuidese IJ, Faateh M, Nejim BJ, et al. Risks Associated With Primary and Redo Carotid Endarterectomy in the Endovascular Era. JAMA Surg 2018;153(3):252.
[103] Elsayed N, Ramakrishnan G, Naazie I, et al. Outcomes of Carotid Revascularization in the Treatment of Restenosis After Prior Carotid Endarterectomy. Stroke 2021;52(10):3199–208.
[104] Elsayed N, Yei KS, Naazie I, et al. The impact of carotid lesion calcification on outcomes of carotid artery stenting. J Vasc Surg 2022;75(3):921–9.
[105] Elsayed N, Khan MA, Moacdieh MP, et al. Carotid lesion length independently predicts stroke and death after transcarotid artery revascularization and transfemoral carotid artery stenting. J Vasc Surg 2022;76(6):1615–23.e2.
[106] Health C for D and R. ENROUTE transcarotid stent system – P140026/S016. FDA. 2022. Available at: https://www.fda.gov/medical-devices/recently-approved-devices/enroute-transcarotid-stent-system-p140026s016. [Accessed 9 October 2023].
[107] Silk Road Medical. Post-Approval Study of Transcarotid Artery Revascularization in Standard Risk Patients With Significant Carotid Artery Disease. The ROADSTER 3 Study. clinicaltrials.gov. 2023. Available at: https://clinicaltrials.gov/study/NCT05365490. [Accessed 31 December 2022].
[108] Liang P, Cronenwett JL, Secemsky EA, et al. Risk of Stroke, Death, and Myocardial Infarction Following Transcarotid Artery Revascularization vs Carotid Endarterectomy in Patients With Standard Surgical Risk. JAMA Neurol 2023;80(5):437–44.

Advances in Surgery 58 (2024) 191–202

ADVANCES IN SURGERY

ELSEVIER
MOSBY

Is the Supraclavicular Approach Effective in Treating Patients with Thoracic Outlet Syndrome?

Nikhil Panda, MD, MPH[a], Dean M. Donahue, MD[a,b,*]

[a]Division of Thoracic Surgery, Department of Surgery, Massachusetts General Hospital, 55 Fruit Street, Austen 7, Boston, MA 02114, USA; [b]Thoracic Outlet Syndrome Program, 55 Fruit Street, Austen 7, Boston, MA 02114, USA

Keywords

• Thoracic outlet syndrome • Supraclavicular approach
• Health-related quality of life

Key points

- Thoracic outlet syndrome is a rare clinical condition resulting from compression of the brachial plexus, subclavian vein, or subclavian artery at sites of anatomic narrowing within the thoracic outlet.
- A critical component of the management of patients with thoracic outlet syndrome is surgical decompression of the thoracic outlet.
- The supraclavicular approach to thoracic outlet decompression represents a safe operative exposure that, in experienced centers, produces durable improvements in patient health-related quality of life.

INTRODUCTION

Thoracic outlet syndrome (TOS) encompasses a set of clinical conditions resulting from compression of the brachial plexus, subclavian vein, or subclavian artery within the cervicothoracic or thoracobrachial anatomic spaces. Each of these neurovascular structures may become compressed within the posterior neck in the interscalene triangle, or else within the costoclavicular or subcoracoid spaces. Clinicians often consider neurogenic TOS (nTOS; brachial plexus compression), venous TOS (vTOS; subclavian vein compression), and arterial

*Corresponding author. Massachusetts General Hospital, 55 Fruit Street, Austen 7, Boston, MA 02114. *E-mail address:* ddonahue@mgh.harvard.edu
Twitter: @NikhilPanda_MD (N.P.)

https://doi.org/10.1016/j.yasu.2024.04.011

TOS (aTOS; subclavian artery compression) as distinct clinical entities. However, patients frequently present with overlapping symptoms. Without treatment, the clinical phenotypes resulting from TOS are associated with a significant impact on patients' functional status. As such, careful evaluation, accurate diagnosis, and appropriate management strategies provide surgical care teams with an opportunity to improve patients' overall health-related quality of life [1].

Once a diagnosis of TOS is made and the site of compression is localized, an important component of the multidisciplinary management is operative decompression. When the site of compression is within the interscalene triangle or costoclavicular spaces, thoracic outlet decompression includes a variable degree of first rib resection with or without scalenectomy, brachial plexus neurolysis, subclavian venolysis and venoplasty, subclavian arteriolysis, or vascular reconstruction. There are various operative approaches to achieving decompression of the thoracic outlet, including supraclavicular, infraclavicular, transaxillary, open transthoracic, and minimally invasive transthoracic exposures [2–4]. There is no clear gold standard for operative approach. The purpose of this study is to present and review the experience of a dedicated, high-volume, TOS center where thoracic outlet decompression occurs via a supraclavicular operative approach. The data presented here support the safety and efficacy of this operative approach as a component of the multidisciplinary management of patients with TOS.

OPERATIVE TECHNIQUE: SUPRCLAVICULAR THORACIC OUTLET DECOMPRESSION

Our clinical approach to patients with TOS begins with an in-person history and physical examination. Elements of the history focus on antecedent trauma and repetitive motion or overuse injury. The physical examination includes stress maneuvers to reproduce symptoms. Patients presenting with vTOS undergo venography with catheter-direct thrombolysis followed by therapeutic anticoagulation [5]. Additional axial imaging for patients with vTOS is helpful, but not necessary. Patients with nTOS and aTOS undergo axial imaging to delineate the anatomy of the thoracic outlet and select patients with nTOS to undergo botulinum toxin injection as a diagnostic and potentially therapeutic intervention. Based on the results of the physical examination, imaging, and botulinum toxin injection, patients undergo transaxillary pectoralis minor tenotomy if compression is localized in the subcoracoid space or a near-complete supraclavicular decompression if compression is localized in the interscalene triangle or costoclavicular space. A summary of our clinical approaches to patients with nTOS and vTOS are shown in Figs. 1 and 2, respectively.

The goal of operative intervention for patients with TOS is decompression of the thoracic outlet. This typically involves resection of the first thoracic rib, bony abnormalities of the C7 vertebra (eg, C7 apophysomegaly), and anterior and middle scalenectomy. We aim to perform a near-complete resection of the first thoracic rib, leaving the head of the rib to avoid disruption of the

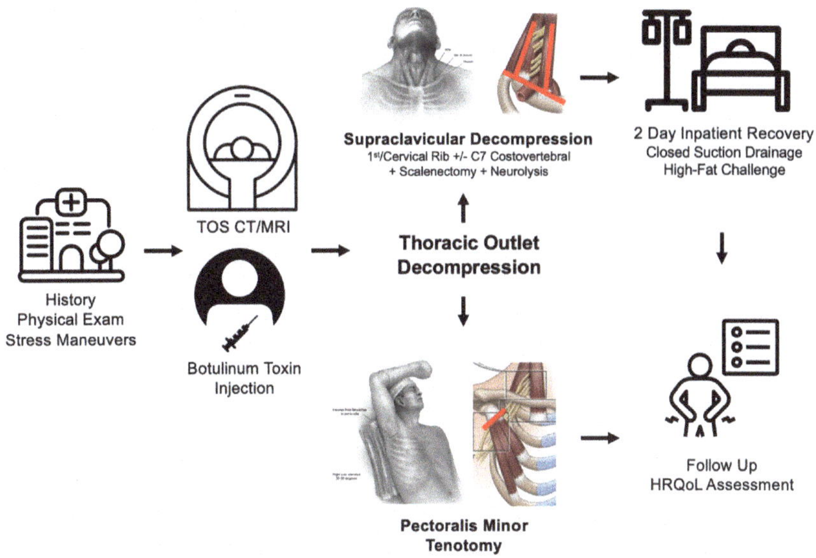

Fig. 1. Clinical approach to patients presenting with nTOS.

stellate ganglion and sympathetic trunk. Intraoperative observations during revisional thoracic outlet decompression after prior partial rib resection demonstrate dense callous formation and scar tissue between the partially divided first rib and the brachial plexus, subclavian vein, and subclavian artery. In addition to first thoracic rib resection, additional neurolysis, venolysis, and/or arteriolysis with or without vascular reconstruction are also performed depending on the patient's clinical presentation and TOS subtype. In our experience, the

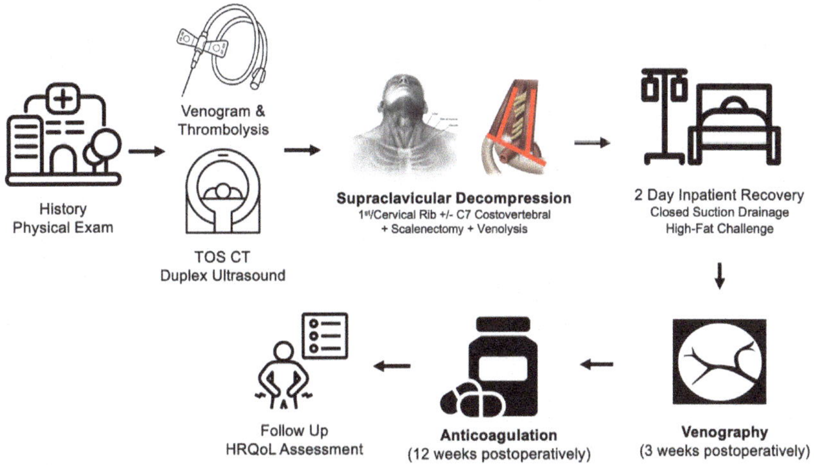

Fig. 2. Clinical approach to patients presenting with vTOS.

supraclavicular approach offers the best exposure to the scalene musculature and contents of the interscalene triangle to allow for adequate thoracic outlet decompression and release of scar tissue.

The learning curve and operative technique of the supraclavicular thoracic outlet decompression has been previously described in detail and is summarized here [4,6]:

- Preoperative preparation: Patients are instructed to eat a high-fat meal the evening prior to their operation to identify disrupted lymphatics more easily both intra and early postoperatively.
- Surgeon equipment: The surgeon and assistant wear 3.5x loupe magnification.
- Anesthetic considerations: Patients are induced with general anesthesia with the use of short-acting paralytics for the purposes of endotracheal intubation. Absent paralysis allows for the use of an electrical nerve stimulator during the case to assist in identification of nerves and confirm intact conduction following dissection and neurolysis.
- Positioning: The patient is placed in modified semi-Fowler's position with both arms tucked and padding over all pressure points. Towels are used to elevate the shoulder of the affected side 6 inches anteriorly to open the costoclavicular space for dissection of the anterior first rib and subclavian venolysis. The neck and chest are prepped and draped allowing for access to perform a median sternotomy should a major vascular injury warrant proximal vascular control (Fig. 3).
- Exposure: The skin is incised 1 cm medial to the lateral border of the clavicular head of the sternocleidomastoid muscle and carried 5 cm laterally one fingerbreadth above the clavicle (Fig. 4). The subcutaneous tissue and platysma are divided and 2 cm subplatysmal flaps are raised. The scalene fat pad is mobilized from lateral border of the sternocleidomastoid muscle, preserving a lateral pedicle, any sensory nerves, and vessels. Deep to the scalene fat pad, the omohyoid muscle is preserved, mobilized, and retracted with a vessel loop.
- Anterior scalenectomy: Using bipolar electrocautery, the fat deep to the omohyoid muscle is dissected to expose the anterior scalene muscle. The phrenic nerve is identified anterior to the anterior scalene muscle. Again, absent paralysis, a nerve stimulator placed on the phrenic nerve can generate diaphragmatic contraction to confirm its location and integrity throughout

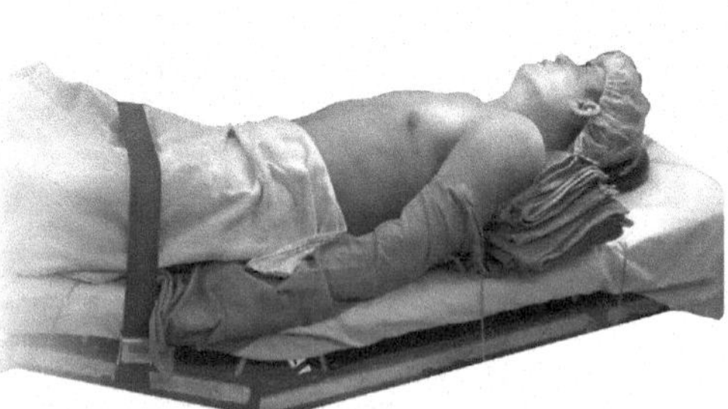

Fig. 3. Patient positioning in modified semi-Fowler's position. Note the elevation of the left shoulder anteriorly to increase space between the clavicle and first thoracic rib. (Dean M. Donahue, Supraclavicular First Rib Resection, Operative Techniques in Thoracic and Cardiovascular Surgery, 16 (4), 2011, 252-266, https://doi.org/10.1053/j.optechstcvs.2012.02.001.)

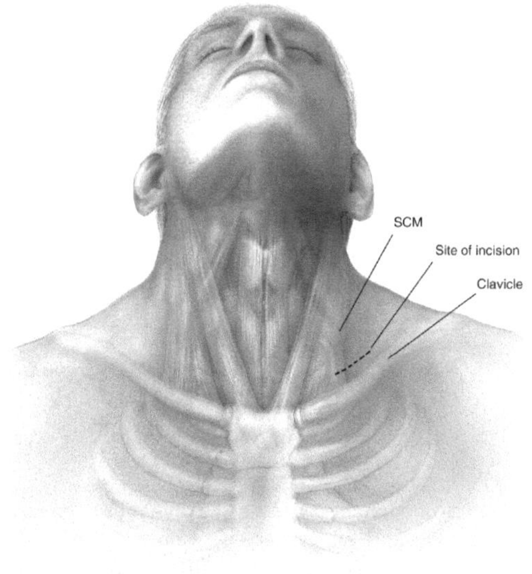

Fig. 4. Identification of surface musculoskeletal anatomy aids in planning an approximately 5 cm incision (*dotted line*) for a left supraclavicular thoracic outlet decompression. (Dean M. Donahue, Supraclavicular First Rib Resection, Operative Techniques in Thoracic and Cardiovascular Surgery, 16 (4), 2011, 252-266, https://doi.org/10.1053/j.optechstcvs.2012.02.001.)

dissection. Tissue adjacent to the phrenic nerve is used to retract and mobilize the nerve medially from the anterior scalene muscle. The medial and lateral borders of the anterior scalene muscle are dissected cephalad and caudad to the muscle's insertion onto the first thoracic rib, partially dividing medial and lateral attachments to the rib (Fig. 5). During this process, it is common to encounter communicating muscular bands between the anterior and middle scalene muscles, which are representative of their common embryologic origin and development. The anterior scalene muscle is then divided as far cephalad as possible and then completely resected from the scalene tubercle of the first thoracic rib.

- Neurolysis, arteriolysis, and middle acalenectomy: The subclavian artery and brachial plexus trunks are then mobilized, which requires a combination of sharp and bipolar electrocautery dissection of scar tissue. The mobilized brachial plexus trunks are gently retracted medially to expose the middle scalene muscle fibers overlying the posterior first thoracic rib (Fig. 6). The middle scalene muscle fibers are then divided off the cephalad and lateral surfaces of the first thoracic rib.
- Dissection of and resection first thoracic rib: The inner and undersurfaces of the first thoracic rib are then dissected from the underlying Sibson's fascia (Fig. 7). The intercostal fibers between the first and second thoracic ribs are then divided from the lateral surface of the first thoracic rib (Fig. 8). The first thoracic rib is divided first posteriorly at the neck of the rib. Depressing the partially divided

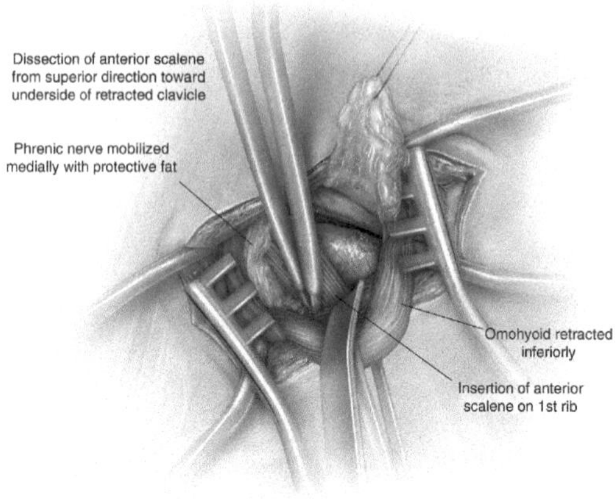

Fig. 5. Dissection of medial and lateral borders of the anterior scalene muscle. Note the mobilized pedicled scalene fat pad (lateral), preserved omohyoid muscle (inferior), and phrenic nerve (medial). (Dean M. Donahue, Supraclavicular First Rib Resection, Operative Techniques in Thoracic and Cardiovascular Surgery, 16 (4), 2011, 252-266, https://doi.org/10.1053/j.optechstcvs.2012.02.001.)

rib caudally provides exposure to the subclavius muscle and anterior rib. The attachments of the subclavius muscle to the first thoracic rib are divided and the anterior rib is divided medial to the scalene tubercle.

- Venolysis and closure: With the first thoracic rib removed, the surgical field is evaluated for hemostasis. For patients with vTOS, removal of the first thoracic rib

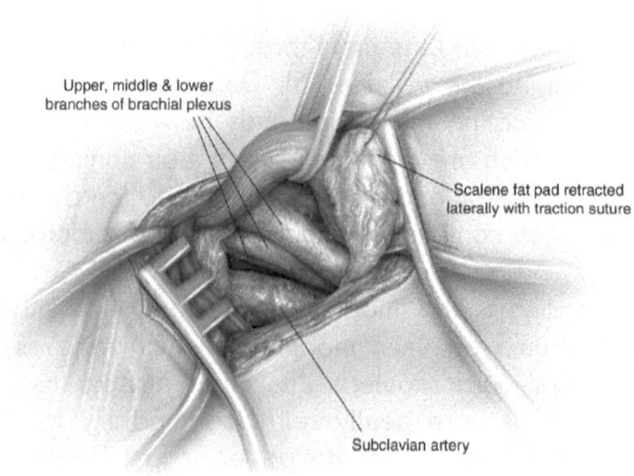

Fig. 6. Resection of the anterior scalene muscle exposes the underlying upper, middle, and lower trunks of the brachial plexus, as well as the subclavian artery. Neurolysis, arteriolysis, and mobilization of these structures allow for exposure of the underlying middle scalene muscle and first thoracic rib. (Dean M. Donahue, Supraclavicular First Rib Resection, Operative Techniques in Thoracic and Cardiovascular Surgery, 16 (4), 2011, 252-266, https://doi.org/10.1053/j.optechstcvs.2012.02.001.)

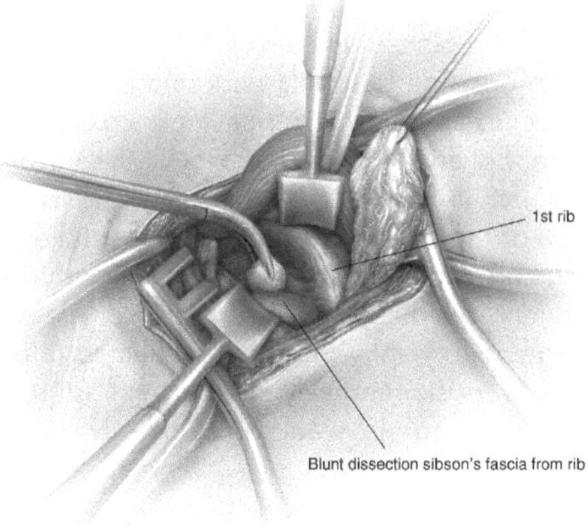

Fig. 7. Division of the middle scalene muscle fibers expose the inner and undersurfaces of the first thoracic rib for blunt dissection of Sibson's fascia. (Dean M. Donahue, Supraclavicular First Rib Resection, Operative Techniques in Thoracic and Cardiovascular Surgery, 16 (4), 2011, 252-266, https://doi.org/10.1053/j.optechstcvs.2012.02.001.)

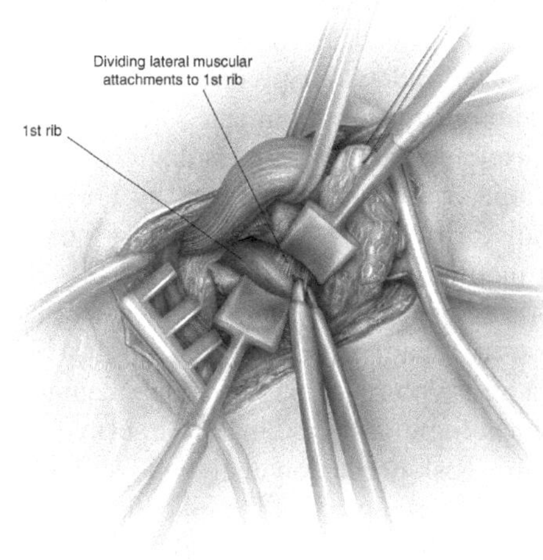

Fig. 8. Intercostal muscle fibers between the first and the second thoracic ribs are exposed on the posterior lateral surface of the first thoracic rib. Division of these muscle fibers then allows for division of the first thoracic rib posteriorly lateral to the C8 spinal nerve root. Anteriorly additional serratus anterior fibers are dissected before division of the first thoracic rib anteriorly near the costochondral junction. (Dean M. Donahue, Supraclavicular First Rib Resection, Operative Techniques in Thoracic and Cardiovascular Surgery, 16 (4), 2011, 252-266, https://doi.org/10.1053/j.optechstcvs.2012.02.001.)

provides excellent exposure for adequate venolysis and venoplasty. Following this, the integrity of the phrenic nerve is confirmed with the nerve stimulator, and a closed suction drain is placed. In the event of pleural space entry, a saline leak test with a positive pressure breath is performed and a red rubber catheter is inserted into the pleura to evacuate a pneumothorax at skin closure.

- Postoperative care: Patients typically recover in the hospital for 48 hours. The surgical drain is left in place to monitor for air, blood, and particularly lymphatic leakage as the patient consumes a high-fat diet. The drain is removed prior to discharge. All patients are seen in clinic, during which time symptomatic improvement and health-related quality of life are assessed. Patients with vTOS undergo venography of both the affected and contralateral subclavian veins 3 weeks postoperatively. If the vein is patent or dilated, anticoagulation is continued for 12 weeks postoperatively.

OUTCOMES FOLLOWING SUPRACLAVICULAR THORACIC OUTLET DECOMPRESSION

We recently reported the Massachusetts General Hospital experience from 2007 to 2021, during which time 2,869 patients were evaluated for nTOS, vTOS, and aTOS [7]. Among this cohort, 1,032 patients underwent surgery for predominantly nTOS (75.4%) and vTOS (23.4%), including 864 supraclavicular thoracic outlet decompression operations. Notable characteristics of the cohort included a median age of 36 years (interquartile range [IQR] 26, 46), a female predominance (70%), and 40% of patients reported prior mechanical trauma or overuse injury. Six percent of patients had undergone prior operations for TOS and remained with persistent or recurrent symptoms. Among patients with nTOS, 93% underwent preoperative botulinum toxin injection and 56% reported symptomatic improvement. The median time to supraclavicular thoracic outlet decompression from consultation was 225 days (IQR 136, 495). Composite perioperative morbidity was 20%. The most common complication was postoperative chyle leak (8%), the majority of which was managed with temporary diet modification.

Follow-up health-related quality of life data were available for 75% of the study cohort. There were 4 patients among 864 supraclavicular thoracic outlet decompression operations who required revisional decompression and 93% reported clinically meaningful symptomatic improvement after surgery compared with baseline. Risk prediction analysis identified 4 factors associated with differential health-related quality of life following surgery. First, older age was associated with a lower odds of symptomatic improvement, potentially due to a longer duration of symptoms or concurrent musculoskeletal disease. Second, patients with a history of repetitive motion trauma had a greater odds of symptomatic improvement following surgery. It is possible that repetitive motion unmasks symptoms in patients anatomically predisposed to TOS; as such, these patients may present earlier prior to the development of irreversible nerve injury. Third, a lack of symptomatic improvement following botulinum toxin was associated with worse odds of symptomatic improvement, underscoring the importance of this preoperative diagnostic and potentially therapeutic intervention. Fourth, patients undergoing revisional thoracic outlet decompression had a lower odds of symptomatic improvement following revisional surgery, underscoring the importance of a near-complete surgical decompression at the time of the index operation.

The opportunity to review this 15 year experience offered several lessons learned. First, the supraclavicular decompression is not only safe, but also effective in terms of achieving symptomatic improvement among patients with TOS. Second, approximately one-third of patients who were evaluated for potential TOS ultimately underwent an operation. Similarly, the median time from consultation to operation was nearly 4 months. During this time, patients underwent multiple in-person clinic visits, dedicated TOS axial imaging, and–for nTOS–selective botulinum toxin injection, where symptomatic improvement may take months to occur. These data emphasize the importance of careful patient selection for surgical decompression and avoiding potentially unnecessary intervention or harm for patients who have alternative diagnoses. Third, there were 4 patients within the operative cohort who required revisional thoracic outlet decompression, supporting our opinion that a supraclavicular approach allows for optimal exposure for resection of a greater amount of the first rib, abnormalities of the C7 vertebral body, scalenectomy, and lysis of scar tissue surrounding the brachial plexus, subclavian vein, and subclavian artery.

It is also important to acknowledge prior series of supraclavicular thoracic outlet decompression from high-volume centers caring for patients with TOS. In 1996, Hempel and colleagues published the Baylor University Medical Center series of 770 supraclavicular scalenectomy and first rib resections for patients with nTOS, vTOS, and aTOS [8]. Acceptable health-related quality of life outcomes were achieved in 86% of patients with a 2% reoperation rate. Like our experience at the Massachusetts General Hospital, the results of this series underscore the importance of careful patient selection for operative thoracic outlet decompression. It is worth noting that the patients in Hempel and colleagues's series were treated in an era marked by differences in epidemiology and health care technology. First, the prevalence of conditions with symptom complexes mimicking TOS (eg, cervical disk disease, complex regional pain syndrome), especially within an aging population, is increasing. Second, current high-resolution cross-sectional imaging is more readily available and, when used to assist in the diagnosis of TOS, can help delineate the anatomy of the thoracic outlet and evaluate for concurrent musculoskeletal disease. For example, our TOS team designed and implemented a dedicated TOS-protocol CT scan of the neck and chest with thin (ie, 5 mm) sectional images, a timed multiphase contrast injection, and 3-dimensional reconstruction [9]. Third, the use of botulinum toxin emerged and was popularized in the last two decades, with a growing body of data supporting its predictive and prognostic role in the management of patients with TOS [10,11]. Lastly, as the quality of surgical care delivery for patients with TOS continues to improve, outcome assessment is centered around patient-reported outcome (PROM) and experience measures.

Most PROM instruments used in the care of patients with TOS have been adapted from other musculoskeletal or extremity conditions. There is currently no dedicated PROM instrument specific to patients with TOS.

ALTERNATIVE OPERATIVE APPROACHES TO THORACIC OUTLET DECOMPRESSION

In the hands of experienced surgeons at other high-volume centers, alternative operative approaches have demonstrated safety and efficacy in terms of patient symptomatic improvement (Table 1). Urschel and Kourlis published the largest series of 5,102 patients with TOS, which included predominantly transaxillary decompressions, and achieved good health-related quality of life outcomes in 85% of patients with less than 1% morbidity rate [12]. A more contemporary series from the Johns Hopkins of 538 transaxillary decompressions was reported by Orlando and colleagues [13]. Among these patients, 95% reported positive health-related quality of life following thoracic outlet decompression. There are no prospective randomized trials comparing safety and efficacy of different operative approaches for thoracic outlet decompression. However, the results from these large prior series and our data at the Massachusetts General Hospital illustrate that when patients are cared for at high-volume TOS centers, thoracic outlet decompression provides durable results for patients.

There remain many opportunities for surgical care teams to continue to optimize the multidisciplinary care of patients with TOS. First, TOS remains a rare condition treated by surgical care teams across general, thoracic, vascular, neurosurgical, orthopedic, and plastic surgery. This leads to large heterogeneity in diagnostic approaches and treatment algorithms. There will always be an art in caring for patients with TOS. Nevertheless, there is an opportunity for surgeons to work toward standardization in evaluation, diagnostic approaches, patient selection, and response to nonoperative and operative treatment. In 2016, the Society of Vascular Surgery published reporting standards for TOS on behalf of a committee of experts, representing the first step toward achieving

Table 1
Summary of prior large series reporting health-related quality of life and perioperative outcomes following various operative approaches to thoracic outlet decompression

Experience	Operative approach	Outcomes
Baylor University Hempel et al, [8] 1996	Supraclavicular decompression (n = 770)	86% acceptable HRQoL 2% reoperations
Baylor University Urschel and Kourlis [12] 2007	Majority transaxillary decompression (n = 5,102)	85% good HRQoL <1% morbidity
Johns Hopkins Orlando et al, [13] 2015	Transaxillary decompression (n = 538)	95% positive HRQoL 29% morbidity
Massachusetts General Hospital 2023	Majority supraclavicular decompression (n = 1,032)	93% improvement HRQoL 19.8% morbidity 0.4% reoperations

Abbreviation: HRQoL, health-related quality of life.

standardization around this condition [14]. Second, there is a paucity of data around successful nonoperative management of patients with TOS, especially nTOS. High-volume TOS centers are referred many patients with suspected TOS; only a fraction of these patients ultimately will undergo thoracic outlet decompression. Comparative health-related quality of life outcomes data from not only patients with nTOS who underwent operative decompression, but also among a nonoperative cohort are needed to further understand the benefit of thoracic outlet decompression, botulinum toxin injection, and patient selection. Lastly, health-related quality of life assessment among patients with TOS remains an ongoing challenge. The symptom complex associated with nTOS is difficult to measure, including response to operative and nonoperative interventions. The design, validation, and implementation of a TOS-specific PROM instrument are needed. Our team is also evaluating novel methods of functional outcome assessment using mobile health care technology (eg, wearables, digital phenotyping), which may offer a passive and unobtrusive method for longitudinal health measurement [15].

SUMMARY

TOS remains a rare condition, which if left untreated, leads to a significant detriment to the health-related quality of life of affected patients. When a diagnosis of TOS is made, a critical component of management is complete thoracic outlet decompression, including a near-complete resection of the first thoracic rib, anterior and middle scalenectomy, and lysis of scar tissue around the brachial plexus, subclavian artery, and subclavian. In our experience, the supraclavicular approach is safe, provides optimal exposure for a complete thoracic outlet decompression, and produces durable improvements in health-related quality of life. Future efforts to improve the quality-of-care delivery for patients with TOS will ideally focus on improving measurement of health-related quality of life.

CLINICS CARE POINTS

- A thorough history, physical examination, and diagnostic testing are essential before considering operative decompression for TOS. Many patients may be referred to surgeons with a symptom complex more consistent with alternative diagnoses and/or amenable to alternative treatment options.
- The goal of surgery for TOS is decompression of the thoracic outlet including near-complete resection of the first thoracic rib, anterior and middle scalenectomy, and additional neurolysis, venolysis, arteriolysis, and/or reconstruction, when indicated.
- Results from a high-volume, dedicated TOS center demonstrate that the supraclavicular approach offers excellent exposure for adequate thoracic outlet decompression and results in few complications, rare revisional thoracic outlet decompression, and durable improvements in health-related quality of life.

Acknowledgments

The authors and patients are indebted to the Massachusetts General Hospital Thoracic Outlet Program clinic and operating room teams.

Disclosure

The authors have nothing to disclose.

References

[1] Donahue DM, Auchincloss HG. Challenges in the evaluation and management of thoracic outlet syndrome. Thorac Surg Clin 2021;31(1):xi; https://doi.org/10.1016/j.thorsurg.2020.09.009.

[2] Burt BM, Palivela N, Karimian A, et al. Transthoracic robotic first rib resection: Twelve steps. JTCVS Tech 2020;1(March):104–9; https://doi.org/10.1016/j.xjtc.2020.01.005.

[3] Urschel HC. Transaxillary first rib resection for thoracic outlet syndrome. Operat Tech Thorac Cardiovasc Surg 2005;10(4):313–7; https://doi.org/10.1053/j.optechstcvs.2005.10.002.

[4] Donahue DM. Supraclavicular first rib resection. Operat Tech Thorac Cardiovasc Surg 2011;16(4):252–66; https://doi.org/10.1053/j.optechstcvs.2012.02.001.

[5] Cook JR, Thompson RW. Evaluation and management of venous thoracic outlet syndrome. Thorac Surg Clin 2021;31(1):27–44; https://doi.org/10.1016/j.thorsurg.2020.08.012.

[6] Panda N, Phillips WW, Geller AD, et al. Supraclavicular approach for neurogenic thoracic outlet syndrome: description of a learning curve. Ann Thorac Surg 2021;112(5):1616–23; https://doi.org/10.1016/j.athoracsur.2020.11.010.

[7] Panda N, Hurd J, Madsen J, et al. Efficacy and safety of supraclavicular thoracic outlet decompression. Ann Surg 2023;278(3):417–25; https://doi.org/10.1097/SLA.0000000000005957.

[8] Hempel GK, Shutze WP, Anderson JF, et al. 770 Consecutive Supraclavicular First Rib Resections for Thoracic Outlet Syndrome. Ann Vasc Surg 1996;10(5):456–63; https://doi.org/10.1007/BF02000592.

[9] Donahue D, Khalilzadeh O, Dinkel J, et al. Radiological Assessment of Thoracic Outlet Syndrome: Four Years of Institutional Experience; Radiological Society of North America 2013 Scientific Assembly and Annual Meeting. 2013.

[10] Donahue DM, Godoy IRB, Gupta R, et al. Sonographically guided botulinum toxin injections in patients with neurogenic thoracic outlet syndrome: correlation with surgical outcomes. Skeletal Radiol 2020;49(5):715–22; https://doi.org/10.1007/s00256-019-03331-9.

[11] Jordan SE, Ahn SS, Freischlag JA, et al. Selective botulinum chemodenervation of the scalene muscles for treatment of neurogenic thoracic outlet syndrome. Ann Vasc Surg 2000;14(4):365–9; https://doi.org/10.1007/s100169910079.

[12] Urschel HC, Kourlis H. Thoracic outlet syndrome: a 50-year experience at baylor university medical center. Baylor Univ Med Cent Proc 2007;20(2):125–35; https://doi.org/10.1080/08998280.2007.11928267.

[13] Orlando MS, Likes KC, Mirza S, et al. A decade of excellent outcomes after surgical intervention in 538 patients with thoracic outlet syndrome. J Am Coll Surg 2015;220(5):934–9; https://doi.org/10.1016/j.jamcollsurg.2014.12.046.

[14] Illig KA, Donahue D, Duncan A, et al. Reporting standards of the Society for Vascular Surgery for thoracic outlet syndrome. J Vasc Surg 2016;64(3):e23–35; https://doi.org/10.1016/j.jvs.2016.04.039.

[15] Panda N, Solsky I, Huang EJ, et al. Using smartphones to capture novel recovery metrics after cancer surgery. JAMA Surg 2019;1–7; https://doi.org/10.1001/jamasurg.2019.4702.

Advances in Surgery 58 (2024) 203–221

ADVANCES IN SURGERY

Antibiotic Use in the Surgical Intensive Care Unit

Liza Laquian, MD[a], Philip A. Efron, MD[a,*]

[a]Department of Surgery, University of Florida College of Medicine, Gainesville, FL, USA

Keywords

• Infection • Antibiotics • De-escalation • Antimicrobial resistance • Antimicrobial stewardship • Surgical ICU

Key points

- Empiric antibiotics should be initiated when infection is suspected and should be tailored based on patient factors and local resistance patterns.
- De-escalation to narrower spectrum agents should be based on culture and sensitivity results and should occur ideally no more than 48 to 72 hours of starting empiric antimicrobials. If no infection is confirmed, antibiotics should be discontinued.
- The primary mechanisms of antibiotic resistance involve decreasing drug entry into the cell, increasing drug efflux, modifying antimicrobial targets, and inactivating the antibiotic.
- Antibiotic stewardship consists of collective strategies to optimize antimicrobial selection, dosage, and duration for individual patients while minimizing toxicities and the risk of resistance.

INTRODUCTION

Antimicrobial therapy has been a cornerstone of improving recovery and survival from life-threatening infections. Unfortunately, with expansions in the antimicrobial armamentarium, new mechanisms of resistance and virulence have emerged. Due to the threat of multidrug-resistant (MDR) organisms, infections in the critically ill require judicious antimicrobial use. Providers must weigh the risks and benefits of their antimicrobial selections in the context of each patient's clinical picture. Surgical intensive care unit (SICU) patients are

*Corresponding author. University of Florida Health Science Center, PO Box 100108, Gainesville, FL 32610-0108. *E-mail address:* Philip.Efron@surgery.ufl.edu

https://doi.org/10.1016/j.yasu.2024.04.012

particularly challenging, as their infections may either require operative intervention or be a consequence of previous traumatic injury or surgery. Despite best efforts, up to 30% of critically ill patients on antimicrobial agents are on inappropriate therapy due to indication, regimen, or duration of treatment [1]. Antimicrobial stewardship (AMS), which should be embraced by all surgeons, aims to address these issues in addition to minimizing drug resistance, improving clinical outcomes, and decreasing cost.

PHARMACOKINETICS AND PHARMACODYNAMICS

Optimal antibiotic use in the critically ill extends beyond selection of the appropriate agent. Knowledge of the drug's pharmacokinetics and pharmacodynamics allows dosing that achieves efficacy against the pathogen while minimizing adverse effects. While the modern SICU typically has an intensive care unit (ICU) pharmacist as part of a multidisciplinary approach to every patient, a surgeon still requires an appropriate knowledge of this topic.

Pharmacokinetics describes the relationship between the antimicrobial dose administered and the change in plasma drug concentration over time [2]. This includes the processes of drug absorption, distribution, metabolism, and elimination [3]. An antimicrobial's distribution properties (such as volume of distribution) influence initial dosing since they reflect the likelihood of the drug reaching the site of infection. In contrast, drug clearance represents the elimination phase and, therefore, impacts the antibiotic's maintenance dosing [4].

Pharmacodynamics refers to the relationship between the antimicrobial concentration and its activity against the target pathogen in the body [3]. Antimicrobial killing mechanisms can be time-dependent, concentration-dependent, or a combination of both. Pharmacodynamic parameters quantify the antibiotic exposure needed to maximize killing activity. For example, minimum inhibitory concentration (MIC) represents an antibiotic's potency to kill or inhibit the growth of an organism and is unique to a specific combination of pathogen and antimicrobial [4]. For time-dependent antimicrobials, maximal killing activity occurs when the drug concentration exceeds the MIC. It is optimal to maximize the percentage of time with the antibiotic concentration remains above the MIC. Thus, the appropriate dosing for an individual may not be a typical "q12 or q24" delivery. Often the patient may require adjustment of their dose frequency or conversion to an extended or continuous infusion [3]. Examples of time-dependent antibiotics include beta-lactams and carbapenems. Concentration-dependent antimicrobials have maximal killing activity when they reach a target peak concentration (C_{max}) to MIC ratio. Aminoglycosides are examples of concentration-dependent antibiotics, but they also have postantibiotic effects, which inhibit microbial growth even after concentrations drop below the MIC. Fluoroquinolones, vancomycin, daptomycin, and linezolid are examples of drugs with concentration-dependent killing with time dependence. Their peak killing activity is based on reaching a target area under concentration curve to MIC ratio [3].

Antibiotic dosing in the critically ill is further complicated by concomitant pathophysiologic changes. Volume of distribution and clearance are commonly altered in ICU patients due to renal failure, liver failure, fluid shifts, or hypoalbuminemia. Dose adjustments may also be needed for patients on extracorporeal membrane oxygenation or renal replacement therapy [5]. The modern surgeon and surgical intensivist should work collaboratively with their pharmacists and multidisciplinary team to engender personalized "precision medicine" dosing regimens for their patients that allow the best antibiotic efficacy for that individual.

PROPHYLAXIS

Perioperative antimicrobial prophylaxis aims to prevent intraoperative contamination from intrinsic and extrinsic bacteria from developing into a postoperative surgical site infection [6]. Administration within 60 minutes before skin incision is optimal, except for vancomycin and fluoroquinolones. These agents require 1 to 2 hours for administration, and therefore, they should be started within 2 hours prior to incision. Intraoperative redosing to maintain adequate serum and tissue concentrations is indicated in procedures with large volume blood loss or duration longer than 2 half-lives of the agent. Continuing antimicrobial prophylaxis postoperatively is not necessary for most procedures, but if administered, it should end within 24 hours of the procedure [7]. Minimizing the postoperative duration of prophylactic antibiotics in critically ill patients is particularly essential to decrease the risks of allergic or anaphylactic reactions, *Clostridium difficile* colitis, and MDR infections [6]. Additionally, there is no evidence for continuing postoperative prophylactic antibiotics until all drains, catheters, or tubes are removed [7].

EMPIRIC THERAPY

When infection is evident or strongly suspected, broad-spectrum antimicrobial agents should be promptly initiated. Empiric therapy is ideally limited to 48 to 72 hours while awaiting culture and susceptibility data. Multiple factors should be considered in the selection of empiric therapy, including [8]

1. Most likely source of infection and causative pathogen
2. History of antimicrobial use and prior infections with antimicrobial-resistant organisms
3. Illness severity
4. Optimal delivery of agent to site of infection
5. Drug adverse effects
6. Ecology and resistance profile for specific hospital and ICU

These factors result in an individualized approach for empiric treatment. For example, the standard empiric regimen may be inadequate for patients with MDR infections. Patients should be assessed for risk factors for infection with MDR organisms, including advanced age, diabetes mellitus, renal failure, intravenous drug use, solid organ transplantation, history of prolonged hospitalization, and prior antibiotic exposure [6]. Table 1 lists risk additional factors for specific MDR organisms and options for empiric regimens. Additionally, a patient's allergies or organ dysfunction may limit their antimicrobial options. Finally, the risks of renal, hepatic, or neurologic toxicity may outweigh the benefits of using specific antimicrobial drugs in some patients (Table 2).

Coverage of gram-positive bacteria is indicated for ventilator-associated pneumonia and any suspected infection in which the skin barrier is breached. This includes central venous line and wound infections. Vancomycin is the usual empiric antibiotic due to its efficacy against enterococci, streptococci, and staphylococci, particularly methicillin-resistant *Staphylococcus aureus* (MRSA). If the causative organism is susceptible to penicillin or oxacillin, de-escalation from vancomycin to one of these agents provides superior efficacy with a narrower spectrum [6]. For vancomycin-resistant bacteria, daptomycin or linezolid is the empiric agent of choice (see Table 1). Of note, daptomycin has poor penetration in the lungs, and therefore, linezolid is superior for treating pneumonia from vancomycin-resistant bacteria [6]. It should be noted that using certain polymerase chain reaction (PCR) techniques, rapid discontinuation of empiric MRSA coverage may be possible in the ICU [9,10].

Gram-negative coverage is also indicated for ventilator-associated pneumonia and wound infections associated with abdominal or genitourinary procedures. Options for empiric gram-negative coverage include aminoglycosides, fluoroquinolones, and third-generation cephalosporins such as ceftriaxone and ceftazidime (see Table 2). While local antibiograms differ, cefepime, piperacillin–tazobactam, ceftazidime, aztreonam, meropenem, and imipenem are possible empiric agents for *Pseudomonas aeruginosa* [6,11]. If extended-spectrum beta-lactamase (ESBL)-producing organisms are suspected due to patient risk factors, the empiric antibiotic of choice is a carbapenem [12] (see Table 1).

Surgeons should familiarize themselves with AmpC beta-lactamase-producing Enterobacterales. These bacteria were formerly referred to as "SPACE" organisms (acronym for *Serratia*, *Pseudomonas*, *Acinetobacter*, *Citrobacter*, and *Enterobacter*). They have now been refined based on likelihood of AmpC production and narrowed to species abbreviated as "HECK YES." Enterobacterales at moderate to high risk of clinically significant AmpC production due to inducible *ampC* gene are *Hafnia alvei*, *Enterobacter cloacae*, *Citrobacter freundii*, *Klebsiella aerogenes*, and *Yersinia enterocolitica*. Increased AmpC beta-lactamase production from inducible *ampC* gene expression can result in ceftriaxone and ceftazidime resistance. Unlike these other 2 cephalosporins, cefepime is not susceptible to hydrolysis by AmpC and is therefore the antibiotic of choice for "HECK YES" organisms. If the bacteria are susceptible to carbapenems and the cefepime MIC is 4 μg/mL or above, current guidelines suggest a carbapenem as the preferred agent [12].

Infections associated with the gastrointestinal tract are often polymicrobial and require empiric antibiotics for anaerobes. Metronidazole is commonly used for anaerobic coverage in intra-abdominal infections. Clindamycin is another empiric option with broad anaerobic activity and is used in head

Table 1
Risk Factors for Infection with Multidrug-Resistant Organisms in Intensive Care Unit

Organism	MRSA	VRE	MDR *Pseudomonas aeruginosa*	ESBL Enterobacterales
Risk factors	• MRSA colonization • Age >65 years old • Prior antibiotic exposure • Skin/soft tissue infection • Transfer from long-term care facility • Urinary catheter	• VRE colonization • Exposure to vancomycin or third-generation cephalosporin • Central venous catheter • Hemodialysis	• Exposure to quinolone, carbapenem, or cephalosporin and piperacillin–tazobactam • History of hospitalization • Total parenteral nutrition	• Colonization with ESBL organism • History of hospitalization for at least 48 hours within past 90 days • Broad-spectrum antibiotic therapy within past 90 days
Empiric antibiotic options	• Vancomycin • Linezolid • Daptomycin • Ceftaroline	• Linezolid • Daptomycin	• Piperacillin–tazobactam • Ceftazidime • Cefepime • Aztreonam • Meropenem • Imipenem–cilastatin	• Meropenem • Imipenem–cilastatin

Abbreviations: ESBL, extended-spectrum beta-lactamase; MDR, multidrug-resistant; MRSA, methicillin-resistant *Staphylococcus aureus*; VRE, vancomycin-resistant enterococcus [12,27,28].

Table 2
Antibiotic Classes and Pertinent Spectra of Activity for Intensive Care Unit

Antibiotic class	Mechanism of action	Agent(s)	Spectrum of coverage: Gram-positive	Spectrum of coverage: Gram-negative	Spectrum of coverage: Anaerobes	Clearance	Significant adverse effects
Penicillin	Inhibition of cell wall synthesis	**Penicillin G**	Beta-hemolytic streptococci +++ *Streptococcus pneumoniae* +++ *Enterococcus faecalis* +++ *Listeria monocytogenes* ++ Viridans streptococci +	*Leptospira* sp +++ *Neisseria meningitidis* ++	Peptostreptococci +++ *Actinomyces* sp +++ *Clostridium perfringens* +++ *Fusobacterium necrophorum* + *Prevotella* sp +	Renal	Hypersensitivity/ anaphylaxis
Antistaphylococcal penicillin	Inhibition of cell wall synthesis	**Oxacillin** **Nafcillin**	MSSA +++ *Staphylococcus* sp coagulase negative +++ *Staphylococcus epidermidis* +++ Beta-hemolytic streptococci ++ *S. pneumoniae* ++ Viridans streptococci +	None	None	Renal	Rash; eosinophilia, neutropenia (nafcillin)
Aminopenicillins	Inhibition of cell wall synthesis	**Ampicillin** **Amoxicillin**	*E faecalis* +++ *L monocytogenes* +++ Beta-hemolytic streptococci ++ *S. pneumoniae* ++ Viridans streptococci +	*N meningitidis* +++ *Proteus mirabilis* ++ *Haemophilus influenzae* + *E coli* +	Peptostreptococci +++ *Actinomyces* sp +++ *C perfringens* ++ *F necrophorum* + *Prevotella* sp +	Renal	Hypersensitivity, rash, thrombocytopenia
Aminopenicillins with beta-lactamase inhibitors	Amoxicillin, ampicillin—inhibition of cell wall synthesis Clavulanate, sulbactam—beta-lactamase inhibition	**Amoxicillin–clavulanate** **Ampicillin–sulbactam**	MSSA ++ *E faecalis* ++ *Staphylococcus* sp coagulase negative ++ *S epidermidis* ++ Beta-hemolytic streptococci ++ *L monocytogenes* ++ *S. pneumoniae* ++ Viridans streptococci +	*H influenzae* +++ *Moraxella catarrhalis* +++ *P mirabilis* ++ *E coli* ++ *Klebsiella* sp ++ Same as amoxicillin–clavulanate plus *Acinetobacter baumannii* +	*Bacteroides fragilis* +++ Peptostreptococci ++ *Actinomyces* sp ++ *C perfringens* ++ *F necrophorum* ++ *Prevotella* sp ++	Renal	Hepatotoxicity (clavulanate), hypersensitivity, rash, diarrhea Hypersensitivity, rash, eosinophilia

Antipseudomonal penicillin	Piperacillin—inhibition of cell wall synthesis Tazobactam—beta-lactamase inhibitor	**Piperacillin-tazobactam**	MSSA ++ *E faecalis* ++ *Staphylococcus* sp coagulase negative ++ *S epidermidis* ++ Beta-hemolytic streptococci ++ *L monocytogenes* ++ *S. pneumoniae* ++ Viridans streptococci +	***P aeruginosa*** +++ *E coli* +++ *Citrobacter koseri* +++ *Klebsiella* sp +++ *Morganella morganii* +++ *P mirabilis* ++ *Serratia marcescens* ++ *H influenzae* ++ *M catarrhalis* ++ *N meningitidis* ++	*B fragilis* +++ Peptostreptococci ++ *Actinomyces* sp ++ *C perfringens* ++ *F necrophorum* ++ *Prevotella* sp ++	Renal	Possible increased risk of acute kidney injury when combined with vancomycin, thrombocytopenia
Cephalosporins First generation	Inhibition of cell wall synthesis	**Cefazolin**	MSSA +++ *Staphylococcus* sp coagulase negative +++ *S epidermidis* +++ Streptococci ++	*E coli* ++ *Klebsiella* sp ++ *Proteus* sp ++	Peptostreptococci ++	Renal	Hypersensitivity
Cephalosporins Second generation	Inhibition of cell wall synthesis	**Cefotetan**	MSSA ++ *Staphylococcus* sp coagulase negative ++ *S epidermidis* ++	*E coli* ++ *Klebsiella* sp ++ *Proteus* sp ++ *H influenzae* ++ *M catarrhalis* ++	Peptostreptococci ++ *C perfringens* ++ *F necrophorum* ++ *Prevotella* sp ++ *B fragilis* +	Renal	Hypersensitivity, hemolytic anemia
		Cefoxitin	Streptococci ++		Same as cefotetan plus *Actinomyces* sp ++		Rash, eosinophilia
		Cefuroxime			Peptostreptococci ++		Rash, eosinophilia

(*continued on next page*)

Table 2
(continued)

Antibiotic class	Mechanism of action	Agent(s)	Spectrum of coverage: Gram-positive	Spectrum of coverage: Gram-negative	Spectrum of coverage: Anaerobes	Clearance	Significant adverse effects
Cephalosporins Third generation	Inhibition of cell wall synthesis	**Ceftriaxone**	Viridans streptococci +++ MSSA ++ *Staphylococcus* sp coagulase negative ++ *S epidermidis* ++ Beta-hemolytic streptococci ++ *S. pneumoniae* ++	*H influenzae* +++ *E coli* +++ *Klebsiella* sp +++ *Serratia* sp +++ *N meningitidis* +++ *M morganii* +++ *Leptospira* sp +++ *Proteus* sp ++ *C koseri* ++ *S marcescens* ++ *M catarrhalis* ++	Peptostreptococci ++ *Actinomyces* sp ++ *C perfringens* ++ *F necrophorum* ++	Hepatic	Pseudocholelithiasis, thrombocytopenia
		Ceftazidime	Beta-hemolytic streptococci ++ *S. pneumoniae* ++ Viridans streptococci +	***P aeruginosa*** **+++** *E coli* ++ *Klebsiella* sp ++ *Proteus* sp ++ *C koseri* ++ *M morganii* +++ *S marcescens* ++ *H influenzae* ++ *M catarrhalis* ++	Peptostreptococci ++	Renal	Hypersensitivity, rash, *C difficile* diarrhea
Cephalosporins Fourth generation	Inhibition of cell wall synthesis	**Cefepime**	MSSA ++ *Staphylococcus* sp coagulase negative ++ *S epidermidis* ++ Beta-hemolytic streptococci ++ *S. pneumoniae* ++ Viridans streptococci ++	***P aeruginosa*** **+++** ***Enterobacter cloacae*** **+++** ***C freundii*** **+++** ***Klebsiella aerogenes*** **+++** ***Yersinia enterocolitica*** **+++** *E coli* ++ *Proteus* sp ++ *M morganii* +++ *S marcescens* ++ *H influenzae* ++ *M catarrhalis* ++	Peptostreptococci ++	Renal	Neurotoxicity (nonconvulsive status epilepticus)

Carbapenems	Inhibition of cell wall synthesis	**Imipenem–cilastatin**	MSSA ++ *Staphylococcus* sp coagulase negative ++ *S epidermidis* ++ *E faecalis* ++ Streptococci ++	**ESBL *E coli*** +++ **ESBL *Klebsiella* sp** +++ *Nocardia* sp +++ ***P aeruginosa*** ++ *E cloacae* ++ *C freundii* ++ *K aerogenes* ++ *E coli* ++ *Serratia* sp ++ *Acinetobacter* sp ++ *H influenzae* ++	*B fragilis* +++ Peptostreptococci ++ *Actinomyces* sp ++ *C perfringens* ++ *F necrophorum* ++ *Prevotella* sp ++	Renal	Neurotoxicity (seizures)
		Meropenem	MSSA ++ *Staphylococcus* sp coagulase negative ++ *S epidermidis* ++ Streptococci ++	**ESBL *E coli*** +++ **ESBL *Klebsiella* sp** +++ ***C freundii*** +++ ***P aeruginosa*** +++ *E cloacae* ++ *K aerogenes* ++ *E coli* ++ *Proteus* sp ++ *M morganii* +++ *S marcescens* ++ *H influenzae* ++ *M catarrhalis* ++	*B fragilis* +++ Peptostreptococci ++ *Actinomyces* sp ++ *C perfringens* ++ *F necrophorum* ++ *Prevotella* sp ++	Renal	Neurotoxicity (seizures)
		Ertapenem	MSSA ++ *Staphylococcus* sp coagulase negative ++ *S epidermidis* ++ Streptococci ++	**ESBL *E coli*** +++ **ESBL *Klebsiella* sp** ++ *E cloacae* ++ *C freundii* ++ *K aerogenes* ++ *E coli* ++ *Proteus* sp ++ *M morganii* +++ *S marcescens* ++ *H influenzae* ++ *M catarrhalis* ++	*B fragilis* +++ Peptostreptococci ++ *Actinomyces* sp ++ *C perfringens* ++ *F necrophorum* ++ *Prevotella* sp ++	Renal	Neurotoxicity (seizures)

(continued on next page)

Table 2
(*continued*)

Antibiotic class	Mechanism of action	Agent(s)	Spectrum of coverage			Clearance	Significant adverse effects
			Gram-positive	Gram-negative	Anaerobes		
Monobactams	Inhibition of cell wall synthesis	**Aztreonam**	None	***P aeruginosa*** ++ *E coli* ++ *Klebsiella* sp ++ *Proteus* sp ++ *M morganii* ++ *S marcescens* ++ *H influenzae* ++ *M catarrhalis* ++ *C koseri* +	None	Renal	Rash, eosinophilia
Glycopeptides	Inhibition of cell wall synthesis	**Vancomycin**	MSSA/**MRSA** +++ *S epidermidis* +++ *E faecalis* +++ Streptococci +++ *Enterococcus faecium* +	None	Peptostreptococci ++ *Clostridium* sp ++	Renal	Nephrotoxicity, Red man syndrome
Lipopeptides	Membrane depolarization	**Daptomycin**	MSSA/**MRSA/VISA/VRSA** +++ *E faecalis/E faecium/* **VRE** +++ Beta-hemolytic streptococci ++ *S. pneumoniae* +	None	Peptostreptococci ++ *C perfringens* +	Renal	Skeletal muscle myopathy, eosinophilic pneumonia, peripheral neuropathy
Oxazolidinones	Inhibition of bacterial protein synthesis (binds 50S ribosomal subunit)	**Linezolid**	MSSA/**MRSA/VISA/VRSA** +++ *E faecalis/E faecium/* **VRE** +++ Streptococci +++	None	Peptostreptococci ++ *Actinomyces* sp ++ *C perfringens* ++	Hepatic	Optic/peripheral neuropathy, thrombocytopenia, serotonin syndrome

Aminoglycosides	Inhibition of bacterial protein synthesis (binds to 30S ribosomal subunit)	**Amikacin** **Tobramycin** **Gentamicin**	None Synergy only	***P aeruginosa*** ++ *Citrobacter* sp ++ *E cloacae* ++ *E coli* ++ *Klebsiella* sp ++ *M morganii* ++ *Proteus* sp ++ *S marcescens* ++	None	Renal	Nephrotoxicity, ototoxicity, neuromuscular blockade (rare)
Fluoroquinolones	Inhibition of bacterial DNA synthesis (inhibits DNA gyrase in gram-negative bacteria and topoisomerase IV in gram-positive bacteria)	**Ciprofloxacin**	Streptococci +	*M catarrhalis* +++ *E coli* +++ *Proteus* sp +++ *Klebsiella* sp +++ *Serratia* sp +++ *Enterobacter* sp +++ *Citrobacter* sp +++ *Legionella* sp +++ ***P aeruginosa*** ++ ESBL *E coli* +	None	Renal	Tendon rupture, neurotoxicity, neuropathy, QT prolongation
		Levofloxacin	Streptococci +++	Same as ciprofloxacin plus *H influenzae* +++	Peptostreptococci ++ *Prevotella* sp +	Renal	
		Moxifloxacin	Streptococci ++ MSSA ++ *Staphylococcus* sp coagulase negative ++ *S epidermidis* ++ *E faecalis* ++	*H influenzae* +++ *Legionella* sp +++ *Enterobacter* sp +++ *Citrobacter* sp +++ *Klebsiella* sp +++ *E coli* +++ *Proteus* sp +++ *Serratia* sp +++ *M catarrhalis* +++	Peptostreptococci ++ *Prevotella* sp ++ *B fragilis* +	Hepatic	
Lincosamides	Inhibition of protein synthesis	**Clindamycin**	MSSA ++ *Staphylococcus* sp coagulase negative ++ *S epidermidis* ++ Beta-hemolytic streptococci ++ *S. pneumoniae* ++ Viridans streptococci + MRSA +	*Capnocytophaga* sp +++	*Actinomyces* sp +++ Peptostreptococci ++ *C perfringens* ++ *F necrophorum* ++ *Prevotella* sp ++	Hepatic	*C difficile* colitis, hypersensitivity, rash

(*continued on next page*)

Table 2
(continued)

Antibiotic class	Mechanism of action	Agent(s)	Spectrum of coverage: Gram-positive	Gram-negative	Anaerobes	Clearance	Significant adverse effects
Other	DNA strand breakage; loss of DNA helical structure; inhibition of protein synthesis	**Metronidazole**	None	None	*B fragilis* +++ *F necrophorum* +++ *Prevotella* sp +++ *C perfringens* ++ Peptostreptococci +	Renal	Uncommon: neurotoxicity (neuropathy, seizures, encephalopathy)
	Inhibition of folate synthesis	**Trimethoprim-sulfamethox azole**	MSSA/**MRSA** +++ *S epidermidis* +++ *Streptococcus pyogenes* +++ *S. pneumoniae* +	*Stenotrophomonas maltophilia* +++ *E coli* ++ ESBL *E coli* ++ *Klebsiella* sp ++ *Serratia* sp ++ *Proteus* sp ++	None	Renal	Increased serum creatinine/acute kidney injury, drug-induced liver injury (rare), hypersensitivity, thrombocytopenia, anemia

Boldface text in "Agent(s)" column is intended to make antibiotic names stand out from rest of text. Boldface text in "Spectrum of coverage" columns are to emphasize the organisms that specific antibiotics are effective against (basically highlights the most clinically relevant data in the chart)

Abbreviations: +, variable or limited activity; ++, good activity (potential alternative or second-line therapy); +++, first-line therapy or excellent activity; ESBL, extended-spectrum beta-lactamase; MRSA, methicillin-resistant *Staphylococcus aureus;* MSSA, methicillin-sensitive *Staphylococcus aureus;* VISA, vancomycin-intermediate *Staphylococcus aureus;* VRE, vancomycin-resistant Enterococcus; VRSA, vancomycin-resistant *Staphylococcus aureus* [12,27,29,30].

and neck infections as well as aspiration pneumonia. An empiric regimen for these polymicrobial infections would include either metronidazole or clindamycin in combination with antibiotics for gram-negative and gram-positive coverage. A carbapenem or piperacillin–tazobactam are alternative empiric regimens for mixed aerobic and anaerobic infections, especially those involving resistant gram-negative bacteria [6].

DE-ESCALATION

De-escalation is defined as replacing broad-spectrum antimicrobials with agents of a narrower spectrum or lower ecologic impact. This includes stopping components of empiric therapy targeting organisms not isolated in cultures and discontinuing agents intended for double coverage of specific pathogens. Ideally, de-escalation should occur within 24 hours of definitive culture (including PCR) and susceptibility results [13]. In the absence of confirmed infection, discontinuation of antimicrobials is fundamental, despite exclusion from the formal definition of de-escalation. The benefits of decreasing patient exposure to broad-spectrum therapy include reducing risk of antibiotic resistance, adverse effects, and cost.

ANTIMICROBIAL RESISTANCE

Over time bacteria have acquired a wide array of mechanisms for antimicrobial resistance. One MDR organism may have multiple mechanisms of resistance, which can be intrinsic, acquired, or both. Inherent resistance stems from traits encoded in the species' genome, while acquired mechanisms are the result of integration of new genetic material or sporadic mutations in intrinsic genes. Examples of common mechanisms of resistance include alteration of cell membrane permeability, transformation of the antimicrobial target, inactivation of the drug, and expulsion of the antibiotic from the cell [14].

Decreasing cell membrane permeability blocks antimicrobial entry into the cell and interaction with its intended target. One of the many resistance mechanisms of MRSA is its ability to tightly bind extracellular antimicrobials, which impedes drug uptake into the cell. Other bacteria have alterations in the membrane pore proteins that control influx of an antibiotic and decrease the intracellular drug concentration. In MDR *P aeruginosa*, decreased expression of the pore protein for imipenem is an intrinsic mechanism of resistance. Acquired mutations or changes in *Klebsiella pneumoniae* pore proteins prevent antimicrobial absorption and contribute to resistance [15].

Modification of antimicrobial targets is another mechanism of resistance in bacteria such as MRSA, *K pneumoniae*, and *E coli*. The main methicillin resistance mechanism in *S aureus* is acquired via incorporation of the *mecA* gene. This gene is carried on a mobile genetic element and encodes an alternative penicillin-binding protein (PBP2a), which has a low affinity for almost all beta-lactams, with ceftaroline as one of the rare exceptions. Compared to native penicillin-binding proteins, PBP2a has a less-accessible active site, which hinders beta-lactam binding [16,17]. *K pneumoniae* illustrates another example of resistance due to changes in target proteins. Aminoglycosides exert their bactericidal effect by binding the 30S subunit of ribosomes and thereby inhibiting bacterial protein synthesis. Mutations in *K pneumoniae* ribosome proteins interfere with binding of aminoglycosides, resulting in resistance. Similarly, fluoroquinolone resistance can develop in *E coli* if mutations modify their target enzymes such as DNA gyrases or topoisomerases [15].

Inactivation of antimicrobials is a widespread resistance mechanism, and beta-lactamases are among the most common enzymes involved. These enzymes inactivate beta-lactam antibiotics through hydrolysis of the beta-lactam ring, which prevents binding to their target proteins. Beta-lactamase production may be intrinsic or acquired via plasmids. Enterobacterales such as the "HECK YES" organisms have inducible *ampC* gene expression that can increase AmpC beta-lactamase production and result in resistance to penicillin and cephalosporins, including third-generation antimicrobials [12]. Some MDR bacteria such as *K pneumoniae* and *E coli* may produce ESBLs, which can broaden resistance to include all cephalosporins [14].

Active expulsion of antibiotics is another mechanism of resistance that decreases the intracellular concentration of the drug. This is accomplished by efflux pumps, which may be intrinsically expressed or induced by mutations. MDR *P aeruginosa*'s intrinsic resistance to aminoglycosides, fluoroquinolones, and cephalosporins can be partly attributed to overexpression of its efflux pumps. Acquired point mutations can also induce overexpression of these pumps in *Acinetobacter baumannii*, resulting in resistance to cephalosporins and carbapenems. Upregulated expression of efflux pumps in combination with downregulated expression of pore proteins are associated with aminoglycoside resistance in MDR *E coli*. Expelling antimicrobials via this pump system also plays a significant role in resistance for MRSA and *K pneumoniae* [15].

Antimicrobial resistance can arise from 3 sources: emergence, spread, and influx. It can emerge under the combined influence of several selective factors, including the specific antimicrobial agent or concurrent drug therapy. Resistance can spread on a cellular level (among the bacteria of one host) or among hosts (by contact with mutual staff or equipment). An influx can occur when an undetected antimicrobial-resistant organism is introduced into the ICU by a new patient or staff [6]. Understanding the complexities of resistance mechanisms and their spread is essential to the prevention and targeted treatment of MDR infections.

SOURCE CONTROL

Achieving source control is paramount in treating surgical infections. This involves removal of the source of infection and any infected material [8]. Examples range from removal of an infected organ (appendectomy for appendicitis, cholecystectomy for cholecystitis) to incision and drainage of pus and debridement of necrotic infected tissue (as in abscesses and necrotizing soft tissue infections). In most cases, the need for source control is urgent or emergent. Depending on the patient's clinical condition and the etiology of the infection, interventions may not be strictly operative and require multidisciplinary cooperation.

Examples include percutaneous drainage of intra-abdominal abscesses and endoscopic retrograde cholangiopancreatography for ascending cholangitis.

SPECIAL PATIENT POPULATIONS

Patient populations who deserve special consideration in antimicrobial selection include children, pregnant women, and immunocompromised patients, including organ transplant recipients. In pregnancy, the risks of adverse effects on both the patient and the fetus must be weighed with the benefits. Additionally, the physiologic changes of pregnancy complicate dosing due to changes in volume of distribution and clearance of certain medications [6].

Following organ transplant, the patient's immunocompromised status requires careful consideration. Early diagnosis of infection is paramount but can be challenging since fever and other signs of infection may be absent or attenuated. Due to their increased risk of opportunistic infections, transplant patients may be on daily antimicrobials as prophylaxis, such as trimethoprim-sulfamethoxazole for *Pneumocystis jirovecii* [18]. Furthermore, they may require broader empiric coverage compared to immunocompetent patients. Drug interactions with their immunosuppression regimen may also influence antimicrobial selection.

The most common infection in lung transplant recipients is a respiratory tract infection. In the immediate posttransplant period, prophylactic antibiotics are directed by donor and recipient bronchial cultures. This is particularly important in lung transplant recipients with a history of cystic fibrosis, who are often colonized with MDR bacteria before transplant [19]. Bacterial pneumonia can be caused by nosocomial, community-acquired, or opportunistic organisms. Compared to immunocompetent patients, transplant patients require a more intensive evaluation for infection due to the wider spectrum of possible pathogens. Depending on history and exposure, workup for fungal, viral, and more obscure bacterial etiologies such as *Legionella pneumophila* and nontuberculous mycobacteria should be pursued. Early pneumonia after lung transplant is primarily caused by nosocomial bacteria or previous colonization of the donor or recipient. Examples of early pneumonia pathogens include *S aureus*, Enterobacteriaceae, *P aeruginosa*, and *Burkholderia*. Over 6 months after transplant, community-acquired bacteria like *Streptococcus pneumoniae* and *Haemophilus influenzae* are the predominant cause of pneumonia [20]. An empiric antibiotic regimen will depend on time from transplant, immunosuppression, history of colonization, recent exposures, and local susceptibilities.

Following kidney transplantation, the most common infection is a urinary tract infection (UTI). *Enterococcus* sp and *Escherichia coli* are the leading causative agents [19]. Depending on prior UTI organisms and susceptibilities, a broad-spectrum beta-lactam agent or carbapenem may serve as empiric therapy [21]. In the case of other infections in kidney transplant recipients, the nephrotoxicity of some agents such as vancomycin and aminoglycosides should be carefully weighed when selecting antimicrobial therapy. When combined with a calcineurin inhibitor such as tacrolimus, these antibiotics' toxicity to the graft is compounded. Other significant interactions between tacrolimus and antibiotics involve alterations in metabolism. For example, rifampin induces the metabolism of tacrolimus by the cytochrome P-450 system, leading to a reduction in the plasma concentration of tacrolimus and, therefore, increasing the risk of rejection. In contrast, macrolides (with the exception of azithromycin) inhibit tacrolimus metabolism, which can lead to elevated levels and an increased risk of toxicity [22].

The most common infections after liver transplant are similar to those in nontransplant SICU patients: pneumonia, surgical site infection, intra-abdominal fluid collections, UTI, and blood stream infections. Unlike their nontransplant peers, over half of liver transplant recipients develop major infections [23]. Therefore, a high index of suspicion must be maintained throughout all posttransplant phases. In the first month after transplant, most bacterial infections are from nosocomial organisms or the recipient's normal flora, but close monitoring for donor-derived pathogens is imperative. Postoperative complications like bile leaks, hepatic artery thrombosis, biliary ductal stenosis, and anastomotic strictures can lead to peritonitis, abscess (intrahepatic or abdominal), and acute cholangitis [19]. *Enterococcus* sp and *E coli* are the most common bacteria, but vancomycin-resistant enterococcus (VRE), anaerobes, and other gram-negative bacilli should be considered. Empiric antibiotics for liver abscess or cholangitis may consist of metronidazole, an anti-MRSA agent, and either a broad-spectrum beta-lactam or a carbapenem. Of note, in the case of an infected biloma, antifungal coverage is warranted. The same regimen can be utilized for intra-abdominal abscess or peritonitis, but antipseudomonal and antifungal coverage should be added. Additionally, linezolid or daptomycin should be used for both VRE and MRSA coverage [21]. Surgeons and intensivists should seek the expertise of infectious disease physicians specialized in transplant to ensure the proper workup, prophylaxis, empiric regimen, and de-escalation are implemented in these high-risk patients.

ANTIMICROBIAL STEWARDSHIP

AMS is "the optimal selection, dosage, and duration of antimicrobial treatment that results in the best clinical outcome for the treatment or prevention of infection, with minimal toxicity to the patient and minimal impact on subsequent resistance" [24]. More simply, it aims for "the right antibiotic for the right indication, the right patient, at the right time, with the right dose and route, causing the least harm to the patient and future patients" [25]. Through collective efforts to minimize inappropriate antibiotic use, antimicrobial stewardship programs can also help decrease health care costs.

Due to the accelerated rise of MDR organisms, AMS has become a priority. The Centers for Disease Control and Prevention (CDC) recommends the establishment of an AMS program at all hospitals. On an institutional level, the core elements of an AMS program have been defined by the CDC as [26]

1. Leadership commitment, or dedicating human, financial, and information technology resources

2. Accountability, which entails appointing a physician or pharmacist as a leader
3. Pharmacy expertise in the form of an appointed pharmacist leader
4. Action, which means implementing at least one recommended AMS strategy, such as preauthorization or prospective audit and feedback
5. Tracking antibiotic prescribing, resistance patterns, and the impact of interventions
6. Reporting on antibiotic use and resistance on a regular basis
7. Education of prescribers, pharmacists, and nurses about optimal antibiotic use, adverse effects, and resistance

Specifically in the ICU, the components of AMS can be broken down into 3 stages: before, during, and after treatment. The first phase consists of considering local antibiotic resistance rates and a patient's specific risk factors for infection with MDR organisms. It also includes accelerating time to diagnosis and excluding antibiotics when treating fever of noninfectious etiologies. During antimicrobial treatment, the priorities include achieving source control, considering the pharmacokinetic and pharmacodynamic properties of the regimen, reassessing clinical symptoms and culture data daily, and de-escalating or stopping antimicrobial agents as soon as appropriate. The final phase involves reducing unnecessary antibiotic use through automatic stop-orders or "time-outs" to mandate re-evaluation for continuing or changing agents such as meropenem or vancomycin. The "after treatment" stage also requires ongoing collaboration and communication among the multitude of clinical team members who contribute to the AMS effort: infectious disease physicians, intensivists, clinical pharmacists, microbiologists, nurses, and infection control staff [27].

Implementing optimal antibiotic practices in the ICU faces multiple challenges. First, the acuity of some patients, such as those admitted in shock, may outweigh the benefits of postponing or stopping antibiotics. Second, management of infections in complex ICU patients requires specialized expertise and collaboration that may be unavailable or limited at some centers. Continuity of care by the same ICU team may also be a barrier to consistency in antimicrobial selection, duration, and de-escalation [5]. Despite these obstacles, antibiotic stewardship must be prioritized to achieve the best outcomes for patients, both individually and as a whole.

SUMMARY

Surgeons and intensivists should lead a collaborative effort to use antibiotics judiciously in the ICU. Evaluations for infection should include careful consideration of a patient's history, such as prior infections or immunocompromised status. If infection is evident or strongly suspected, prompt initiation of empiric antibiotics is vital, particularly for patients who present in shock. The surgeon must decide if source control is indicated and feasible, as well as the optimal approach and timing. De-escalation from broad-spectrum agents to more targeted narrower spectrum antimicrobials should occur as soon as culture and susceptibility results are available. In the absence of confirmed infection, antibiotics should be stopped. Antibiotic stewardship should be a priority in the SICU in order to optimize antibiotic regimens for individual patients while minimizing resistance for future patients.

CLINICS CARE POINTS

- Ensure perioperative prophylactic antibiotics are given within 60 minutes of skin incision (for most antibiotics), appropriately re-dosed intraoperatively, and stopped within 24 hours after the procedure.
- When infection is strongly suspected, promptly send cultures (according to source) and start empiric antimicrobials. Utilize culture and sensitivity data to de-escalate empiric antimicrobials as soon as possible.
- Urgent or emergent source control is a priority in surgical infections. This is not always strictly operative and may require a multidisciplinary approach.
- Integrate the collaborative input of surgeons, intensivists, pharmacists, and infectious disease experts to select and optimize individualized antibiotic therapy for complex ICU patients.

Disclosure

The authors have nothing to disclose.

References

[1] Trivedi KK, Bartash R, Letourneau AR, et al. Opportunities to improve antibiotic appropriateness in U.S. ICUs: a multicenter evaluation. Crit Care Med 2020;48(7):968–76.

[2] Varghese JM, Roberts JA, Lipman J. Antimicrobial pharmacokinetic and pharmacodynamic issues in the critically ill with severe sepsis and septic shock. Crit Care Clin 2011;27(1): 19–34.

[3] Jarrell AS, Kruer RM, Johnson D, et al. Antimicrobial pharmacokinetics and pharmacodynamics. Surg Infect (Larchmt) 2015;16(4):375–9.

[4] Parker SL, Sime FB, Roberts JA. Optimizing dosing of antibiotics in critically ill patients. Curr Opin Infect Dis 2015;28(6):497–504.

[5] Luyt CE, Bréchot N, Trouillet JL, et al. Antibiotic stewardship in the intensive care unit. Crit Care 2014;18(5):480.

[6] Duncan R. Antimicrobial use in surgical intensive care. In: JM OD, FE N, editors. Surgical intensive care medicine. 2010. 2010. p. 361–8.

[7] Bratzler DW, Dellinger EP, Olsen KM, et al. Clinical practice guidelines for antimicrobial prophylaxis in surgery. Am J Health Syst Pharm 2013;70(3):195–283.

[8] Kisat M, Zarzaur B. Antibiotic therapy in the intensive care unit. Surg Clin North Am 2022;102(1):159–67.

[9] Parente DM, Cunha CB, Mylonakis E, et al. The clinical utility of methicillin-resistant Staphylococcus aureus (MRSA) nasal screening to rule out MRSA pneumonia: a diagnostic meta-analysis with antimicrobial stewardship implications. Clin Infect Dis 2018;67(1):1–7.

[10] Tenover FC, Tickler IA. Detection of Methicillin-Resistant Staphylococcus aureus Infections Using Molecular Methods. Antibiotics (Basel) 2022;11(2):239.

[11] Niederman MS, Baron RM, Bouadma L, et al. Initial antimicrobial management of sepsis. Crit Care 2021;25(1):307.

[12] Tamma PD, Aitken SL, Bonomo RA, et al. Infectious Diseases Society of America 2023 Guidance on the Treatment of Antimicrobial Resistant Gram-Negative Infections. Clin Infect Dis 2023;ciad428.
[13] Tabah A, Bassetti M, Kollef MH, et al. Antimicrobial de-escalation in critically ill patients: a position statement from a task force of the European Society of Intensive Care Medicine (ESICM) and European Society of Clinical Microbiology and Infectious Diseases (ESCMID) Critically Ill Patients Study Group (ESGCIP). Intensive Care Med 2020;46(2):245–65.
[14] Reygaert WC. An overview of the antimicrobial resistance mechanisms of bacteria. AIMS Microbiol 2018;4(3):482–501.
[15] Teng J, Imani S, Zhou A, et al. Combatting resistance: understanding multi-drug resistant pathogens in intensive care units. Biomed Pharmacother 2023;167:115564.
[16] Lakhundi S, Zhang K. Methicillin-resistant Staphylococcus aureus: molecular characterization, evolution, and epidemiology. Clin Microbiol Rev 2018;31(4).
[17] Peacock SJ, Paterson GK. Mechanisms of methicillin resistance in Staphylococcus aureus. Annu Rev Biochem 2015;84:577–601.
[18] Fishman JA. Infection in organ transplantation. Am J Transplant 2017;17(4):856–79.
[19] Timsit JF, Sonneville R, Kalil AC, et al. Diagnostic and therapeutic approach to infectious diseases in solid organ transplant recipients. Intensive Care Med 2019;45(5):573–91.
[20] Joean O, Welte T, Gottlieb J. Chest infections after lung transplantation. Chest 2022;161(4): 937–48.
[21] Kaviani A, Ince D, Axelrod DA. Management of antimicrobial agents in abdominal organ transplant patients in intensive care unit. Curr Transplant Rep 2020;7(1):1–11.
[22] Paterson DL, Singh N. Interactions between tacrolimus and antimicrobial agents. Clin Infect Dis 1997;25(6):1430–40.
[23] Kim SI. Bacterial infection after liver transplantation. World J Gastroenterol 2014;20(20): 6211–20.
[24] Gerding DN. The search for good antimicrobial stewardship. Jt Comm J Qual Improv 2001;27(8):403–4.
[25] Obe DN, editor. Antimicrobial stewardship: from principles to practice. British Society for antimicrobial chemotherapy. 2018. Available at: https://www.bsac.org.uk/antimicrobialstewardshipebook/BSAC-AntimicrobialStewardship-FromPrinciplestoPractice-eBook.pdf. [Accessed 14 November 2023] 2018.
[26] Core elements of hospital antibiotic stewardship programs. 2019. Available at: https://www.cdc.gov/antibiotic-use/core-elements/hospital.html. [Accessed 14 November 2023].
[27] Ture Z, Güner R, Alp E. Antimicrobial stewardship in the intensive care unit. J Intensive Med 2023;3(3):244–53.
[28] Sartelli M, Coccolini F, Kluger Y, et al. WSES/GAIS/SIS-E/WSIS/AAST global clinical pathways for patients with intra abdominal infections. World J Emerg Surg 2021;16(1):49.
[29] Eyler RF, Shvets K. Clinical pharmacology of antibiotics. Clin J Am Soc Nephrol 2019;14(7):1080–90.
[30] The Sanford Guide to Antimicrobial Therapy, Gilbert DN, Saag MS, Pavia AT, Boucher HW, et al. Antimicrobial therapy, Inc. 2023. Available at: https://webedition.sanfordguide.-com/. [Accessed 10 December 2023].

Advances in Surgery 58 (2024) 223–234

ADVANCES IN SURGERY

The Role of Surgery for Stage IV Melanoma

Amanda M. Dann, MD[a,*], Charlotte Ariyan, MD, PhD[b]

[a]Division of Surgical Oncology, Department of Surgery, University of Texas Southwestern, 5323 Harry Hines Boulevard, Dallas, TX 75390-8548, USA; [b]Department of Surgical Oncology, Memorial Sloan Kettering Cancer Center, 1275 York Avenue, New York, NY 10065, USA

Keywords

• Melanoma • Metastatic melanoma • Metastatectomy • Palliative resection • Immunotherapy

Key points

- Surgery has a long-standing historical and evolving role in the management of stage IV melanoma.
- Prior to modern therapies, surgical resection was the primary option for management of metastatic disease and was associated with improved survival in selected patients.
- With improved systemic therapies, metastatectomy is still frequently employed and associated with durable long-term survival, though current guidelines and indications for surgery remain poorly defined.
- In addition to its role in disease control, surgical resection can be effectively used for symptom palliation and tissue procurement for novel individualized therapies.

INTRODUCTION

Melanoma remains the most fatal cutaneous malignancy accounting for nearly 8000 annual deaths in the United States [1]. While the vast majority of melanomas present at an early stage, approximately 5% of melanomas will present as stage IV disease [1]. Additionally, many patients initially treated with surgical resection will go on to develop distant metastases [2].

Prior to the development of more effective systemic therapies, overall 5 year survival for patients with stage IV melanoma was only 6% [3]. In the era of modern treatments, 5 year survival for patients in the United States with stage IV disease has increased to 30% [1], and can be 50% in patients receiving dual

*Corresponding author. *E-mail address:* Amanda.Dann@utsouthwestern.edu

https://doi.org/10.1016/j.yasu.2024.04.013
0065-3411/24/Published by Elsevier Inc.

checkpoint blockade [1,4]. This improvement in the efficacy of medical therapies has led to a substantial increase in the number of patients surviving with stage IV disease and a commensurate increase in the population potentially eligible for metastatectomy. This study reviews the historical role of surgical resection of melanoma metastases and its current role in the multimodality treatment of this disease.

ROLE OF SURGERY BEFORE EFFECTIVE SYSTEMIC THERAPIES

Prior to the emergence of targeted therapy and immune checkpoint blockade, surgery represented the only potential option for long-term survival in metastatic melanoma [5–7]. However, it must be noted that the potential survival benefit of surgical intervention in this setting is difficult to quantify as most studies present retrospective, observational results, rather than randomized trial data, allowing for selection bias when comparing surgical and nonsurgical cohorts.

Table 1 presents a summary of results from retrospective, largely single-center studies reporting survival figures in patients with stage IV melanoma who underwent metastatectomy prior to the introduction of targeted therapies and immune checkpoint blockade. As prognosis varies between stage M1a (distant, skin, subcutaneous tissue, lymph nodes), M1b (pulmonary metastasis), M1c (non-pulmonary visceral metastases), and M1d (central nervous system [CNS] metastases), these studies are stratified by site of metastatic disease. Taken together, these studies present significantly longer median overall survivals and higher 5 year survival rates than the contemporary figures for all patients with stage IV melanoma.

Several retrospective studies specifically reported survival data in patients who underwent surgical resection compared to those who did not with an attempt to control for other factors associated with prognosis. Coleman and colleagues evaluated the role of surgical resection of bony metastases and found a median survival of 11.8 months compared to 4.8 months in the nonoperative group, and on regression analysis found resection to be an independent variable associated with improved survival (hazard ratio [HR]: 0.53) [3,8]. Faries and colleagues evaluated a similar question for hepatic metastases and found a median overall survival of 24.8 months in the resection groups versus 8 months in the medical therapy group. They also found completeness of resection to be an independent predictor of improved overall survival [9]. Wasif and colleagues used the SEER database for a similar analysis and reported improved median and 5 year overall survival for patients undergoing metastatectomy and again found metastatectomy to be an independent predictor of survival (HR: 0.59) [10]. Additional studies have cited improved outcomes in patients undergoing resection when there is a long disease-free interval between initial resection and development of metastases, metastases are unifocal or confined to one organ, and metastases can be fully resected [5,11]. These results demonstrate the ability to select for a group of patients who do better with surgery. However, the complex selection criteria and underlying tumor biology that permitted this selection are not well clarified.

Table 1
Survival figures in patients with stage IV melanoma who underwent metastatectomy prior to the introduction of targeted therapies and immune checkpoint blockade

Authors	Institution (year)	# Of patients undergoing resection	Median survival (mo.)	5 y overall survival (%)
M1a				
Eton et al [30], 1988	MDACC (1988)	57	10	5
Barth et al [3], 1995	JWCI (1995)	281	15	14
Essner et al [31], 2004	JWCI (2004)	260	NR	25
M1b				
Pogrebniak et al [32], 1988	NCI (1988)	49	13	NR
Gorenstein et al [33] 1991	MDACC (1991)	56	18	25
Tafra et al [34], 1995	JWCI (1995)	106	18	27
Leo et al [35], 2000	IRLM (2000)	282	19	22
Essner et al [31], 2004	JWCI (2004)	364	28.1	21
Andrews et al [36], 2006	Moffitt (2006)	86	35	33
Neuman et al [37], 2007	MSKCC (2007)	26	40	29
Petersen et al [38], 2007	Duke (2007)	249	19	21
M1c				
Ollila et al [27], 1996	JWCI (1996)	46	48.9	41
Agrawal et al [39], 1999	MSKCC (1999)	68	8.2	18
Haigh et al [40], 1999	JWCI (1999)	27	18.6	NR
Rose et al [41], 2001	JWCI, SMU (2001)	18	18.2	23
Wood et al [42], 2002	JWCI (2002)	60	15	24
Mittendorf et al [43], 2008	MDACC (2008)	20	20.7	NR
Collinson et al [44], 2008	SMU (2008)	23	16	NR
M1d				
Patchell et al [45], 1990	UK (1990)	25	9.2	NR
Wronski et al [46], 2000	MSKCC (2000)	91	6.7	7
Fife et al [47], 2004	Sydney (2004)	205	8.9	NR
Mixed				
Karakousis et al [6], 1994	Roswell Park (1994)	114	19	22

(*continued on next page*)

Table 1
(*continued*)

Authors	Institution (year)	# Of patients undergoing resection	Median survival (mo.)	5 y overall survival (%)
Fletcher et al [48], 1998	OHSU (1998)	77	13	10
Meyer et al [11], 2000	Erlangen, Germany (2000)	174	7	16% (2 y)

Abbreviations: IRLM, International Registry of Lung Metastases; JWCI, John Wayne Cancer Institute; MDACC, MD Anderson cancer center; MSKCC, Memorial Sloan Kettering Cancer Center; NCI, National Cancer Institute; NR, not reported; OHSU, Oregon Health Sciences University.

There are also prospective, multicenter trials that have evaluated the role of metastatectomy for stage IV melanoma in the era prior to targeted immunotherapies. In 2011, the Southwest Oncology Group presented a phase II multicenter, prospective trial of surgical resection in stage IV melanoma and found a 4 year overall survival rate of 31% in patients with complete resection [12]. MSLT-1, a randomized phase III trial designed to examine the role of sentinel lymph node biopsy in patients with stage I and II melanoma also reported on outcomes of patients who ultimately developed distant disease. They identified 291 patients who developed distant metastases, and noted 151 (55%) patients underwent surgical resection with or without systemic therapy. They reported a median survival of 15.8 months and a 4 year overall survival of 20.8% in the surgery group compared to 6.9 months and 7% in the systemic therapy alone group. However, they note these groups were not directly comparable as those undergoing surgery were more likely to have fewer involved organ sites and fewer metastatic lesions [13]. The MMAIT-IV trial reported the most promising outcome data for patients with resected stage IV melanoma in the preimmunotherapy era. This was a prospective, phase III randomized, control trial looking at the efficacy of adjuvant BCG versus BCG plus canvaxin, an allogenic melanoma vaccine, following complete resection of distant metastases. While this study failed to show efficacy of canvaxin over BCG alone, they reported a 5 and 10 year overall survival of greater than 40% and 30% in both arms of the trial, concluding metastatectomy can provide favorable long-term disease control. The improved outcomes of this group provide early data of a possible synergy between immunotherapy (BCG alone or in combination with canvaxin) with surgery [14]. In aggregate, the survival figures in these studies suggest a role for metastatectomy in well-selected patents in the absence of other effective therapies.

There are also limited data on repeat metastatectomy in recurrent stage IV disease. Ollila and colleagues presented data for the role of metastatectomy for recurrent metastases after initial complete surgical resection for distant disease and found a median survival of 18.2 months for those who were completely resected, compared to 12.5 months for those who underwent palliative resection or 5.9 months for those with nonsurgical management. They concluded that repeat metastatectomy can prolong survival even in those patients with recurrent stage IV disease if they can be completely resected [7]. Similarly, in the analysis of patients with stage IV disease from the MLST-1 trial, of the 161 patients who underwent surgical resection, 67 (42%) patients had more than one operation and this group exhibited a 21 month median survival and 25% 4 year survival, which was actually superior to those who only underwent one operation [13]. Following MSLT-1, a prospective, randomized phase III trial of initial surgical resection versus best medical therapy (NCT01013623) was opened, but failed to accrue, in part do to the emergence of checkpoint blockade.

KEY POINTS

- Significantly better long-term survival rates were observed in well-selected patients for metastatectomy compared to results with contemporary systemic therapy alone; however, the direct contribution of surgical resection is not well defined.

ROLE OF SURGERY IN THE MODERN ERA

In the era of effective checkpoint blockade and targeted therapy, patients with stage IV melanoma are experiencing survival rates well above what was historically observed. As discussed in the previous section, evidence has demonstrated that surgery may have a role in well-selected patients. This is reflected by current NCCN guidelines, which recommend consideration of surgical resection in selected patients with oligometastatic disease, either as initial treatment or following systemic therapy. However, there currently is no standardized approach to patient selection and clinicians are challenged with decision of if and when to employ surgical resection. This section will review available data and considerations for metastatectomy for patients with stage IV melanoma in the era of modern therapies. As the majority of available data assessing the role of surgery in conjunction with modern systemic therapies is with immunotherapy, this section will focus on that cohort of patients.

Timing of surgery

Upfront resection with adjuvant systemic therapy

Recently, several randomized trials have been published on outcomes of patients with advanced melanoma undergoing resection with adjuvant immunotherapy. The IMMUNED trial was a randomized, phase II trial comparing adjuvant nivolumab plus ipilimumab, ipilimumab and placebo following resection or radiation to no evidence of disease (NED) in patients with stage IV melanoma. They found 4 year recurrence-free survival rates of 64.2%, 31.4% and 15% in these groups, respectively [15], suggesting a favorable and durable response can be achieved with surgical resection and adjuvant immune checkpoint blockade, while the vast majority of patients treated with resection alone will recur in this time. CheckMate-238 evaluated the efficacy of nivolumab versus ipilimumab following resection of stage IIIB–IV disease and found 4 year recurrence-free survival rates of 52% and 41% in the study arms. While this study was not designed to compare adjuvant systemic therapy to resection alone, and the study population was only approximately 20% stage IV disease, it still reflects the long-term disease control achievable with resection and systemic therapy in advanced disease [16]. Similar findings were seen in the CheckMate-915 trial evaluating nivolumab plus ipilimumab versus nivolumab in the same study population [16,17].

Nelson and colleagues sought to more directly assess the effect of upfront resection on outcomes of patients with stage IV disease in those receiving modern systemic therapy. They performed a retrospective match-paired analysis of patients who underwent resection followed by adjuvant therapy, versus systemic therapy alone and found a significantly higher 5 year melanoma-specific survival in those who underwent initial resection (58.8% vs 38.9%) [18]. While the authors attempted to match for known relevant prognostic factors, these results are limited by the retrospective nature of the study. Taken together, these studies show the possibility of durable, long-term survival in patients with advanced disease with surgical resection followed by effective systemic therapy.

Initial systemic therapy with subsequent metastatectomy

The previously described studies suggest surgery as a component of care can lead to effective disease control in patients with advanced melanoma. However, they also highlight the importance of the systemic agents in achieving these results and there are several benefits to strategies pursuing upfront systemic therapy followed by surgical resection. One important factor is the notion of using systemic therapy to select patients most likely to benefit from surgical resection. Most studies have focused on the role of immunotherapy and surgery, which is described in the later section.

Klemen and colleagues evaluated patterns of treatment failure of patients with stage IV melanoma treated with immune checkpoint inhibitors. They identified a cohort of patients who survived at least 6 months while on checkpoint inhibitor therapy, but exhibited progression, incomplete responses, or progression after initial response. Around 18% of these patients went on to receive local therapy to achieve NED or be resected to non-progressive residual disease. They found a 3 year disease-specific survival of 60% in those patients resected to NED and found the best outcomes in those with a single site of progression [19].

Similarly, Bello and colleagues evaluated outcomes of patients with advanced melanoma who underwent surgery stratified by their response to immunotherapy. They found that patients with stable or responding disease to immunotherapy had superior survival to those with isolated progression (90% vs 60% 5 year survival). Patients who do not respond to immunotherapy have multisite progression, and had a dismal 5 year survival of 6%, similar to historical groups of patients with stage IV melanoma. Selecting patients able to be rendered NED by resection, identified a group with better survival than those with residual disease after surgery (75 vs 15% 5 year overall survival) [20]. However, patients with stable disease or partial response who only had a progressing lesion resected still had a 30% 5 year survival, suggesting that metastatectomy is an option for escape lesions.

Li and colleagues evaluated patients with disease progression on systemic therapy and found salvage metastatectomy could provide patients with an overall 5 year survival of 52% and a local disease control rate of 61%. Patients resected to NED performed best, followed closely by those with residual but non-progressive disease, while those with residual progressive disease had only an 8% 5 year survival [21]. Versulis and colleagues report data from a multicenter, international retrospective review of patients who had local treatment (55% surgical resection) for a solitary site of progression during or following response to immune checkpoint blockade therapy. Their cohort was diverse in terms of location of progression, timing of progression and immunotherapy regimens received. Estimated 3 year overall survival was 79% and 44% of patients treated for a solitary site of progression had no subsequent disease progression (median follow-up time 43 months) [22]. These studies suggest pursuing upfront immunotherapy and assessing response may allow us to more discerningly identify the patients who will benefit most from surgical resection of their disease.

In addition to the ability to allow for better patient selection, there are more emerging data from translational and clinical data to suggest immunotherapy may have enhanced efficacy when employed in a neoadjuvant setting. SWOG 1801 was a randomized phase II trial that sought to evaluate the role of neoadjuvant plus adjuvant pembrolizumab versus adjuvant pembrolizumab in resected stage IIIB to IVC melanoma. They found there was a significantly higher 2 year event-free survival (defined as disease progression, drug toxicity precluding surgery, inability to resect all gross disease, surgical or treatment complications prevent initiation of adjuvant therapy, melanoma recurrence, or death) in the neoadjuvant–adjuvant group, compared to the adjuvant only group (72% vs 49%). Patients with stage IV disease only accounted for 9% of the study population, but the trend favoring the neoadjuvant–adjuvant group was also seen in this subgroup [23]. These studies suggest resection can reasonably be considered in those with responding, stable, or oligo-progressing metastatic disease.

KEY POINTS

- Surgical resection plus effective systemic therapy can afford durable, long-term disease control in metastatic melanoma
- Assessing response to systemic therapy may help identify patients most likely to derive a survival benefit from surgery, though there are currently no established guidelines to guide these treatment decisions

Utilization of surgery for stage IV melanoma and associated outcomes

Studies have evaluated the utilization of surgical resection for stage IV melanoma. The previously mentioned study by Nelson and colleagues also sought to evaluate trends in the use of resection for stage IV melanoma at their high-volume center. They evaluated over 2300 patients with resectable stage IV disease in their database from 1965 to 2015 and found 45.2% of patients underwent surgical resection. This was 44.7% in the "early" era (prior to 2008) and increased slightly to 54.5% in the later era. They found that in the modern era, younger age was the only independent factor associated with the receipt of therapy [18].

Follow up from prospective randomized trials of systemic treatment has also demonstrated the increased use of surgery in stage IV disease. The long-term follow up of Checkmate 067, evaluating the efficacy of nivolumab plus ipilimumab and nivolumab and ipilimumab monotherapies in initially unresectable stage III and IV disease demonstrated a remarkable survival of 42% to 49% at 6.5 years of follow-up for patients treated with CTLA-4/PD1 or PD1 blockade alone. However, 66% to 79% of these patients progressed or recurred during the study period and over 20% underwent surgery at time of relapse [4].

A recent meta-analysis by Lwin and colleagues used the National Cancer Database to evaluate outcomes and factors associated with the use of surgery in patients with stage IV melanoma. They evaluated a total of 9800 patients who received immunotherapy, surgery, or both. Overall, 22% of patients underwent surgery. Those undergoing surgery were younger, had better performance status, and were less likely to have received immunotherapy. Receipt of surgery was also associated with nonclinical factors including undergoing treatment at an academic/research program, having private insurance and higher median patient income [24]. The authors found the longest median overall survival in patients who received immunotherapy and surgery, compared to immunotherapy or surgery alone (50.9 vs 22.4 vs 20.5 months). While this study is limited both by the granularity of the data in the National Cancer Database and the retrospective nature of the analysis, it does confirm that metastatectomy is a frequently used tool in the treatment armamentarium and that appropriate patient selection seems to be possible at the national level.

ADDITIONAL INDICATIONS FOR SURGICAL RESECTION IN METASTATIC DISEASE

Palliation

In addition to providing surgical disease control in conjunction with modern systemic therapies, surgical resection continues to have a role for palliation for symptomatic systemic disease refractory to alternative therapies. Surgical resection can provide effective palliation even in patients with progressive disease or unfavorable tumor biology. Symptom relief with palliative intent surgery has been reported in 77% to 100% of metastatic melanoma cases depending on the site of metastasis [25]. Surgery can be particularly effective for patients with symptoms related to gastrointestinal (GI) bleeding or obstruction. Series reporting on resection of GI metastases report a 79% to 97% success rate in relieving presenting symptoms [26,27]. With the continuing advent of less invasive and less morbid surgical techniques, the potential risks of surgical intervention versus the potential benefits in the palliative setting will likely continue to support resection in certain settings.

Metastatectomy for adoptive cell therapy

While less commonly performed, an additional indication for metastatectomy is in the development of personalized adoptive cell therapies. This therapeutic strategy was developed by Dr. Rosenberg at the National Cancer Institute (NCI) in the 1980s and involves the use of adoptive cell transfer of tumor-infiltrating lymphocytes (TILs), usually in a highly individualized approach. This strategy requires surgical resection of metastatic sites for harvesting of the TILs and relies on surgeons to appropriately select patients and metastatic lesions amenable to low morbidity resection.

This approach allows for antitumor lymphocytes to be expanded and selected ex vivo and then be reintroduced to the host to ideally select the lymphocytes with the most antitumor activity and tumor-specific antigen avidity. Initial studies from the NCI showed response rates of up to 55% and complete regressions in 22% of patients [28]. A recent, phase III randomized trial out of the Netherlands compared the results of TIL therapy versus ipilimumab in patients with advanced melanoma, the majority of whom had progressed on anti-PD1, and found a higher objective response rate with TIL therapy (49% vs 21%) and longer median overall (25.8 vs 18.9 months) and progression-free survival (3.1 vs 7.2 months) [29]. This technology has previously only been available in a few specialized centers worldwide; however, there are now several commercial companies working to expand access to this therapy and continue to refine the technology.

SUMMARY

Surgery has an increasingly important role in the overall treatment strategy of patients with stage IV melanoma. Metastatectomy in patients with well-controlled systemic disease who undergo complete resection can have very long-term disease control and survival. Metastatectomy can also be safely and effectively employed in the palliative setting for symptomatic disease. Furthermore, with the expansion of TIL therapy, metastatectomy has a therapeutic role for personalized development of novel therapeutics. While further studies prospectively evaluating how to best utilize resection in stage IV melanoma are needed, it is clear surgeons will continue to play a pivotal role in this disease.

CLINICS CARE POINTS

- Surgical resection should be considered as part of the treatment strategy for patients with stage IV melanoma in certain clinical contexts.

Disclosures

Dr A.M. Dann has no disclosures. Dr C. Ariyan owns stock in Pfizer and sits on the ad board of Iovance and Merck.

References

[1] Siegel RL, Miller KD, Wagle NS, et al. Cancer statistics, 2023. CA Cancer J Clin 2023;73(1):17–48.
[2] Morton DL, Thompson JF, Cochran AJ, et al. Final Trial Report of Sentinel-Node Biopsy versus Nodal Observation in Melanoma. N Engl J Med 2014;370(7):599–609.
[3] Barth A, Wanek LA, Morton DL. Prognostic factors in 1,521 melanoma patients with distant metastases. J Am Coll Surg 1995;181(3):193–201.
[4] Wolchok JD, Chiarion-Sileni V, Gonzalez R, et al. Long-Term Outcomes With Nivolumab Plus Ipilimumab or Nivolumab Alone Versus Ipilimumab in Patients With Advanced Melanoma. J Clin Oncol 2022;40(2):127–37.
[5] Wong JH, Skinner KA, Kim KA, et al. The role of surgery in the treatment of nonregionally recurrent melanoma. Surgery 1993;113(4):389–94.
[6] Karakousis CP, Velez A, Driscoll DL, et al. Metastasectomy in malignant melanoma. Surgery 1994;115(3):295–302.
[7] Ollila DW, Hsueh EC, Stern SL, et al. Metastasectomy for recurrent stage IV melanoma. J Surg Oncol 1999;71(4):209–13.
[8] Colman MW, Kirkwood JM, Schott T, et al. Does metastasectomy improve survival in skeletal melanoma? Melanoma Res 2014;24(4):354–9.
[9] Faries MB, Leung A, Morton DL, et al. A 20-year experience of hepatic resection for melanoma: is there an expanding role? J Am Coll Surg 2014;219(1):62–8.
[10] Wasif N, Bagaria SP, Ray P, et al. Does metastasectomy improve survival in patients with Stage IV melanoma? A cancer registry analysis of outcomes. J Surg Oncol 2011;104(2):111–5.
[11] Meyer T, Merkel S, Goehl J, et al. Surgical therapy for distant metastases of malignant melanoma. Cancer 2000;89(9):1983–91.
[12] Sosman JA, Moon J, Tuthill RJ, et al. A phase 2 trial of complete resection for stage IV melanoma: results of Southwest Oncology Group Clinical Trial S9430. Cancer 2011;117(20):4740-4706.
[13] Howard JH, Thompson JF, Mozzillo N, et al. Metastasectomy for distant metastatic melanoma: analysis of data from the first Multicenter Selective Lymphadenectomy Trial (MSLT-I). Ann Surg Oncol 2012;19(8):2547–55.
[14] Faries MB, Mozzillo N, Kashani-Sabet M, et al. Long-Term Survival after Complete Surgical Resection and Adjuvant Immunotherapy for Distant Melanoma Metastases. Ann Surg Oncol 2017;24(13):3991–4000.
[15] Livingstone E, Zimmer L, Hassel JC, et al. Adjuvant nivolumab plus ipilimumab or nivolumab alone versus placebo in patients with resected stage IV melanoma with no evidence of disease (IMMUNED): final results of a randomised, double-blind, phase 2 trial. Lancet 2022;400(10358):1117–29.
[16] Ascierto PA, Del Vecchio M, Mandalá M, et al. Adjuvant nivolumab versus ipilimumab in resected stage IIIB-C and stage IV melanoma (CheckMate 238): 4-year results from a multicentre, double-blind, randomised, controlled, phase 3 trial. Lancet Oncol 2020;21(11):1465–77.
[17] Weber JS, Schadendorf D, Del Vecchio M, et al. Adjuvant Therapy of Nivolumab Combined With Ipilimumab Versus Nivolumab Alone in Patients With Resected Stage IIIB-D or Stage IV Melanoma (CheckMate 915). J Clin Oncol 2023;41(3):517–27.
[18] Nelson DW, Fischer TD, Graff-Baker AN, et al. Impact of Effective Systemic Therapy on Metastasectomy in Stage IV Melanoma: A Matched-Pair Analysis. Ann Surg Oncol 2019;26(13):4610–8.

[19] Klemen ND, Feingold PL, Goff SL, et al. Metastasectomy Following Immunotherapy with Adoptive Cell Transfer for Patients with Advanced Melanoma. Ann Surg Oncol 2017;24(1):135–41.
[20] Bello DM, Panageas KS, Hollmann T, et al. Survival Outcomes After Metastasectomy in Melanoma Patients Categorized by Response to Checkpoint Blockade. Ann Surg Oncol 2020;27(4):1180–8.
[21] Li AT, Vakharia K, Lo SN, et al. Survival Outcomes of Salvage Metastasectomy After Failure of Modern-Era Systemic Therapy for Melanoma. Ann Surg Oncol 2021;28(11):6109–23.
[22] Versluis JM, Hendriks AM, Weppler AM, et al. The role of local therapy in the treatment of solitary melanoma progression on immune checkpoint inhibition: A multicentre retrospective analysis. Eur J Cancer 2021;151:72–83.
[23] Patel SP, Othus M, Chen Y, et al. Neoadjuvant–Adjuvant or Adjuvant-Only Pembrolizumab in Advanced Melanoma. N Engl J Med 2023;388(9):813–23.
[24] Lwin TM, Kaelberer Z, Ruan M, et al. Surgical Utilization and Outcomes for Patients with Stage IV Melanoma in the Modern Immunotherapy Era. Ann Surg Oncol 2023;30(8): 5005–12.
[25] Wornom IL 3rd, Smith JW, Soong SJ, et al. Surgery as palliative treatment for distant metastases of melanoma. Ann Surg 1986;204(2):181–5.
[26] Khadra MH, Thompson JF, Milton GW, et al. The justification for surgical treatment of metastatic melanoma of the gastrointestinal tract. Surg Gynecol Obstet 1990;171(5):413–6.
[27] Ollila DW, Essner R, Wanek LA, et al. Surgical resection for melanoma metastatic to the gastrointestinal tract. Arch Surg 1996;131(9):975–9, 979-980.
[28] Rosenberg SA, Restifo NP. Adoptive cell transfer as personalized immunotherapy for human cancer. Science 2015;348(6230):62–8.
[29] Rohaan MW, Borch TH, van den Berg JH, et al. Tumor-Infiltrating Lymphocyte Therapy or Ipilimumab in Advanced Melanoma. N Engl J Med 2022;387(23):2113–25.
[30] Eton O, Legha SS, Moon TE, et al. Prognostic factors for survival of patients treated systemically for disseminated melanoma. J Clin Oncol 1998;16(3):1103–11.
[31] Essner R, Lee JH, Wanek LA, et al. Contemporary surgical treatment of advanced-stage melanoma. Arch Surg 2004;139(9):961–6 [discussion 966-7].
[32] Pogrebniak HW, Stovroff M, Roth JA, et al. Resection of pulmonary metastases from malignant melanoma: results of a 16-year experience. Ann Thorac Surg 1988;46(1):20–3.
[33] Gorenstein LA, Putnam JB, Natarajan G, et al. Improved survival after resection of pulmonary metastases from malignant melanoma. Ann Thorac Surg 1991;52(2):204–10.
[34] Tafra L, Dale PS, Wanek LA, et al. Resection and adjuvant immunotherapy for melanoma metastatic to the lung and thorax. J Thorac Cardiovasc Surg 1995;110(1):119–28 [discussion 129].
[35] Leo F, Cagini L, Rocmans P, et al. Lung metastases from melanoma: when is surgical treatment warranted? Br J Cancer 2000;83(5):569–72.
[36] Andrews S, Robinson L, Cantor A, et al. Survival after surgical resection of isolated pulmonary metastases from malignant melanoma. Cancer Control 2006;13(3):218–23.
[37] Neuman HB, Patel A, Hanlon C, et al. Stage-IV melanoma and pulmonary metastases: factors predictive of survival. Ann Surg Oncol 2007;14(10):2847–53.
[38] Petersen RP, Hanish SI, Haney JC, et al. Improved survival with pulmonary metastasectomy: an analysis of 1720 patients with pulmonary metastatic melanoma. J Thorac Cardiovasc Surg 2007;133(1):104–10.
[39] Agrawal S, Yao TJ, Coit DG. Surgery for melanoma metastatic to the gastrointestinal tract. Ann Surg Oncol 1999;6(4):336–44.
[40] Haigh PI, Essner R, Wardlaw JC, et al. Long-term survival after complete resection of melanoma metastatic to the adrenal gland. Ann Surg Oncol 1999;6(7):633–9.
[41] Rose DM, Essner R, Hughes TM, et al. Surgical resection for metastatic melanoma to the liver: the John Wayne Cancer Institute and Sydney Melanoma Unit experience. Arch Surg 2001;136(8):950–5.

[42] Wood TF, DiFronzo LA, Rose DM, et al. Does complete resection of melanoma metastatic to solid intra-abdominal organs improve survival? Ann Surg Oncol 2001;8(8):658–62.

[43] Mittendorf EA, Lim SJ, Schacherer CW, et al. Melanoma adrenal metastasis: natural history and surgical management. Am J Surg 2008;195(3):363–8 [discussion 368-9].

[44] Collinson FJ, Lam TK, Bruijn WMJ, et al. Long-term survival and occasional regression of distant melanoma metastases after adrenal metastasectomy. Ann Surg Oncol 2008;15(6):1741–9.

[45] Patchell RA, Tibbs PA, Walsh JW, et al. A randomized trial of surgery in the treatment of single metastases to the brain. N Engl J Med 1990;322(8):494–500.

[46] Wroński M, Arbit E. Surgical treatment of brain metastases from melanoma: a retrospective study of 91 patients. J Neurosurg 2000;93(1):9–18.

[47] Fife KM, Colman MH, Stevens GN, et al. Determinants of outcome in melanoma patients with cerebral metastases. J Clin Oncol 2004;22(7):1293–300.

[48] Fletcher WS, Pommier RF, Lum S, et al. Surgical treatment of metastatic melanoma. Am J Surg 1998;175(5):413–7.

Advances in Surgery 58 (2024) 235–247

ADVANCES IN SURGERY

Stem Cell Therapy for Wound Healing in Ischemic Limbs

Is It Effective?

Li Ting Tan, MBBS[a], Farzad Mokhtari-Esbuie, MD[b], Niloufar Shababi, MD[b], John W. Harmon, MD[b,*]

[a]Department of Surgery, The Johns Hopkins Hospital, Blalock 658, 600 North Wolfe Street, Baltimore, MD 21287, USA; [b]Department of Surgery, Johns Hopkins University, Surgery A Building 5th Floor, 4940 Eastern Avenue, Baltimore, MD 21224, USA

Keywords

• Stem cell therapy • Critical limb ischemia • Mesenchymal stem cells • Mononuclear stem cells • Bone marrow-derived cells

Key points

- Stem cell therapy has emerged as a promising option for patients with critical limb ischemia where revascularization is no longer an option.
- The preliminary results of randomized clinical trials have shown that stem cell therapy may aid in wound healing, improvement of symptoms, and possibly reduce amputation rates.
- Multiple options of stem cell therapy include allogeneic or autologous sources harvested from bone marrow, adipose tissue, or human placental and umbilical cord.
- A more recent combination therapy of AMD3100 and low-dose tacrolimus mobilizes stem cells into the intravascular space that negates the need for cell harvest.

INTRODUCTION

As the general population grows older, the prevalence of patients with peripheral arterial disease (PAD) continues to increase. Patients with PAD now encompass about 3% to 10% of the population. A subset of these patients would then continue to progress in severity, resulting in chronic limb-threatening ischemia (CLI) or sometimes known as critical limb ischemia. This is an important clinical

*Corresponding author. *E-mail address:* jharmon@jhmi.edu

https://doi.org/10.1016/j.yasu.2024.04.014
0065-3411/24/

entity to be aware of due to its association with high cardiovascular risk, as well as its increased morbidity and mortality rates. CLI is defined as PAD with the presence of intractable rest pain, gangrene, or ulcerations.

CLI can be devastating to patients due to the significant impact on their quality of life, affected by rest pain and poor wound healing. It also places a significant burden on the health care system due to high treatments costs and poor prognosis associated with the current available treatments. For patients who are not candidates for revascularization options, major amputation might be their only option to prevent progression of infected wounds. Major amputation rates have been reported to be as high as 40% in patients with CLI.

Over the past few decades, researchers have studied the role of cellular therapy for patients with CLI for which revascularization is no longer an option. There have been numerous published studies over the past few years showing promising results, which may be beneficial for this patient population. The various options of cellular therapy that have been studied include hematopoietic stem cell transplantation and mesenchymal stem cells. Numerous preclinical studies have shown that the use of these cells can promote tissue repair by promoting the release of anti-inflammatory factors, regeneration of ischemic tissues, as well as in promoting angiogenesis.

SOURCES OF STEM CELLS

Various sources of stem cells have been proposed and studied for the purpose of tissue regeneration, including different sites of harvest and types of cells isolated. These include bone marrow-derived cells, peripheral blood-derived cells, cells derived from adipose tissue, and the human placenta and umbilical cord (Fig. 1). Each source has certain advantageous properties and associated risks. More recently, mesenchymal stem cells have generated interest among clinicians and researchers alike over recent years due to their multipotent capacity to

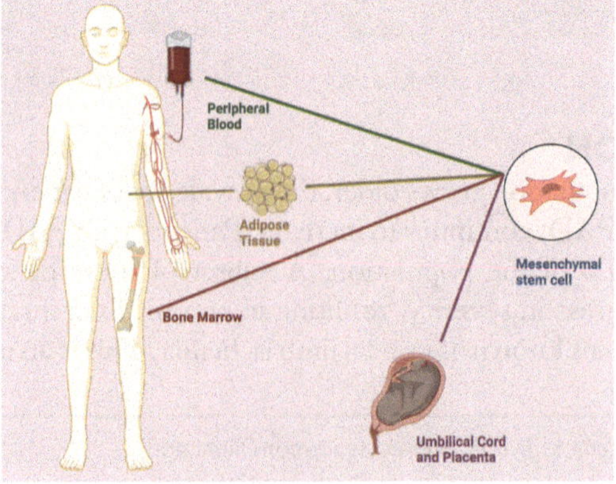

Fig. 1. Sources of stem cells. (Created with BioRender.com.)

differentiate into different cell lines including bone, muscle, cartilage, tendons, ligaments, and fat. In addition, their angiogenic properties are promising for wound healing, especially for ischemic tissue for which blood supply is important. In addition, both allogeneic and autologous cells have been studied. The autologous source of cells is preferable due to the avoidance of immunologic rejection against foreign cells.

Bone marrow-derived stem cells

Bone marrow-derived stem cells can be harvested from different sites including the iliac crest, femoral bone, sternum, and vertebral body. Bone marrow not only provides a high-yield resource of hematopoietic stem cells but also has self-regenerative capacity that makes it a common source of autologous cellular therapy. The downside of bone marrow-derived stem cells is the invasive nature of the cell collection, which requires the patient to be subjected to either local, regional, or sometimes even general anesthesia. Strict aseptic techniques should also be implemented during cell harvest. The blood harvested then undergoes processing including centrifugation, expansion, and isolation of desired cell types prior to administration to patients.

Peripheral blood-derived stem cells

Hematopoietic stem cells have also been discovered to travel in the bloodstream, which has garnered interest due to the less-invasive collection technique. With autologous derivation of stem cells from the peripheral blood, this negates the need for additional anesthesia. Prior to cell collection, patients are administered granulocyte-colony-stimulating factor subcutaneously daily for several days, which has been shown to mobilize stem cells into the bloodstream to increase the yield.

Adipose tissue-derived cells

Adipose tissue-derived cells have recently gained popularity in studies as a substitute for bone marrow-derived cells due to their constant regenerative property. Cells are harvested via liposuction of the abdominal wall adipose tissue under local anesthesia. Similarly, the harvested adipose tissue then undergoes processing to expand the cells and isolate the desired mesenchymal cell type prior to injection. Both allogeneic sources of adipose tissue collected from healthy donors and autologous cells have been studied.

Placenta and umbilical cord-derived cells

A few years ago, the use of embryonic stem cells garnered widespread interest due to its pluripotent capabilities to differentiate into a wide array of cell lineages. However, it soon generated controversy due to ethical concerns surrounding abortion and the use of human embryos. Additionally, clinicians and researchers have raised concerns regarding the possibility of their tumorigenic properties. Instead, studies are now geared toward other forms of fetal stem cells, harvested from the human umbilical cord or placenta. The harvesting process typically occurs at the time of delivery from healthy mothers that have consented for donation.

STEM CELL DELIVERY METHODS

In addition to the multitude of cell types that have been studied, there are also numerous methods of delivery of these cells proposed, and subsequently studied. These include local injection of cells into the subcutaneous space or intramuscular tissue, and intra-arterial injection of the target limb. Intramuscular injection into the gastrocnemius muscle is the preferred method of cell delivery in the literature. This is understandable as intra-arterial injection is more expensive, invasive, and may require additional anesthetics which pose an additional risk to patients. Local intramuscular injection ensures direct implantation of cells into the target ischemic area, while there may be a more widespread delivery of cells via the intra-arterial method of delivery. However, the degree of circulation access to ischemic areas by intra-arterial injection is unclear [1].

For intramuscular injection, patients are often given local anesthesia to relieve pain prior to injection of cells [2]. Cells are then injected into the target limb over multiple sites approximately 2 to 3 cm apart. To ensure safety, patients then undergo monitoring of their vital signs, injection sites, and overall symptoms for side effects.

Angiographic guidance is utilized for intra-arterial injection of cell therapy. Patients will be given moderate sedation during the start of the procedure, while general anesthesia is rarely required. Local anesthesia is then given at the access site prior to either direct hand injection or slow infusion. Arterial delivery into the common femoral artery is preferred for more proximal wounds, while the distal superficial femoral artery may be considered to treat more distal wound sites [3,4]. Similarly, patients then undergo observation for a few hours to monitor for side effects. Although there is the added risk of complications related to vascular access, hence the site of injection should be monitored as well. These patients typically require preoperative heparin to reduce the risk of intra-arterial thrombus.

Several studies have been conducted to compare the outcomes of intramuscular or intra-arterial injection, which have shown that both approaches were not only safe, but there were no significant differences in the effectiveness of the treatment [5,6]. In a study done by Klepanec and colleagues, the authors randomized 41 patients with advanced CLI to treatment with autologous bone marrow cells through either local intramuscular ($n = 21$) or selective intra-arterial infusion ($n = 20$) with the same amount of stem cells delivered [6]. The authors found that there were no significant differences in prevalence of limb salvage at 6 months and wound healing in both groups.

PUBLISHED EXPERIENCE

The possibility of treating CLI with cellular therapy has resulted in numerous clinical trials being conducted, with interesting, published results. Initial phase 1 trials listed in Table 1 have shown the safety and feasibility of this approach.

Table 1
Summary of phase 1 clinical trials to study the safety and feasibility

Study	Sample	Intervention	Allogeneic vs autologous	Route	Number of cells	Follow-up	Conclusion
Kirana et al [7], 2012	24	BM-MNC	Autologous	IM	50×10^6	52 wk	Transplantation of BM-MNC was safe and feasible, and shown to improve microcirculation and wound healing.
Das et al [8], 2013	8	BM-MSC	Allogeneic	IA	2×10^6 cells/kg body weight	6 mo	It was concluded that intra-arterial BM-MSC could be safely administered to patients with CLI.
Lasala et al [9], 2010	10	BM-MNC and BM-MSC	Autologous	IM	Unclear	10 mo	Safe, feasible, and appears effective.
Shirbaghaee et al [10], 2023	8	Placenta-MSC	Allogeneic	IM	20 or 60×10^6	6 mo	Safe and well tolerated and may dramatically improve physical performance and minimize inflammatory conditions in patients with CLI.

Abbreviations: BM-MNC, bone marrow-derived mononuclear cells; BM-MSC, bone marrow-derived mesenchymal cells; CLI, chronic limb-threatening ischemia; IA, intra-arterial; IM, intramuscular.

In these early studies, patients were monitored closely via assessment of their vital signs, symptoms, and blood chemistry analysis after cell therapy administration. In a study by Lasala and colleagues [9], the authors demonstrated the absence of immediate and short-term clinical complications with local intramuscular injection of bone marrow-derived cells, which showed the safety of this approach. The patients were followed further for up to 10 ± 2 months, where the authors were able to note improvements in hemodynamics and clinical symptoms even in these early phase 1 studies. Researchers were also exploring different methods of cell administration, as described earlier.

Since then, there have been multiple randomized, controlled trials that have been performed to try to determine the efficacy of stem cell therapy. Seventeen of these studies reported in the literature have been compiled in Tables 2 and 3 to showcase the methods and results of these trials. Examples of parameters that have been studied include amputation rates, rest pain, ulcer healing, ankle–brachial index, pain-free walking distance, transcutaneous oxygen pressure measurements (TcO_2), and quality of life assessment. In addition, there are more than a hundred trials listed in clinicaltrials.gov that are in various stages of development, which shows the general interest from clinicians and researchers alike regarding this new therapeutic method.

The results of these published randomized clinical trials have been variable. Many of the smaller, earlier trials have shown positive results for most of the parameters measured. Unfortunately, the current largest, double-blinded, placebo-controlled trial, JUVENTAS, done in the Netherlands which included 160 patients failed to show a benefit in any of the outcome measures. It is important to note that the authors have concluded that their study's failure to show benefit does not prove futility of the approach, as there may yet be discovered benefits of other cell sources or subpopulations, different administration methods or in patients with milder disease.

While the safety of cellular therapy has been demonstrated, it is important to note that the strategies differ widely among the numerous studies published, which could influence the study results. These include the cell dose, the number of treatments whether single or repeated, intervals between treatments if multiple administered and cell source and type. Further study is warranted to investigate the best outcomes from the different cellular therapy strategies.

FUTURE OPTIONS: THE ROLE OF ENDOGENOUS STEM CELLS

Most of the autologous options discussed involved harvesting of cells either from the bone marrow, adipose tissue, or even peripheral blood which subjects these patients to an additional procedure, sometimes under either local or general anesthesia. Moreover, these harvested cells will have to undergo additional processing in order to isolate and expand the desired cell type, which can be expensive and time consuming. An alternative option is medical treatment to release endogenous stems cells into the circulation where they can then travel to areas of inflammation.

Table 2
Summary of randomized, controlled trials to study efficacy

Study	Sample (T/C)	Intervention		Allogen vs autologous	Route	Number of cells	Number of treatments
		Treatment	Control				
Gupta et al [11], 2013	18 (8/10)	BM-MSC	Placebo	Allogeneic	IM	2×10^9	1
Debin et al [2], 2008	45 (22/23)	BM-MSC	Standard care	Autologous	IM	7.32×10^8–5.61×10^9	1
Dash et al [12], 2009	24 (12/12)	BM-MSC	Standard care	Autologous	IM	4.5–6.0×10^7	1
Skora et al [13], 2015	32 (16/16)	BM-MNC + VEGF	Pentoxifylline	Autologous	IM	0.77–3.83×10^9	1
Pignon et al [14], 2017- BALI	36 (17/19)	BM-MNC	Placebo	Autologous	IM	1.3×10^9–33.5×10^6	1
Arai et al [15], 2006	25 (13/12)	BM-MNC	Standard care	Autologous	IM	1–3×10^9	1
Li et al [16], 2013	58 (29/29)	BM-MNC	Placebo	Autologous	IM	5×10^8 - 1.2×10^9	1
Huang et al [17], 2005	28 (14/14)	G-CSF-mobilized PB-MNC	Prostaglandin E1	Autologous	IM	3×10^9	2 (40 d intervals)
Ozturk et al [18], 2012	40 (20/20)	G-CSF-mobilized PB-MNC	Standard care	Autologous	IM	2.48×10^7	1
Mohammadzadeh et al [19], 2013	21 (7/14)	G-CSF-mobilized PB-MNC	Placebo	Autologous	IM	2×10^7	1
Szabo et al [20], 2013	20 (10/10)	VesCell, PB-stem cells	Standard care	Autologous	IM	$66.4 \pm 19.2 \times 10^6$	1
Benoit et al [21], 2011	48 (34/14)	BM-stem cells (unspecified)	Placebo	Autologous	IM	Unclear	1
Jain et al [22], 2011	48 (25/23)	BM-stem cells (unspecified)	Placebo	Autologous	IM, topical	Unclear	1
Powell et al [23], 2012	72 (48/24)	BM-stem cells (unspecified)	Standard care	Autologous	IM	0.35–2.95×10^8	1
Teraa et al [24], 2015—JUVENTAS	160 (81/79)	BM-MNC	Placebo	Autologous	IA	5×10^8	3 (3 wk intervals)
Walter et al [25], 2011—PROVASA	40 (19/21)	BM-MNC	Placebo	Autologous	IA	1.53–1.65×10^8	1

Abbreviations: BM, bone marrow; BM-MNC, bone marrow-derived mononuclear cells; BM-MSC, bone marrow-derived mesenchymal cells; C, control; G-CSF, granulocyte colony–stimulating factor; PB, peripheral blood; PB-MNC, peripheral blood mononuclear cells; T, treatment; VEGF, vascular endothelial growth factor.

Color shades: It groups the different published papers into type of intervention given and route of intervention for ease of interpretation of the table/results.

Table 3
Results of randomized controlled trials from Table 2

Study	Follow-up	ABI	Rest pain	Pain-free walking distance	TcO2	Major amputation rates	Angiographic	Ulcer healing
Gupta et al [11], 2013	6 mo	1	2	n/a	n/a	0	n/a	2
Debin et al [2], 2008	3 mo	1	1	1	n/a	1	n/a	1
Dash et al [12], 2009	3 mo	n/a	1	1	n/a	n/a	n/a	1
Skora et al [13], 2015	3 mo	1	1	n/a	n/a	1	1	1
Pignon et al [14], 2017- BALI	6 mo	0	0	n/a	2	1	n/a	0
Arai et al [15], 2006	1 mo	1	1	n/a	1	n/a	n/a	1
Li et al [16], 2013	6 mo	1	1	n/a	n/a	0	n/a	1
Huang et al [17], 2005	3 mo	1	1	1	n/a	1	1	1
Ozturk et al [18], 2012	3 mo	1	2	2	1	0	0	1
Mohammadzadeh et al [19], 2013	3 mo	1	n/a	1	n/a	1	n/a	1
Szabo et al [20], 2013	3 mo	1	1	n/a	1	1	n/a	1
Benoit et al [21], 2011	26 wk	0	n/a	n/a	n/a	0	n/a	n/a
Jain et al [22], 2011	3 mo	n/a	n/a	n/a	n/a	n/a	n/a	1
Powell et al [23], 2012	12 mo	n/a	n/a	n/a	n/a	0	n/a	n/a
Teraa et al [24], 2015 - JUVENTAS	6 mo	2	2	n/a	2	0	n/a	2
Walter et al [25], 2011 - PROVASA	3 mo	0	1	n/a	0	0	n/a	1

Abbreviations: ABI, ankle-brachial index; n/a, not assessed; TcO2, transcutaneous oxygen pressure measurements; 0, no improvement in treatment group; 1, improvement in treatment group with significant difference; 2, improvement in both groups without significant difference.

A promising therapy of this type is being developed at the Johns Hopkins Hospital. Early therapeutic benefits are seen in a combination therapy of 2 Food and Drug Administration (FDA)-approved drugs. One of which is AMD3100, used to release hematopoietic stem cells to facilitate bone marrow transplantation for cancer therapy. The other drug in the combination therapy is tacrolimus which is commonly used for immunosuppression. When AMD3100 and tacrolimus are used in combination, also known as AF combination therapy, tacrolimus is given at a low dose that does not cause immunosuppression. At this dose, it converts the population of stem cells released into the circulation to a regenerative phenotype that is rich in CD133+ cells.

In a double-blinded randomized animal study by Lin and colleagues, the authors studied the effects of the AF combination therapy on the duration of complete healing of full-thickness wounds in mice [26]. They have divided the surgically wounded mice randomly into 4 groups, receiving either (1) saline as the control group; (2) low-dose tacrolimus; (3) AMD3100 every other day; and (4) combination of low-dose tacrolimus and AMD3100. They have found that monotherapy with either AMD3100 or low-dose tacrolimus exhibited moderate, faster healing time of 11 days compared to 12 days in the control group. Astonishingly, the group of mice treated with the AF combination therapy showed a 25% reduction in complete healing time, down to 9 days. In fact, Tolar described that "very few articles have the potential to change clinical practice; this one does," in a commentary article of this study in noting the clinical implications of this combination therapy [27]. In addition, Lin and colleagues also found an increase in hair follicle regeneration and reduced scar formation in mice receiving the AF combination therapy, as shown in Fig. 2.

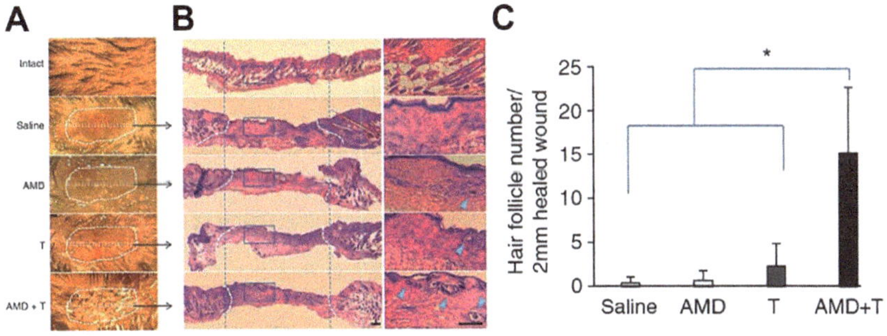

Fig. 2. AF combination therapy promotes hair follicle regeneration in healed skin of mice. (*A*) Macroscopic appearance of re-epithelialized wounds on day 15. (*B*) Microscopic sections from the middle of scars showing new hair follicles within healed wounds, with the scarred area outlined by broken lines. (*C*) Graphical presentation of the number of hair follicles per 2 mm healed wound. Data represent mean and standard error of mean (n = 9). **P*<.01. (Figures reproduced with permission from study done by Lin Q, Wesson RN, Maeda H, et al. Pharmacological Mobilization of Endogenous Stem Cells Significantly Promotes Skin Regeneration after Full-Thickness Excision: The Synergistic Activity of AMD3100 and Tacrolimus. Journal of Investigative Dermatology. 2014;134(9):2458-2468. doi:https://doi.org/10.1038/jid.2014.162.)

In a subsequent study published a few years later, the authors aimed to investigate the role of tacrolimus (FK506) in wound healing by substituting FK506 with a non-immunosuppressive FK506 analog named FKVP.[28] FKVP, like FK506 binds to FK506-binding protein 12 which then goes on to activate the bone morphogenetic protein-signaling pathway. However, FKVP does not have the immunosuppressive calcineurin-inhibiting effects that are present in FK506. The investigators performed an animal study to determine the wound healing effect of FKVP on a rat model of type 2 diabetes with 4 full-thickness wounds each. Wounded rats were divided randomly into 3 groups, receiving subcutaneous injections of either (1) saline, (2) AMD3100 plus FK506 (AF group), or (3) AMD3100 plus FKVP (AV group). The authors found that the AV group displayed a shorter average healing time of 20 days to reach complete re-epithelialization compared to 26 days in the saline group, equivalent to the AF group of 21 days. Fig. 3 shows photographic and graphical comparison of wound healing time among type 2 diabetic rats between each group. These are initial animal studies, further safety clinical trials are required as the next step to further study this promising therapy.

CURRENTLY AVAILABLE STEM CELL THERAPY

To conclude this study, we find it important to describe some of the commercially available stem cell products. A quick online search for stem cell therapies yields

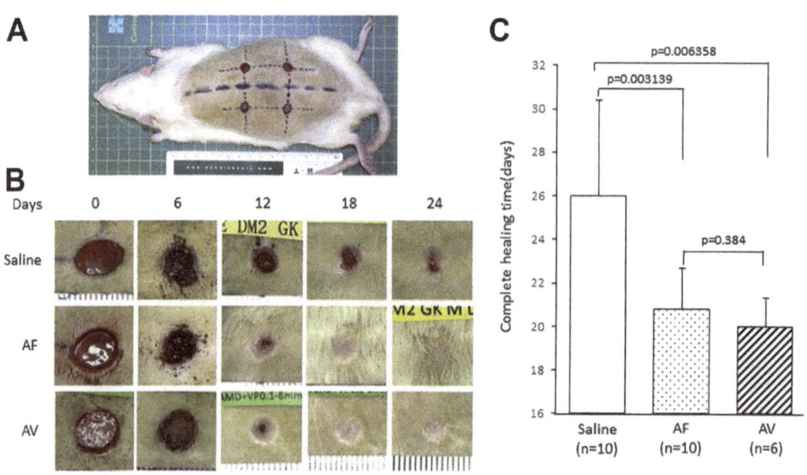

Fig. 3. Comparison of wound healing between AF combination therapy, AV combination therapy, or saline as a control. (*A*) Wound model of 4 full-thickness wounds with a diameter of 8 mm created on type 2 diabetic rats. (*B*) Photographic comparison between each group, showing accelerated wound healing in the AV and AF groups. (*C*) Graphical presentation comparing complete healing time between groups. (*Figures reproduced with permission from study done by* Peiffer BJ, Qi L, Ahmadi AR, et al. Activation of BMP Signaling by FKBP12 Ligands Synergizes with Inhibition of CXCR4 to Accelerate Wound Healing. *Cell Chem Biol.* 2019;26(5):652-661.e4. https://doi.org/10.1016/j.chembiol.2019.01.011.)

multiple entries, some targeted specifically toward patients with non-healing wounds as a result of CLI. Several online write-ups have asserted that stem cell therapies have been observed to be beneficial in wound healing, including "the association with a major reduction in amputation rate with 41% fewer patients needing amputation than the control group" and "the significantly increased probability of ulcer healing, improved symptoms like pain and difficulty walking."

We know from our careful review of the literature that the current evidence is conflicting and do not currently prove the absolute benefit of stem cell therapy for CLI yet. In fact, the use of stem cell therapy for CLI has not been approved by the FDA. With this, the cost of stem cell treatments is high and not covered by insurance, which could amount up to US$15,000 at the time of writing. The final assessment is that continued trials are needed in search of a more effective stem cell therapy type and delivery system.

CLINICS CARE POINTS

- Stem cell therapy is a promising option for patients with critical limb ischemia where revascularization is no longer an option.
- Stem cell therapy have been shown to aid in wound healing, improvement of symptoms, and possibly reduce amputation rates.
- Options for stem cell therapy inclide allogeneic or autologous sources harvested from bone marrow, adipose tissue, or human placental and umbilical cord. However, current evidence is conflicting and do not currently prove the absolute benefit of stem cell therapy for critical limb ischemia yet.
- The cost of stem cell treatments is high, and not currently FDA-approved.

Disclosure

Dr J.W. Harmon is a founding member of MedRegen Baltimore, Maryland, which was established to develop a therapeutic to mobilize endogenous stem cells for wound healing.

References

[1] Chavakis E, Aicher A, Heeschen C, et al. Role of β2-integrins for homing and neovascularization capacity of endothelial progenitor cells. J Exp Med 2004;201(1):63–72.

[2] Debin L, Youzhao J, Ziwen L, et al. Autologous transplantation of bone marrow mesenchymal stem cells on diabetic patients with lower limb ischemia★ ★Supported by the Clinical Research Fund of Southwest Hospital at Third Military Medical University (SWH2005A109). J Med Coll PLA 2008;23(2):106–15.

[3] Lenk K, Adams V, Lurz P, et al. Therapeutical potential of blood-derived progenitor cells in patients with peripheral arterial occlusive disease and critical limb ischaemia. Eur Heart J 2005;26(18):1903–9.

[4] Chochola M, Pytlík R, Kobylka P, et al. Autologous intra-arterial infusion of bone marrow mononuclear cells in patients with critical leg ischemia. Int Angiol 2008;27(4):281–90. Available at: http://europepmc.org/abstract/MED/18677289.

[5] quan GUY, ZHANG J, GUO L rui, et al. Transplantation of autologous bone marrow mononuclear cells for patients with lower limb ischemia. Chin Med J (Engl) 2008;121(11). Available at: https://journals.lww.com/cmj/fulltext/2008/06010/transplantation_of_autologous_bone_marrow.1.aspx.
[6] Klepanec A, Mistrik M, Altaner C, et al. No Difference in Intra-Arterial and Intramuscular Delivery of Autologous Bone Marrow Cells in Patients with Advanced Critical Limb Ischemia. Cell Transplant 2012;21(9):1909–18.
[7] Kirana S, Stratmann B, Prante C, et al. Autologous stem cell therapy in the treatment of limb ischaemia induced chronic tissue ulcers of diabetic foot patients. Int J Clin Pract 2012;66(4): 384–93.
[8] Das AK, Abdullah BB, Dhillon SS, et al. Intra-arterial Allogeneic Mesenchymal Stem Cells for Critical Limb Ischemia are Safe and Efficacious: Report of a Phase I Study. World J Surg 2013;37(4):915–22.
[9] Lasala GP, Silva JA, Gardner PA, et al. Combination stem cell therapy for the treatment of severe limb ischemia: safety and efficacy analysis. Angiology 2010;61(6):551–6.
[10] Shirbaghaee Z, Heidari Keshel S, Rasouli M, et al. Report of a phase 1 clinical trial for safety assessment of human placental mesenchymal stem cells therapy in patients with critical limb ischemia (CLI). Stem Cell Res Ther 2023;14(1):174.
[11] Gupta PK, Chullikana A, Parakh R, et al. A double blind randomized placebo controlled phase I/II study assessing the safety and efficacy of allogeneic bone marrow derived mesenchymal stem cell in critical limb ischemia. J Transl Med 2013;11(1):143.
[12] Dash NR, Dash SN, Routray P, et al. Targeting nonhealing ulcers of lower extremity in human through autologous bone marrow-derived mesenchymal stem cells. Rejuvenation Res 2009;12(5):359–66.
[13] Skóra J, Pupka A, Janczak D, et al. Clinical research
Combined autologous bone marrow mononuclear cell and gene therapy as the last resort for patients with critical limb ischemia. Arch Med Sci 2015;11(2):325–31.
[14] Pignon B, Sevestre MA, Kanagaratnam L, et al. Autologous bone marrow mononuclear cell implantation and its impact on the outcome of patients with critical limb ischemia — results of a randomized, double-blind, placebo-controlled trial. Circ J 2017;81(11):1713–20.
[15] Arai M, Misao Y, Nagai H, et al. Granulocyte colony-stimulating factor. Circ J 2006;70(9): 1093–8.
[16] Min L, Hua Z, Xing J, et al. Autologous bone marrow mononuclear cells transplant in patients with critical leg ischemia: preliminary clinical results. Experimental and Clinical Transplantation 2013;11(5):435–9.
[17] Huang P, Li S, Han M, et al. Autologous transplantation of granulocyte colony–stimulating factor–mobilized peripheral blood mononuclear cells improves critical limb ischemia in diabetes. Diabetes Care 2005;28(9):2155–60.
[18] Ozturk A, Kucukardali Y, Tangi F, et al. Therapeutical potential of autologous peripheral blood mononuclear cell transplantation in patients with type 2 diabetic critical limb ischemia. J Diabet Complicat 2012;26(1):29–33.
[19] Mohammadzadeh SH, Keshavarzi A, Alimoghaddam K, et al. Therapeutic outcomes of transplanting autologous granulocyte colony-stimulating factor-mobilised peripheral mononuclear cells in diabetic patients with critical limb ischaemia. Exp Clin Endocrinol Diabetes 2013;121(01):48–53.
[20] Szabó GV, Kövesd Z, Cserepes J, et al. Peripheral blood-derived autologous stem cell therapy for the treatment of patients with late-stage peripheral artery disease—results of the short- and long-term follow-up. Cytotherapy 2013;15(10):1245–52.
[21] Benoit E, O'Donnell TF, Iafrati MD, et al. The role of amputation as an outcome measure in cellular therapy for critical limb ischemia: implications for clinical trial design. J Transl Med 2011;9(1):165.

[22] Jain P, Perakath B, Jesudason MR, et al. The effect of autologous bone marrow-derived cells on healing chronic lower extremity wounds: results of a randomized controlled study. Wound Manag Prev 2011;57(7):38–44.
[23] Powell RJ, Marston WA, Berceli SA, et al. Cellular therapy with ixmyelocel-t to treat critical limb ischemia: the randomized, double-blind, placebo-controlled RESTORE-CLI Trial. Mol Ther 2012;20(6):1280–6.
[24] Teraa M, Sprengers RW, Schutgens REG, et al. Effect of repetitive intra-arterial infusion of bone marrow mononuclear cells in patients with no-option limb ischemia. Circulation 2015;131(10):851–60.
[25] Walter DH, Krankenberg H, Balzer JO, et al. Intraarterial administration of bone marrow mononuclear cells in patients with critical limb ischemia. Circ Cardiovasc Interv 2011;4(1): 26–37.
[26] Lin Q, Wesson RN, Maeda H, et al. Pharmacological mobilization of endogenous stem cells significantly promotes skin regeneration after full-thickness excision: the synergistic activity of AMD3100 and tacrolimus. J Invest Dermatol 2014;134(9):2458–68.
[27] Tolar J, McGrath JA. Augmentation of cutaneous wound healing by pharmacologic mobilization of endogenous bone marrow stem cells. J Invest Dermatol 2014;134(9):2312–4.

Advances in Surgery 58 (2024) 249–273

ADVANCES IN SURGERY

Use of Extracorporeal Membrane Oxygenation for Patients with Coronavirus Disease 2019 Infection

Jessica M. Ruck, MD, PhD[a], Errol L. Bush, MD[a,*]

[a]Division of Thoracic Surgery, Department of Surgery, Johns Hopkins University School of Medicine, Baltimore, MD, USA

Keywords

• Extracorporeal membrane oxygenation • COVID-19 • Coronavirus
• Cardiac failure • Respiratory failure • VV ECMO

Key points

- The best available evidence suggests that ECMO initiation reduces mortality in patients with severe COVID-19 infection complicated by hypoxemia.
- Clinical management of patients on ECMO for severe COVID-19 should follow criteria established prior to the pandemic with severe respiratory disease.
- Lung transplantation is a viable treatment option for patients on prolonged ECMO for severe COVID-19 infection, and selection criteria continue to evolve.

INTRODUCTION

The coronavirus disease 2019 (COVID-19) pandemic was a cataclysmic event that infected over 772 million and killed over 6.9 million people worldwide [1]. The pandemic pushed hospitals and society to their limits and resulted in incredibly severe respiratory disease in millions of people. This severe respiratory disease often necessitated maximum medical therapy, including the use of extracorporeal membrane oxygenation (ECMO). While our understanding of COVID-19 and its treatment continue to evolve, we review the current evidence to guide the care of patients with severe COVID-19 infection.

*Corresponding author. Johns Hopkins Medical Institutions, Blalock 240, 600 North Wolfe Street, Baltimore, MD 21287. *E-mail address:* errol.bush@jhu.edu

https://doi.org/10.1016/j.yasu.2024.05.003
0065-3411/24/

EXTRACORPOREAL MEMBRANE OXYGENATION

ECMO is a technique used to support patients during episodes of severe respiratory and/or cardiac failure unresponsive to optimal medical management and conventional therapies. Veno-venous (VV) ECMO provides gas exchange and is used to manage severe respiratory failure, while veno-arterial (VA) ECMO both provides gas exchange and augments native cardiac output and is therefore used to manage severe cardiac failure [2]. In VV ECMO, deoxygenated blood is drained from a large-diameter (ie central) vein and circulated through a membrane in which gas exchange occurs, removing carbon dioxide and adding oxygen. The oxygenated blood is then reinfused into a central vein for circulation throughout the body. In VA ECMO, deoxygenated blood is similarly removed from a central vein before undergoing gas exchange, but oxygenated blood is returned into the arterial system.

HISTORIC AND CURRENT USE OF EXTRACORPOREAL MEMBRANE OXYGENATION

Use of ECMO for the treatment of respiratory and cardiac failure has increased over the last several decades, with a dramatic increase in use over the past several years due to the COVID-19 pandemic. Prior to the COVID-19 pandemic, interest in ECMO increased in 2009 during the influenza A (H1N1) pandemic [3,4]. That same year, the Conventional ventilatory support versus Extracorporal membrane oxygenation for Severe Adult Respiratory failure multicenter randomized controlled trial evaluated adult patients with severe respiratory failure and found that transfer to an ECMO center was associated with significantly lower risk of mortality or severe disability at 6 months [5]. Criticisms of the study noted that this benefit might be due to the experience and specialized care at these centers, as not all patients transferred to ECMO centers received ECMO [6]. Nearly a decade later, a second randomized controlled trial was designed to better define the role of ECMO in the management of severe acute respiratory distress syndrome (ARDS). The 2018 ECMO to Rescue Lung Injury in Severe ARDS (EOLIA) trial randomized patients either to ECMO or to standard of care [7], which was defined as protocolized mechanical ventilation [8]. The study was terminated early for futility at a prespecified interim analysis. At that time, the 11% mortality benefit (35% vs 46%) observed at 60 days did not reach statistical significance. However, subsequent re-evaluations of the data using Bayesian analysis found a significant survival benefit associated with the early initiation of ECMO [9]. The inclusion criteria used in the EOLIA trial continue to guide evaluations of ECMO candidacy in patients with severe ARDS. These criteria include a ratio of arterial oxygen partial pressure to fractional inspired oxygen (PaO_2/FiO_2 ratio) lower than 50 mm Hg for more than 3 hours, a PaO_2/FiO_2 ratio lower than 80 mm Hg for more than 6 hours, and a pH lower than 7.25 with a partial pressure of carbon dioxide ($PaCO_2$) greater than or equal to 60 mm Hg for more than 6 hours [8,10].

Of note, technological improvements in ECMO circuit parts, including pumps, tubing, and membrane lungs, have improved gas exchange and reduced complications. For example, polymethylpentene membranes have been introduced and are replacing silicone rubber polymer and polypropylene membranes [11]. Additionally, the centrifugal pumps within the circuit require smaller filling volumes than the previous roller pumps [12].

SEVERE CORONAVIRUS DISEASE 2019-RELATED DISEASE

While COVID-19 infection can affect multiple organs, it most commonly caused respiratory symptoms [13,14]. In severe infections, this led to the development of ARDS, resulting in an increase in anatomic shunt and a reduction of functional lung size. The physiologic shunt observed was due to both a loss of hypoxic pulmonary vasoconstriction and an increase in dead space secondary to pulmonary vascular microthrombi [15,16]. While the ARDS picture was the most common severe lung disease phenotype observed, a progressive fibrotic phenotype was also noted and was potentially more common among people who had underlying lung disease. Notably, the post-COVID-19 pulmonary fibrosis phenotype developed later than the ARDS phenotype, typically 4 to 12 weeks after initial infection, and was seen among patients with all stages of severity of their initial COVID-19 infection, including among patients who did not require mechanical ventilation [17].

In addition to respiratory disease, a minority of patients with severe disease developed right ventricular dysfunction secondary to massive pulmonary embolus or other causes, COVID-19 myocarditis, stress cardiomyopathy, arrhythmias, or acute coronary syndrome and required VA ECMO [18–22]. Unless otherwise noted, the focus of this study will be on VV ECMO, on which there is substantially greater evidence given the greater requirement for and use of VV ECMO versus VA ECMO for the treatment of severe COVID-19 infection.

EARLY CORONAVIRUS DISEASE 2019 EXTRACORPOREAL MEMBRANE OXYGENATION EXPERIENCE

Early in the COVID-19 pandemic, the recognition that severe COVID-19 infection resulted in ARDS prompted immediate consideration of ECMO for treatment. This otherwise young and healthy patient population was, in many ways, similar to what was seen in the H1N1 pandemic [3,4] and met EOLIA criteria. However, 2 early studies of ECMO use for the treatment of severe COVID-19 infection found high mortality rates, resulting in initial hesitancy to use ECMO given poor results and strains on hospital resources [23,24]. Later, a retrospective cohort study from France reported a 31% 50 day mortality and 36% 90 day mortality in 83 patients supported with VV ECMO for COVID-19-related ARDS from March 8, 2020 through May 2, 2020 [25]. These results were similar to the 35% 60 day mortality observed in the ECMO arm of the 2018 EOLIA trial and prompted renewed interest in ECMO–particularly VV ECMO–for the treatment of severe COVID-19-related disease [8]. Cohort studies from the United States, South America, Europe, and the Middle East soon followed and reported overall similar results [25–30]. These studies of the so-called first wave of COVID-19 reported a 90 day mortality rate of 36% to 47% [25–28]. The regional nature of these early studies, which might have been influenced by differences in patient casemix and degree of resource strain, prompted evaluation of global data from the Extracorporeal Life Support Organization (ELSO) registry. Reassuringly, an ELSO study of 213 hospitals across 36 countries estimated a 90 day cumulative in-hospital mortality of 37.4% for this "first wave," consistent with the prior studies [27] and with the EOLIA trial [7].

However, there were signs of higher mortality rate in some cohort studies, such as a study of 302 patients in Paris, France, between March 2020 and June 2020 (54.3% 90 day mortality) and a study of 3397 patients in Germany from March 2020 through May 2021 (68% overall in-hospital mortality) [31,32]. Unlike the other studies, the German study had the only unselected national cohort, making it a sort of "pragmatic" trial of ECMO for COVID-19 and possibly a more realistic reflection of outcomes [33]. ECMO use in Germany is neither regulated nor restricted, allowing any hospital to start an ECMO program, if it chooses [33].

EVOLVING CORONAVIRUS DISEASE 2019 EXTRACORPOREAL MEMBRANE OXYGENATION EXPERIENCE

Multiple analyses noted an increase in mortality for patients with COVID-19 on ECMO as the pandemic progressed, with absolute increases in mortality of 12% to 18% noted [34–36]. This was confirmed by an evaluation of EuroELSO [34] as well as an updated study from ELSO including 4812 COVID-19 ECMO patients with ECMO initiation in 2020 [37]. This ELSO analysis found a 36.9% 90 day mortality for patients cannulated on or before May 1, 2020, a 51.9% 90 day mortality for patients cannulated after May 1, 2020 at those same centers, and a 58.9% 90 day mortality for patients cannulated after May 1, 2020 at other centers [37]. This underscores that the increase in mortality was seen even at centers with lower initial mortality but also suggests that mortality was even higher at centers that were later to adopt ECMO for the treatment of patients with COVID-19. More recently, an analysis by Jacobs and colleagues divided the pandemic into 4 time periods and assigned patients to a time period by ECMO cannulation date. They found that the odds of survival decreased after the "first wave" and have varied significantly between subsequent time periods, reflecting the dynamic nature of the pandemic [38].

Numerous potential explanations have been put forth to explain the variable mortality risk observed between different studies as well as between time periods during the pandemic. These include differences in patient selection, treatment selection, treatment course (ie longer use of noninvasive ventilation prior to ECMO cannulation, allowing self-inflicted injury or inclusion of more patients with refractory disease), superinfection secondary to increased use of immunosuppression, viral variant, experience of centers using of ECMO, and resource limitations [33,39].

EFFECTIVENESS OF EXTRACORPOREAL MEMBRANE OXYGENATION FOR THE TREATMENT OF CORONAVIRUS DISEASE 2019

There are no randomized controlled trials of ECMO for the treatment of severe COVID-19 infection. Therefore, reviewing the data on the effectiveness of ECMO requires a recognition that these observational trials are uncontrolled and, therefore, may suffer from selection bias and unmeasured confounding even with appropriately-applied statistical techniques. However, the observational studies that exist include nationally representative cohorts in the United States using the National Inpatient Sample (NIS) database. Unfortunately, these have provided conflicting results (Table 1), with Ahmad and colleagues finding that VV ECMO was associated with 33% lower risk of mortality (adjusted HR [aHR] 0.67, 95% confidence interval [CI] 0.57–0.79, $P < .0001$) but Watanabe and colleagues finding no association between the use of ECMO and mortality (adjusted odds ratio [aOR] 1.03, 95% CI 0.86–1.24) [40,41]. Given that the same database was used for these 2 studies, this underscores the challenge of answering the question of effectiveness of ECMO with observational data and the influence that differences in statistical analysis (ie, model type and covariates) can have on the study results. Several groups have attempted to circumvent these issues using propensity score-matched analyses and meta-analyses, with Intrambarya and colleagues and Stessel and colleagues both finding higher mortality associated with ECMO [42,43], though there are lingering concerns that these studies do not consider the temporal changes in COVID-19 and ECMO-associated mortality over the course of the pandemic.

To date, the best evidence regarding the effectiveness of ECMO comes from emulated target trials. While these include patient populations drawn from diverse regions and from different time periods during the pandemic, these studies consistently find that ECMO is associated with a mortality benefit, albeit at different time points [44–47]. Shaefi and colleagues concluded that ECMO initiation was associated with a 45% reduction in 60 day hospital mortality (HR 0.55, 95%CI 0.40–0.77) among patients with severe hypoxemia (PaO_2/FiO_2 <80 mm Hg) [45]. A multicenter European COVID-ICU study found that ECMO initiation was associated with improved survival at 7 days but inferior survival at 90 days; however, the inferior results at 90 days were attenuated after restriction of the analysis to high-volume centers [46]. Finally, a study by the COVID-19 Critical Care Consortium Investigators found that ECMO was associated with lower 60 day mortality than mechanical ventilation alone for COVID-19 patients with severe hypoxemia [47]. Specifically, they found lower mortality among patients who were younger (<65 years), with severe hypoxemia (PaO_2/FiO_2 <80 mm Hg), had shorter duration of invasive mechanical ventilation ($\leq$10 days), and had higher driving pressures (>15 cm H_2O) for their mechanical ventilation. Most recently, Whitmore and colleagues found that adjusted in-hospital mortality was lower in patients receiving ECMO versus mechanical ventilation only (38.8% vs 60.1%, $P < .001$) [44]. They found that ECMO was associated with higher likelihood of liberation from mechanical

Table 1
Effectiveness of veno-venous extracorporeal membrane oxygenation for treatment of coronavirus disease 2019

Authors	Study period	Population/Data source	N	Notes	Outcome	Estimate (95% CI) ECMO vs non-ECMO
Ahmad et al [41], 2023	*Not explicitly stated*	US Healthcare Cost and Utilization Project 2020 National Inpatient Sample	98,528 mechanically ventilated patients with a primary diagnosis of COVID-19	Included patients on VV and VA ECMO	All-cause inpatient mortality	aHR 0.67 (0.57–0.79), $P < .0001$
Watanabe et al [40], 2023	January 1, 2020 to December 31, 2020	US National Inpatient Sample	72,415 mechanically ventilated patients with COVID-19 ARDS	Included patients on VV and VA ECMO	In-hospital mortality	VV ECMO: aOR 1.03 (0.86–1.24) VA ECMO: aHR 1.18 (0.64–2.15)
Indrambarya et al [42], 2023	Articles published December 2019 to December 2020	Pooled from 57 studies	7035 patients with severe acute respiratory syndrome-related coronavirus 2 (SAR-COV-2) infection	Meta-analysis	Mortality	Pooled odds ratio (OR) 4.47 (2.39–8.35), $P < .001$
Stessel et al [43], 2023	March 13, 2020 to July 31, 2021	Single-center cohort study in Belgium	86 eligible patients admitted to ICU and requiring mechanical ventilation	Propensity-matched analysis	ICU mortality 3 mo mortality	OR 4.23 (1.11–16.17), $P = .02$ OR 5.91 (1.55–22.58), $P < .01$

Shaefi et al [45], 2021	March 1, 2020 to July 1, 2020	Multicenter cohort study (68 US hospitals)	1297 critically ill adults with COVID-19	Emulated target trial of ECMO receipt	60 d hospital mortality Among patients with PaO_2/FiO_2<80 mm Hg	HR 0.55 (0.41–0.74) HR 0.55 (0.50–0.77)
Hajage et al [46], 2022 (COVID-ICU Investigators group)	Admission date February 25, 2020 to May 4, 2020	Multicenter European cohort study including patients admitted to 30 ICUs in France, Belgium, and Switzerland	1235 critically ill adults (≥16 y) with COVID-19	Emulated target trial of ECMO receipt	14 d mortality 28 d mortality 60 d mortality 90 d mortality among patients on ECMO at high-volume vs low-volume centers	1.14 (0.85–1.54) 1.66 (1.12–2.46) 3.00 (1.52–5.94) 22% vs 36%
Urner et al [47], 2022 (COVID-19 Critical Care Consortium Investigators group)	January 3, 2020 to August 29, 2021	Multicenter cohort study (30 countries)	7345 critically ill adults with suspected or confirmed COVID-19	Comparative effectiveness study	Adherence-adjusted hospital mortality	26% vs 33.2% RR 0.78 (0.75–0.82)
Whitmore et al [44], 2023	March 1, 2020 to October 31, 2021	Multicenter retrospective cohort study within a large US hospital network	2332 adults with severe hypoxemia secondary to COVID-19	Matched analysis	Adjusted in-hospital mortality	38.8% vs 60.1% aOR 0.43 (0.33–0.56), $P < .001$

ventilation, discharge from the ICU, and "favorable" discharge location [44]. Together, these studies support the use of ECMO for the treatment of severe COVID-19, particularly in patients who are younger, have had a limited course of mechanical ventilation, and have more severe hypoxemia requiring more intensive mechanical ventilation for adequate oxygenation. However, the results of these studies might still be affected by unmeasured confounding and selection bias. Additionally, COVID-19 care continues to evolve with greater uptake of vaccination and boosters, more widespread natural immunity, the development of new viral variants, and the rise of concomitant infections including influenza and respiratory syncytial virus (RSV). Under these circumstances, the group of people who are developing COVID-19 ARDS and requiring ECMO is also likely changing. Changes in patient casemix could affect the efficacy of ECMO as treatment, meaning that the outcomes and efficacy of ECMO for the treatment of COVID-19 requires ongoing evaluation.

CLINICAL MANAGEMENT

The current consensus is that indications for ECMO and management of the ECMO-related care for patients with severe COVID-19 should follow the criteria established prior to the pandemic for patients with severe respiratory disease [48–51]. Despite the importance of ECMO as a treatment modality in the care of COVID-19, optimization of mechanical ventilation and other interventions such as prone positioning should be prioritized prior to consideration of ECMO whenever possible.

There have been numerous studies exploring how optimal ECMO for COVID-19 might differ from optimal ECMO for other indications. As stated earlier, the management of the ECMO circuit should be overall similar to in the pre-COVID-19 era. In the following sections, we explore the evidence to support different aspects of the management of patients with severe COVID-19 infections requiring ECMO.

Prone positioning

Prone positioning should be used both to help patients avoid ECMO initiation as well as once patients are on ECMO, unless contraindicated. This is supported by a meta-analysis of 13 studies of prone positioning in 1836 patients with non-COVID-19-related ARDS on ECMO, which found that prone positioning was associated with an improved 28 day survival (74% vs 58%; relative risk [RR] 1.31, 95% CI 1.21–1.41, $P < .0001$) [52]. This has also been supported by retrospective observational studies in patients on ECMO for COVID-19 [53]. Finally, the results of the Prone ECMO study (PRONECMO) randomized trial, which compared prone versus supine position among patients receiving VV ECMO for severe ARDS, were recently published. Among the 170 patients enrolled, 159 (94%) had COVID-19-related ARDS. The trial found that prone positioning did not significantly reduce time to ECMO weaning within the first 90 days (subhazard ratio 1.11, 95% CI 0.71–1.75, $P = .64$) [54].

Ventilatory strategies

Noninvasive ventilation strategies evolved over the course of the pandemic to include more positive pressure ventilation (eg, high-flow nasal cannula). Attempts to use noninvasive ventilatory strategies with ECMO, instead of invasive mechanical ventilation prior to or during ECMO, has limited evidence. A retrospective case series found that 14 out of 18 patients (78%) were eventually intubated and had higher mortality than the patients who did not require intubation [55]. However, advocates for "awake ECMO" have also published their experience with ECMO without invasive mechanical ventilation precannulation or concurrent with ECMO. They used awake ECMO in 6.8% of their ECMO cannulations and found that 36% of these patients remained awake without requiring sedation or intubation during their intensive care unit (ICU) stay [56]. However, providing invasive mechanical ventilation prior to initiating ECMO remains the more traditional strategy. Evaluations of optimal mechanical ventilation strategy prior to and during ECMO include the reevaluation of systemic early neuromuscular blockade (ROSE) trial, which found no significant benefit of neuromuscular blockade on outcomes [57]. However, the use of neuromuscular blockade is still indicated for patients who are otherwise unable to safely be proned, whose respiratory drive creates suboptimal ventilatory mechanics, or who otherwise have breathing patterns that increase the risk of ventilator-induced lung injury [58]. Regarding other ventilatory parameters, there is not sufficient evidence to change from non-COVID-19 ECMO mechanical ventilation guidelines, including the use of lung-protective ventilation.

Cannulation

As with other aspects of COVID-19 ECMO care, current recommendations are for conventional cannulation strategies [51]. These include either a 2-site or a single-site dual lumen cannulation, with the option to add arterial support in patients that develop concomitant cardiogenic shock. Studies of outcomes by cannulation site found small difference in likelihood of pneumothorax and bleeding but no differences in long-term outcomes [59]. While there might be hesitation to do a single-site dual lumen cannulation in patients who are unstable given concerns about transporting them to a catheterization laboratory or operating room, our group has shown that single-site cannulation can be safely performed at bedside under transesophageal echocardiogram guidance [60]. Consideration of other cannulation strategies, such as veno-pulmonary artery configurations to attempt sparing of the right ventricle, has insufficient evidence at this time [61].

Cytokine hemoadsorption

Early in the pandemic, there was a significant interest in cytokine hemoadsorption strategies due to early reports of the association of high interleukin-6 levels with high mortality in patients with COVID-19 and case reports, case series, and a multicenter retrospective registry study suggesting benefit of hemoadsorption when combined with continuous renal replacement therapy or ECMO [62–64]. This enthusiasm was dampened after the cytokine adsorption in patients with severe COVID-19 pneumonia requiring extracorporeal membrane oxygenation (CYCOV) randomized controlled trial found no benefit for hemoadsorption initiated within the ECMO circuit during the first 72 hours of ECMO support [65]. As a result, hemoadsorption for patients with COVID-19 on ECMO is not currently recommended for patients outside of clinical trials [33,51]. Despite this, there has been an ongoing interest in the use of hemoadsorption, and additional studies continue to be published suggesting a mortality benefit [66,67]. However, an additional randomized controlled trial found that a 5 day hemoadsorption therapy was associated with lower mortality during the first 5 days but similar mortality at 2 weeks [68], suggesting hemoadsorption might delay but not prevent mortality in severely ill patients with COVID-19. Additionally, a meta-analysis of 3 randomized trials and 11 observational studies found that hemoadsorption was associated with lower mortality in patients with COVID-19 not on ECMO, but it was not associated with a difference in mortality in patients with COVID-19 on ECMO [69]. Therefore, there is still not sufficient evidence to recommend hemoadsorption to lower the mortality risk in patients with COVID-19 on ECMO.

Tracheostomy

Given that the majority of patients with COVID-19 cannulated for ECMO receive invasive mechanical ventilation, often for prolonged periods, timing of tracheostomy has been evaluated in this population. The percutaneous approach has been shown to be safe in small, single-center studies [70,71]. However, these studies disagreed on whether early tracheostomy was associated with benefits such as earlier decannulation [70–72]. Therefore, either the percutaneous or open approach for tracheostomy appears to be safe, but there are limited data to guide optimal timing of tracheostomy.

Patient mobilization

Mobilization of patients on ECMO has been explored in non-COVID-19 patients [73–75], but limited data exist for patients treated with ECMO for COVID-19 ARDS. However, a US cohort of 47 patients on ECMO were extubated and able to participate in active physical rehab [76], suggesting that mobilization is possible and safe in carefully selected patients. Of note, this cohort included patients cannulated for VV ECMO, VA ECMO, and VV ECMO with right ventricular assist device, and their standard cannulation strategy was in the neck (eg, right internal jugular venous cannulation with a dual-lumen single venous cannula for the 83% of patients on VV ECMO) to facilitate this early mobilization.

COMPLICATIONS

There have been concerns regarding potentially higher risk of infection among patients on ECMO for an indication of COVID-19 versus other indications. However, early cohort studies of bacterial and fungal infections in patients on ECMO did not suggest that patients requiring ECMO for the treatment of COVID-19 had an increased risk of infection compared to patients treated for other ECMO indications [77–79]. However, more recently single-center data suggested an increased infectious risk, particularly for fungal infections, with 44% of patients in one study contracting a bloodstream infection [80]. This increased risk of infection, if real, could be due to the higher immunosuppression received by patients on ECMO for COVID-19 compared to other indications. Given the evolution of treatment over the course of the pandemic, this could explain the difference in early versus more recent studies of infection. Regardless, ELSO data suggested that contracting a coinfection after a prolonged (>2 weeks) ECMO run was associated with an increased risk of mortality [37].

Given the known thromboembolic and bleeding events associated with COVID-19 infection [81], there has been concern about these complications in patients with COVID-19 on ECMO [82] and ongoing scrutiny of and experimentation with the anticoagulation regimens received by these patients has been ongoing. However, an ELSO registry study of patients receiving ECMO for COVID-19 found a similar prevalence of bleeding and clotting complications as in patients receiving ECMO for other indications [27]. Centers that have changed anticoagulation targets or changed the anticoagulants used have failed to resolve these bleeding and clotting concerns [83,84]. As a result, guidelines for the use of anticoagulation in patients on ECMO for COVID-19 remain the same as for those on ECMO for other indications [51].

There is a growing literature on neurologic complications in patients with COVID-19 on ECMO, since neurologic complications are associated with higher mortality [85–89] and represent the third most common cause of death in this population [86]. Risk of intracranial hemorrhage has been cited at 4.9% [88] and is more common in patients with COVID-19 on ECMO than in non-COVID-19 patients on ECMO [85,90]. Risk factors included obesity and use of vasopressors pre-ECMO [87]. However, these studies have not found a consistent anticoagulation strategy to reduce the risk associated with the "double hit" of COVID-19 infection and ECMO requirements for anticoagulation [90].

With long COVID-19 ECMO run times—often longer by several weeks than was standard for non-COVID-19 ECMO [91,92]—holistic care considerations have become increasingly important. Schneeweiss-Gleixner and colleagues noted that nutritional goals were met on less than 41% of ECMO run days in their cohort, and that mean energy intake exceeding 70% of goal was associated with lower ICU mortality [93]. Additionally, adverse events such as pressure sores and ulcers and airway-related issues arise with long ECMO run times [94]. As we begin to have longer-term follow-up on patients with COVID-19 treated with ECMO who survive, we must also consider longer-term outcomes. Pozzi and colleagues prospectively followed 34 patients with COVID-19 on ECMO who survived to discharge and found that 67% had muscle weakness that improved over time and 86% were able to return to work by 1 year postdischarge [95]. However, approximately one-quarter of patients had anxiety and an equal number had depression, and this prevalence was stable over time [95], highlighting an area that require further study to improve post-COVID-19 ECMO quality of life.

DISPARITIES

Disparities in access to care and outcomes are seen in many fields of medicine and are similarly seen in ECMO before and during the pandemic. Prior to the start of the COVID-19 pandemic, a national analysis of ECMO use in the United States using claims data showed that patients who were female, had Medicaid insurance, and who lived in the lowest-income neighborhoods were less likely to receive ECMO as part of their care [96]. During the pandemic, a national analysis of ECMO outcomes found that Hispanic patients on ECMO had 39% higher odds of in-hospital mortality compared to White patients on ECMO [97]. Using the same database, Ahmad and colleagues did not observe associations between race or ethnicity and mortality, although they did find that Hispanic patients were overrepresented in ECMO populations. While 20% of all admitted patients with COVID-19 were Hispanic, 34% of patients on ECMO were Hispanic [41]. A more recent analysis found that being of Black race or multiple races was associated with a protective effect on a mortality analysis [98]; the reasons for this are unclear but might include different thresholds for selection in certain populations. Therefore, racial and ethnic disparities in ECMO access and outcomes for the treatment of COVID-19 warrant further investigation. Ahmad and colleagues also found that ECMO was being used for younger patients, possibly due to resource limitations and evidence that ECMO's ability to improve survival decreases with age [41]. The same authors also observed differences in survival by gender, with female gender having a protective effect on mortality [41], consistent with male gender as an independent risk factor for COVID-19 severity [99,100]. These disparities may reflect predispositions to disease severity, influences of comorbidities and limited health care access, fluctuating resource limitations during different phases of the pandemic, and systematic issues that perpetuate disparities in care access and outcomes in our national health care system. Given that patients' lives hang in the balance, it is critical that these disparities be further explored and, when possible, addressed.

PROGNOSTICATION

As we accumulate data on COVID-19 ECMO survival, there have been efforts to improve prognostication on which patients will survive to decannulation and discharge. While these efforts have been limited by a lack of randomized data, observational studies have explored the prognostic utility of diaphragm function assessments, respiratory compliance assessments, and T-cell immune response, as well as retrospective analyses of observational data [101–104]. The current best evidence is from a systematic review and meta-analysis by Tran and colleagues that included 42 observational studies of 17,449 patients [105]. They identified independent risk factors for mortality including older age (aHR 2.27, 1.63–3.16), male sex (unadjusted OR [uOR] 1.34, 1.20–1.49), chronic lung disease (aHR 1.55, 1.20–2.00), longer duration of symptoms precannulation (mean difference 1.51 days, 95% CI 0.36–2.65), longer duration of invasive mechanical ventilation precannulation (uOR 1.94, 95% CI 1.40–2.67), higher $PaCO_2$ precannulation (mean difference 4.04 mm Hg, 95% CI 1.64–6.44), higher driving pressure precannulation (aHR 2.36, 95% CI 1.40–3.97), and less previous experience with ECMO at center (aOR 2.27, 1.28–4.05). However, we have no doubt that our understanding of COVID-19 ECMO prognosis will continue to evolve as treatments change; a recent study by Oh and colleagues found that mortality in patients with COVID-19 on ECMO was lower if they had received the second booster dose of the vaccine, suggesting vaccination might play a role in prognostication [106]. This highlights the importance of considering phase of the pandemic and available treatments in any analysis of ECMO outcomes.

Of note, there has been discussion about the need to differentiate between COVID-19 phenotypes when prognosticating, as the progressive fibrotic phenotype might differ from the ARDS phenotype and might be more common among people with underlying lung disease [17]. The progressive fibrotic phenotype develops 4 to 12 weeks after initial infection in patients with all degrees of initial infection severity and, due to inflammation, results in fibrosis and a restrictive ventilatory defect. Unfortunately, to date, there has been insufficient standardization of these characterizations in studies to allow for differentiation of these phenotypes in prognostication studies.

LUNG TRANSPLANTATION

Lung transplantation has been the gold standard treatment for end-stage lung disease for decades. Patients should be considered for lung transplantation if they do not experience lung recovery on ECMO or are unable to be weaned off the circuit, if they are otherwise appropriate candidates [39]. Initial experiences with lung transplant for COVID-19 had promising short-term outcomes [92,107], but the generalizability of these findings was limited by a lack of clear guidelines for patient selection. This is partially due to prolonged recovery times compared to other causes of ARDS, prompting concerns that some patients might be considered for transplant too early. A study by Kehara and colleagues found that 5 of the 13 patients who underwent single lung transplant had improvement in native lung function over time [108]. Additionally, Levy and colleagues followed patients with COVID-19 on ECMO considered for lung transplantation and found that younger patients had a higher likelihood of recovery without lung transplantation after a median of 59 days on ECMO [91]. Based on this, they argued that referral for lung transplantation should be delayed 8 to 10 weeks after ECMO initiation for patients who are younger and/or felt to have a greater change of spontaneous recovery. However, these are small (<20 patients), single-center studies and should be interpreted with caution. Other authors have suggested criteria for lung transplantation consideration including age less than 65 years, single-organ dysfunction, lack of neurologic or other issues that would prevent participation in rehabilitation, and a period of at least 4 to 6 weeks after onset of respiratory failure [39,109]. With the current limited evidence, these guidelines should be considered by a multidisciplinary team prior to referral for lung transplantation. However, for patients with COVID-19 who go on to receive lung transplants, outcomes continue to be promising. Survival at 90 days posttransplant is similar to historic recipients with non-COVID-19 ARDS (94% vs 90%, $P = .17$) [110], and 1-year mortality was similar to those other lung transplant recipients (aHR 0.73, 95%CI 0.49–1.09, $P = .12$) [111].

VENO-ARTERIAL EXTRACORPOREAL MEMBRANE OXYGENATION

While a venovenous configuration is used for the treatment of greater than 95% of patients with COVID-19 requiring ECMO [27], patients have required other configurations due to COVID-19-related complications. Cardiac manifestations can include heart failure, cardiogenic shock, arrhythmia, and myocarditis, among others [18]. For example, heart failure has occurred due to sepsis, cytokine storm, microvascular thrombosis, and viral cardiomyocyte damage [112–114], requiring the use of a VA ECMO configuration. Furthermore, right ventricular dysfunction is seen in approximately 20% of patients with COVID-related ARDS [112], with a phenotype of impaired radial contraction and spared longitudinal contraction of the right ventricle [115]. Right ventricular dysfunction can lead to consideration of use of a right ventricular assistance device with an oxygenator (ie Oxy-right ventricular assist device [RVAD] configuration), which was associated with lower mortality in a small cohort compared to invasive mechanical ventilation alone [116]. Despite these COVID-19-related indications for VA ECMO, this configuration was used sparingly during the pandemic. It is uncertain how much this low utilization was due to concerns about the high morbidity and mortality observed in patients requiring VA ECMO [117], particularly in the setting of resource strain. A systematic review of COVID-19-related myocarditis found that VA ECMO was used in the treatment of 35% of patients, with an overall mortality of 7.9% among all patients [118]. Other forms of mechanical circulatory support were also used to support patients with COVID-19; this care provided benefit but also was associated with significant morbidity and required a multidisciplinary team with knowledge of the available mechanical circulatory support devices [119]. Other cannulation strategies, such as veno-veno-arterial (VVA) or veno-arterial-venous (VAV), can be considered when severe left cardiac or respiratory failure, respectively, coexist with respiratory failure.

PREGNANCY AND EXTRACORPOREAL MEMBRANE OXYGENATION

Over the course of the pandemic, ARDS was the most frequent cause of admission to the ICU among pregnant women, and pregnancy was an independent risk factor for ARDS [120,121]. Pregnant women may have been more affected by COVID-19-related lung injury due to their reduced residual capacity, increased plasma volume, and increased oxygen demand associated with pregnancy [122]. However, care of these patients was complicated by more limited cannulation sites, as the gravid uterus in late pregnancy makes it difficult to use the femoral vessels; the jugular site is, therefore, preferred for cannulation. Given the alterations in physiology and nuances to ECMO cannulation and management among pregnant women, it is recommended that these patients be transferred to an experienced ECMO center. However, outcomes from pre-pandemic studies have found that pregnant and peripartum patients requiring ECMO have good outcomes that are similar to or better than those of other patients [123], including fewer ECMO-related complications and lower hospital mortality [124]. The current Society for Maternal Fetal Medicine guidelines recommend the use of ECMO for refractory COVID-19 ARDS if the fetus is less than 32 weeks of gestational age to allow for further fetal development [125]. Those same guidelines recommend maintaining maternal SaO_2 greater than 90% to ensure adequate fetal oxygenation and $Paco_2$ at 28 to 32 mm Hg to allow fetal CO_2 elimination, using resting ventilation settings during ECMO to reduce lung injury, and engaging a multidisciplinary team early for delivery planning (ie, timing and method) [125]. A systematic review by Palella and colleagues found that maternal and fetal mortality among those on ECMO were 16.9% and 31.8%, respectively [126]. A recent retrospective multicenter cohort study of 100 pregnant or recently ($\leq$6 weeks) postpartum individuals also found a 16% maternal mortality rate, and they found that 76% of individuals had a serious maternal morbidity event [127]. However, it is important to note that these data were all from observational studies and no control groups were available. Relative contraindications for ECMO cannulation in a pregnant patient include imminent need for delivery, eclamptic seizures, and active bleeding from previa or another cause that requires stabilization before cannulation can occur [128]. It is recommended that the role of fetal monitoring be clearly defined prior to ECMO initiation [128]. In a recent series, the majority (19 of 21) of pregnant patients with COVID-19 on ECMO delivered while still on ECMO therapy; Richley and colleagues found that vaginal delivery was not contraindicated [128]. However, other authors have argued for avoiding anticoagulation at the time of delivery, if possible [129].

PEDIATRIC PATIENTS AND EXTRACORPOREAL MEMBRANE OXYGENATION

Children with severe COVID-19 infections requiring ECMO support represent another special patient population. Children were substantially less likely than adults to develop COVID-19-related ARDS [130], leading many pediatric ECMO centers to open their beds to adult patients during the pandemic when adult centers were overwhelmed [131]. However, when children had severe enough cases of COVID-19 infection to warrant hospital admission, approximately one-quarter of these patients required ICU admission [130], often for indications such as pediatric ARDS (PARDS) or multisystem inflammatory syndrome (MISC). Treatment of PARDS and MISC secondary to COVID-19 is similar to the treatment of these conditions when they are secondary to other causes [132]. A 2015 study of PARDS found that it was associated with a less than 1% risk of mortality in the United States. [133]. However, a 2023 systematic review and meta-analysis by Watanabe and colleagues of outcomes of pediatric patients with COVID-19 on ECMO suggested a higher mortality risk. The systematic review included 18 observational studies with a total of 110 children, a small sample size that emphasizes the limited literature on this topic. They found that 48% of the children were previously healthy, 11% were obese, and 11% had congenital heart disease. 52% received ECMO for MISC, while 40% had ARDS, and 71% of the patients received VA ECMO. In this cohort, the mortality risk was nearly 27%, and 37% had complications including stroke, acute kidney injury, pulmonary edema, and venous thromboembolism [134]. This higher risk of mortality emphasizes the need for ongoing optimization of care and evaluation of outcomes in pediatric patients with COVID-19 requiring ECMO. Additionally, a recent study by Krishnan and colleagues suggested that there might be racial disparities in outcomes of pediatric patients with PARDS [135], which also require further evaluation.

RESOURCE AND HEALTH CARE SYSTEM CONSIDERATIONS

One of the main lessons from the pandemic is that these guidelines are just that–guidelines–and need to be considered in the light of a particular hospital's situation, including resource limitations. While the organization of ECMO systems differ by country, prepandemic and early pandemic data suggested that higher volume was associated with better ECMO outcomes [32,37,136]. However, we saw during the COVID-19 pandemic that higher-volume centers might not have sufficient capacity to address the need for ECMO, and the same may occur during a future COVID-19 surge or another pandemic [137]. A benefit of the pandemic has been a dramatic uptake of virtual communication and e-learning platforms, which can be used to disseminate knowledge to and facilitate communication with new or lower volume ECMO centers. Additional innovations in this space includes the creation of ambulatory ECMO simulators to improve providers' understanding of the treatment with ECMO [138].

The COVID-19 pandemic also highlighted how resource limitations can highlight just how resource-intensive ECMO treatment is in terms of structural resources, consumable equipment, and human resources. As a result, during the height of the pandemic, many centers had to restrict or abandon the use of ECMO, and overall resource limitations were exacerbated by the prolonged run times required by patients with COVID-19 on ECMO [23,139–141]. Iterative assessment of resource strain during future COVID-19 surges or pandemics should take into account these lessons learned.

Some authors have even suggested predesigning triage systems to standardize which patients should receive ECMO depending on the capacity of the system [141].

Finally, the COVID-19 pandemic highlighted the need for crisis management plans that can better manage resources on regional and national scales. In the context of ECMO, this could include the creation of ECMO networks to facilitate referrals to and/or advising by high-volume centers and more experienced practitioners, as occurred in Paris, the United Kingdom, and Chile during the pandemic [29,32,142]. This type of coordination helped to improve resource utilization, patient selection, capacity management, workflow and data collection. ELSO also offers an "ECMO Availability Map" that will be a useful tool in the future to help manage capacity [143].

SUMMARY

The COVID-19 pandemic was dynamic, challenging existing care paradigms and pushing health care systems around the world to their limits. The rise in cases of ARDS secondary to severe COVID-19 infections led to a dramatic rise in demand for ECMO support. As COVID-19 becomes an endemic disease, we continue to learn about its pathophysiology and improve our management of patients with COVID-19 infection. With regard to ECMO, guidelines for COVID-19-related ECMO therapy remain consistent with overall ECMO guidelines, though ongoing research efforts may help to tailor ECMO care for patients with COVID-19 in the future.

CLINICS CARE POINTS

- While there have been no large, randomized controlled trials of ECMO use for management of severe COVID-19 infection, the best available evidence has shown that ECMO initiation is associated with a reduction in mortality compared to continued mechanical ventilation alone.
- Clinical management of patients on ECMO for severe COVID-19 should follow criteria established prior to the pandemic with severe respiratory disease.
- For patients stabilized with ECMO who fail to achieve lung recovery, lung transplantation can be considered as destination therapy.
- We recommend use of a multidisciplinary team in these scenarios, as optimal selection criteria and timing for referral to lung transplantation for patients with severe COVID-19 has not been established.

Disclosure

The authors have nothing to disclose.

Funding

F32AG067642 from the National Institute on Aging (PI: Ruck).

References

[1] (WHO) WHO. WHO Coronavirus (COVID-19) Dashboard. 2023. Available at: https://covid19.who.int/. [Accessed 11 December 2023].
[2] Combes A, Schmidt M, Hodgson CL, et al. Extracorporeal life support for adults with acute respiratory distress syndrome. Intensive Care Med 2020;46(12):2464–76.
[3] Pham T, Combes A, Rozé H, et al. Extracorporeal membrane oxygenation for pandemic influenza A(H1N1)-induced acute respiratory distress syndrome: a cohort study and propensity-matched analysis. Am J Respir Crit Care Med 2013;187(3):276–85.
[4] Peek GJ, Elbourne D, Mugford M, et al. Randomised controlled trial and parallel economic evaluation of conventional ventilatory support versus extracorporeal membrane oxygenation for severe adult respiratory failure (CESAR). Health Technol Assess 2010;14(35):1–46.
[5] Peek GJ, Mugford M, Tiruvoipati R, et al. Efficacy and economic assessment of conventional ventilatory support versus extracorporeal membrane oxygenation for severe adult respiratory failure (CESAR): a multicentre randomised controlled trial. Lancet 2009;374(9698):1351–63.
[6] Sidebotham D. Extracorporeal membrane oxygenation–understanding the evidence: CESAR and beyond. J Extra Corpor Technol 2011;43(1):P23–6.
[7] Sameed M, Meng Z, Marciniak ET. EOLIA trial: the future of extracorporeal membrane oxygenation in acute respiratory distress syndrome therapy? Breathe 2019;15(3):244–6.
[8] Combes A, Hajage D, Capellier G, et al. Extracorporeal membrane oxygenation for severe acute respiratory distress syndrome. N Engl J Med 2018;378(21):1965–75.
[9] Goligher EC, Tomlinson G, Hajage D, et al. Extracorporeal membrane oxygenation for severe acute respiratory distress syndrome and posterior probability of mortality benefit in a post hoc bayesian analysis of a randomized clinical trial. JAMA 2018;320(21):2251–9.
[10] Combes A, Peek GJ, Hajage D, et al. ECMO for severe ARDS: systematic review and individual patient data meta-analysis. Intensive Care Med 2020;46(11):2048–57.
[11] Toomasian JM, Schreiner RJ, Meyer DE, et al. A polymethylpentene fiber gas exchanger for long-term extracorporeal life support. Am Soc Artif Intern Organs J 2005;51(4):390–7.
[12] O'Brien C, Monteagudo J, Schad C, et al. Centrifugal pumps and hemolysis in pediatric extracorporeal membrane oxygenation (ECMO) patients: An analysis of Extracorporeal Life Support Organization (ELSO) registry data. J Pediatr Surg 2017;52(6):975–8.
[13] Guan WJ, Ni ZY, Hu Y, et al. Clinical characteristics of coronavirus disease 2019 in China. N Engl J Med 2020;382(18):1708–20.
[14] Wiersinga WJ, Rhodes A, Cheng AC, et al. Pathophysiology, transmission, diagnosis, and treatment of coronavirus disease 2019 (COVID-19): a review. JAMA 2020;324(8):782–93.
[15] Gattinoni L, Chiumello D, Rossi S. COVID-19 pneumonia: ARDS or not? Crit Care 2020;24(1):154.
[16] Xie Y, Wang X, Yang P, et al. COVID-19 Complicated by Acute Pulmonary Embolism. Radiology Cardiothoracic imaging 2020;2(2):e200067.
[17] Kostopanagiotou K, Schuurmans MM, Inci I, et al. COVID-19-related end stage lung disease: two distinct phenotypes. Ann Med 2022;54(1):588–90.
[18] Shafi AMA, Shaikh SA, Shirke MM, et al. Cardiac manifestations in COVID-19 patients-A systematic review. J Card Surg 2020;35(8):1988–2008.
[19] Kang Y, Chen T, Mui D, et al. Cardiovascular manifestations and treatment considerations in COVID-19. Heart (British Cardiac Society) 2020;106(15):1132–41.
[20] Clerkin KJ, Fried JA, Raikhelkar J, et al. COVID-19 and cardiovascular disease. Circulation 2020;141(20):1648–55.
[21] Maharaj V, Alexy T, Agdamag AC, et al. Right ventricular dysfunction is associated with increased mortality in patients requiring venovenous extracorporeal membrane oxygenation for coronavirus disease 2019. Am Soc Artif Intern Organs J 2022;68(6):772–8.

[22] Bhardwaj A, Kirincich J, Rampersad P, et al. Fulminant myocarditis in COVID-19 and favorable outcomes with VA-ECMO. Resuscitation 2022;175:75–6.
[23] Abrams D, Lorusso R, Vincent JL, et al. ECMO during the COVID-19 pandemic: when is it unjustified? Crit Care 2020;24(1):507.
[24] Henry BM, Lippi G. Poor survival with extracorporeal membrane oxygenation in acute respiratory distress syndrome (ARDS) due to coronavirus disease 2019 (COVID-19): Pooled analysis of early reports. J Crit Care 2020;58:27–8.
[25] Schmidt M, Hajage D, Lebreton G, et al. Extracorporeal membrane oxygenation for severe acute respiratory distress syndrome associated with COVID-19: a retrospective cohort study. Lancet Respir Med 2020;8(11):1121–31.
[26] Lorusso R, Combes A, Lo Coco V, et al. ECMO for COVID-19 patients in Europe and Israel. Intensive Care Med 2021;47(3):344–8.
[27] Barbaro RP, MacLaren G, Boonstra PS, et al. Extracorporeal membrane oxygenation support in COVID-19: an international cohort study of the Extracorporeal Life Support Organization registry. Lancet 2020;396(10257):1071–8.
[28] Lorusso R, De Piero ME, Mariani S, et al. In-hospital and 6-month outcomes in patients with COVID-19 supported with extracorporeal membrane oxygenation (EuroECMO-COVID): a multicentre, prospective observational study. Lancet Respir Med 2023;11(2):151–62.
[29] Diaz RA, Graf J, Zambrano JM, et al. Extracorporeal Membrane Oxygenation for COVID-19-associated Severe Acute Respiratory Distress Syndrome in Chile: A Nationwide Incidence and Cohort Study. Am J Respir Crit Care Med 2021;204(1):34–43.
[30] Rabie AA, Azzam MH, Al-Fares AA, et al. Implementation of new ECMO centers during the COVID-19 pandemic: experience and results from the Middle East and India. Intensive Care Med 2021;47(8):887–95.
[31] Karagiannidis C, Slutsky AS, Bein T, et al. Complete countrywide mortality in COVID patients receiving ECMO in Germany throughout the first three waves of the pandemic. Crit Care 2021;25(1):413.
[32] Lebreton G, Schmidt M, Ponnaiah M, et al. Extracorporeal membrane oxygenation network organisation and clinical outcomes during the COVID-19 pandemic in Greater Paris, France: a multicentre cohort study. Lancet Respir Med 2021;9(8):851–62.
[33] Supady A, Combes A, Barbaro RP, et al. Respiratory indications for ECMO: focus on COVID-19. Intensive Care Med 2022;48(10):1326–37.
[34] Broman LM, Eksborg S, Lo Coco V, et al. Extracorporeal membrane oxygenation for COVID-19 during first and second waves. Lancet Respir Med 2021;9(8):e80–1.
[35] Riera J, Roncon-Albuquerque R Jr, Fuset MP, et al. Increased mortality in patients with COVID-19 receiving extracorporeal respiratory support during the second wave of the pandemic. Intensive Care Med 2021;47(12):1490–3.
[36] Schmidt M, Langouet E, Hajage D, et al. Evolving outcomes of extracorporeal membrane oxygenation support for severe COVID-19 ARDS in Sorbonne hospitals, Paris. Crit Care 2021;25(1):355.
[37] Barbaro RP, MacLaren G, Boonstra PS, et al. Extracorporeal membrane oxygenation for COVID-19: evolving outcomes from the international Extracorporeal Life Support Organization Registry. Lancet 2021;398(10307):1230–8.
[38] Jacobs JP, Stammers AH, St Louis JD, et al. Variation in survival in patients with Coronavirus Disease 2019 supported with extracorporeal membrane oxygenation: A multi-institutional analysis of 594 consecutive patients with Coronavirus Disease 2019 supported with extracorporeal membrane oxygenation at 49 hospitals within 21 states. J Thorac Cardiovasc Surg 2023;165(5):1837–48.
[39] Alessandri F, Di Nardo M, Ramanathan K, et al. Extracorporeal membrane oxygenation for COVID-19-related acute respiratory distress syndrome: a narrative review. Journal of intensive care 2023;11(1):5.

[40] Watanabe A, Malik A, Aikawa T, et al. Extracorporeal membrane oxygenation for COVID-19-associated acute respiratory distress syndrome: A nationwide analysis. J Med Virol 2023;95(7):e28961.
[41] Ahmad R, Abrahamian A, Salih A, et al. Demographics and Outcomes of Extracorporeal Membrane Oxygenation in COVID-19 Patients: National Database Analysis. J Clin Med 2023;12(18).
[42] Indrambarya T, Chaichalothorn M, Sirinawin C, et al. Mortality rate in patients with SAR-COV-2 infection treated with extracorporeal membrane oxygenator: A systematic review and meta-analysis. Heart Lung : J Crit Care 2023;58:204–9.
[43] Stessel B, Bin Saad M, Ullrick L, et al. Extracorporeal membrane oxygenation to support COVID-19 patients: a propensity-matched cohort study. Critical care research and practice 2023;2023:5101456.
[44] Whitmore SP, Cyr KJ, Cohen ES, et al. Extracorporeal membrane oxygenation for acute respiratory failure due to COVID-19: a multicenter matched cohort study. Am Soc Artif Intern Organs J 2023;69(8):734–41.
[45] Shaefi S, Brenner SK, Gupta S, et al. Extracorporeal membrane oxygenation in patients with severe respiratory failure from COVID-19. Intensive Care Med 2021;47(2):208–21.
[46] Hajage D, Combes A, Guervilly C, et al. Extracorporeal membrane oxygenation for severe acute respiratory distress syndrome associated with COVID-19: an emulated target trial analysis. Am J Respir Crit Care Med 2022;206(3):281–94.
[47] Urner M, Barnett AG, Bassi GL, et al. Venovenous extracorporeal membrane oxygenation in patients with acute covid-19 associated respiratory failure: comparative effectiveness study. BMJ 2022;377:e068723.
[48] Gajkowski EF, Herrera G, Hatton L, et al. ELSO guidelines for adult and pediatric extracorporeal membrane oxygenation circuits. Am Soc Artif Intern Organs J 2022;68(2):133–52.
[49] Abrams D, Ferguson ND, Brochard L, et al. ECMO for ARDS: from salvage to standard of care? Lancet Respir Med 2019;7(2):108–10.
[50] Fan E, Beitler JR, Brochard L, et al. COVID-19-associated acute respiratory distress syndrome: is a different approach to management warranted? Lancet Respir Med 2020;8(8):816–21.
[51] Badulak J, Antonini MV, Stead CM, et al. Extracorporeal Membrane Oxygenation for COVID-19: Updated 2021 Guidelines from the Extracorporeal Life Support Organization. Am Soc Artif Intern Organs J 2021;67(5):485–95.
[52] Papazian L, Schmidt M, Hajage D, et al. Effect of prone positioning on survival in adult patients receiving venovenous extracorporeal membrane oxygenation for acute respiratory distress syndrome: a systematic review and meta-analysis. Intensive Care Med 2022;48(3):270–80.
[53] Zaaqoq AM, Barnett AG, Griffee MJ, et al. Beneficial effect of prone positioning during venovenous extracorporeal membrane oxygenation for coronavirus disease 2019. Crit Care Med 2022;50(2):275–85.
[54] Schmidt M, Hajage D, Lebreton G, et al. Prone positioning during extracorporeal membrane oxygenation in patients with severe ARDS: The PRONECMO Randomized Clinical Trial. JAMA 2023;330(24):2343–53.
[55] Mang S, Reyher C, Mutlak H, et al. Awake extracorporeal membrane oxygenation for COVID-19-induced acute respiratory distress syndrome. Am J Respir Crit Care Med 2022;205(7):847–51.
[56] Galante O, Hasidim A, Almog Y, et al. Extracorporal membrane oxygenation in nonintubated patients (Awake ECMO) With COVID-19 adult respiratory distress syndrome: the Israeli experience. Am Soc Artif Intern Organs J 2023;69(8):e363–7.
[57] Moss M, Huang DT, Brower RG, et al. Early neuromuscular blockade in the acute respiratory distress syndrome. N Engl J Med 2019;380(21):1997–2008.
[58] Slutsky AS, Villar J. Early paralytic agents for ARDS? yes, no, and sometimes. N Engl J Med 2019;380(21):2061–3.

[59] O'Gara BP, Tung MG, Kennedy KF, et al. Outcomes with single-site dual-lumen versus multi-site cannulation for adults with COVID-19 respiratory failure receiving venovenous extracorporeal membrane oxygenation. Crit Care Med 2023;51(12):1716–26.
[60] Cha S, Kim BS, Ha JS, et al. How to do it: a safe bedside protocol for dual-lumen right internal jugular cannulation for venovenous extracorporeal membrane oxygenation in COVID-19 patients with severe acute respiratory distress syndrome. Am Soc Artif Intern Organs J 2023;69(1):31–5.
[61] Kopanczyk R, Al-Qudsi OH, Bhatt AM. Extracorporeal Membrane Oxygenation and Coronavirus Disease 2019. JAMA Surgery 2021;156(4):401–2.
[62] Ruan Q, Yang K, Wang W, et al. Clinical predictors of mortality due to COVID-19 based on an analysis of data of 150 patients from Wuhan, China. Intensive Care Med 2020;46(5): 846–8.
[63] Rieder M, Zahn T, Benk C, et al. Cytokine adsorption in a patient with severe coronavirus disease 2019 related acute respiratory distress syndrome requiring extracorporeal membrane oxygenation therapy: A case report. Artif Organs 2021;45(2):191–4.
[64] Song T, Hayanga J, Durham L, et al. CytoSorb therapy in COVID-19 (CTC) patients requiring extracorporeal membrane oxygenation: a multicenter, retrospective registry. Front Med 2021;8:773461.
[65] Supady A, Weber E, Rieder M, et al. Cytokine adsorption in patients with severe COVID-19 pneumonia requiring extracorporeal membrane oxygenation (CYCOV): a single centre, open-label, randomised, controlled trial. Lancet Respir Med 2021;9(7):755–62.
[66] Hayanga JWA, Song T, Durham L, et al. Extracorporeal hemoadsorption in critically ill COVID-19 patients on VV ECMO: the CytoSorb therapy in COVID-19 (CTC) registry. Crit Care 2023;27(1):243.
[67] Wei S, Zhang Y, Zhai K, et al. CytoSorb in patients with coronavirus disease 2019: A rapid evidence review and meta-analysis. Front Immunol 2023;14:1067214.
[68] Jarczak D, Roedl K, Fischer M, et al. Effect of hemadsorption therapy in critically ill patients with COVID-19 (CYTOCOV-19): a prospective randomized controlled pilot trial. Blood Purif 2023;52(2):183–92.
[69] He J, Lin Y, Cai W, et al. Efficacy of supplemental hemoadsorption therapy on severe and critical patients with COVID-19: an evidence-based analysis. Shock 2023;60(3):333–44.
[70] Morosin M, Azzu A, Antonopoulos A, et al. Safety of tracheostomy during extracorporeal membrane oxygenation support: A single-center experience. Artif Organs 2023;47(11): 1762–72.
[71] Staibano P, Khattak S, Amin F, et al. Tracheostomy in critically Ill COVID-19 patients on extracorporeal membrane oxygenation: a single-center experience. Ann Otol Rhinol Laryngol 2023;132(12):1520–7.
[72] Tamargo IA, Creel-Bulos C, Callahan MC, et al. Early tracheostomy may be performed safely in obese COVID-19 patients supported on VV-ECMO. Innovations (Philadelphia, Pa) 2023;18(5):472–8.
[73] Kourek C, Nanas S, Kotanidou A, et al. Modalities of Exercise Training in Patients with Extracorporeal Membrane Oxygenation Support. Journal of Cardiovascular Development and Disease 2022;9(2).
[74] Abrams D, Madahar P, Eckhardt CM, et al. Early mobilization during extracorporeal membrane oxygenation for cardiopulmonary failure in adults: factors associated with intensity of treatment. Annals of the American Thoracic Society 2022;19(1):90–8.
[75] Chatziefstratiou AA, Fotos NV, Giakoumidakis K, et al. The early mobilization of patients on extracorporeal membrane oxygenation: a systematic review. Nursing reports (Pavia, Italy) 2023;13(2):751–64.
[76] George TJ, Sheasby J, Taylor JE, et al. Early mobilization in coronavirus-19 patients treated with extracorporeal membrane oxygenation. J Card Surg 2022;37(12):4536–42.

[77] Fekkar A, Lampros A, Mayaux J, et al. Occurrence of invasive pulmonary fungal infections in patients with severe COVID-19 admitted to the ICU. Am J Respir Crit Care Med 2021;203(3):307–17.
[78] Garcia-Vidal C, Sanjuan G, Moreno-García E, et al. Incidence of co-infections and superinfections in hospitalized patients with COVID-19: a retrospective cohort study. Clin Microbiol Infection 2021;27(1):83–8.
[79] Pickens CO, Gao CA, Cuttica MJ, et al. Bacterial Superinfection Pneumonia in Patients Mechanically Ventilated for COVID-19 Pneumonia. Am J Respir Crit Care Med 2021;204(8): 921–32.
[80] Carelli S, Dell'Anna AM, Montini L, et al. Bloodstream infections in COVID-19 patients undergoing extracorporeal membrane oxygenation in ICU: An observational cohort study. Heart Lung : J Crit Care 2023;62:193–9.
[81] Guo Z, Sun L, Li B, et al. Anticoagulation management in severe coronavirus disease 2019 patients on extracorporeal membrane oxygenation. J Cardiothorac Vasc Anesth 2021;35(2):389–97.
[82] Rostami M, Mansouritorghabeh H. Significance of heparin induced thrombocytopenia (HIT) in COVID-19: a systematic review and meta-analysis. J Thromb Thrombolysis 2023;56(2):241–52.
[83] Seelhammer TG, Rowse P, Yalamuri S. Bivalirudin for maintenance anticoagulation during venovenous extracorporeal membrane oxygenation for COVID-19. J Cardiothorac Vasc Anesth 2021;35(4):1149–53.
[84] Diaz D, Martinez J, Bushman G, et al. Anticoagulation strategies in COVID-19 infected patients receiving ECMO support. J Extra Corpor Technol 2023;55(3):121–9.
[85] Lannon M, Duda T, Greer A, et al. Intracranial hemorrhage in patients treated for SARS-CoV-2 with extracorporeal membrane oxygenation: A systematic review and meta-analysis. J Crit Care 2023;77:154319.
[86] Li CMF, Densy Deng X, Ma YF, et al. Neurologic complications of patients with COVID-19 requiring extracorporeal membrane oxygenation: a systematic review and meta-analysis. Critical care explorations 2023;5(4):e0887.
[87] Zaaqoq AM, Griffee MJ, Kelly TL, et al. Cerebrovascular complications of COVID-19 on venovenous extracorporeal membrane oxygenation. Crit Care Med 2023;51(8): 1043–53.
[88] Kannapadi NV, Jami M, Premraj L, et al. Neurological complications in COVID-19 patients with ECMO support: a systematic review and meta-analysis. Heart Lung Circ 2022;31(2): 292–8.
[89] Kannapadi NV, Jami M, Premraj L, et al. Neurologic injury in patients with COVID-19 who receive VV-ECMO therapy: a cohort study. J Cardiothorac Vasc Anesth 2021;35(11): 3456–61.
[90] Jin Y, Zhang Y, Liu J, et al. Thrombosis and bleeding in patients with COVID-19 requiring extracorporeal membrane oxygenation: a systematic review and meta-analysis. Research and practice in thrombosis and haemostasis 2023;7(2):100103.
[91] Levy L, Deri O, Huszti E, et al. Timing of lung transplant referral in patients with severe COVID-19 lung injury supported by ECMO. J Clin Med 2023;12(12).
[92] Bharat A, Machuca TN, Querrey M, et al. Early outcomes after lung transplantation for severe COVID-19: a series of the first consecutive cases from four countries. Lancet Respir Med 2021;9(5):487–97.
[93] Schneeweiss-Gleixner M, Scheiner B, Semmler G, et al. Inadequate energy delivery is frequent among COVID-19 patients requiring ECMO support and associated with increased ICU mortality. Nutrients 2023;15(9).
[94] Adelsten J, Grønlykke L, Pedersen FM, et al. Use of prone position ventilation in patients with COVID-19 induced severe ARDS supported with V-V ECMO: A danish cohort study with focus on adverse events. Perfusion 2023 2676591231198798.

[95] Pozzi M, Giani M, Andreossi M, et al. Long-term physical, cognitive, and psychological outcomes in severe COVID-19 patients managed with extracorporeal membrane oxygenation: a prospective study. Am Soc Artif Intern Organs J 2023;69(8):e376–83.
[96] Mehta AB, Taylor JK, Day G, et al. Disparities in adult patient selection for extracorporeal membrane oxygenation in the United States: a population-level study. Annals of the American Thoracic Society 2023;20(8):1166–74.
[97] Kopanczyk R, Lisco SJ, Pearl R, et al. Racial and ethnic disparities in veno-venous extracorporeal membrane oxygenation mortality for patients with severe coronavirus disease-2019. ASAIO journal (American Society for Artificial Internal Organs 1992;2023.
[98] Enumah ZO, Etchill EW, Kim BS, et al. Racial disparities among patients on venovenous extracorporeal membrane oxygenation in the pre–Coronavirus Disease 2019 and Coronavirus Disease 2019 eras: A retrospective registry review. JTCVS open.
[99] Gao YD, Ding M, Dong X, et al. Risk factors for severe and critically ill COVID-19 patients: A review. Allergy 2021;76(2):428–55.
[100] Richardson S, Hirsch JS, Narasimhan M, et al. Presenting characteristics, comorbidities, and outcomes among 5700 patients hospitalized with COVID-19 in the New York City Area. JAMA 2020;323(20):2052–9.
[101] Arachchillage DJ, Weatherill A, Rajakaruna I, et al. Thombosis, major bleeding, and survival in COVID-19 supported by veno-venous extracorporeal membrane oxygenation in the first vs second wave: a multicenter observational study in the United Kingdom. J Thromb Haemostasis 2023;21(10):2735–46.
[102] Schäfer VS, Recker F, Kretschmer E, et al. Lung ultrasound in predicting outcomes in patients with COVID-19 treated with extracorporeal membrane oxygenation. Viruses 2023;15(9).
[103] Valentin S, Amalric M, Granier G, et al. Prognostic value of respiratory compliance course on mortality in COVID-19 patients with vv-ECMO. Ann Intensive Care 2023;13(1):54.
[104] Ulakcsai Z, Szabo L, Szabo Z, et al. T cell immune response predicts survival in severely ill COVID-19 patients requiring venovenous extracorporeal membrane oxygenation support. Front Immunol 2023;14:1179620.
[105] Tran A, Fernando SM, Rochwerg B, et al. Prognostic factors associated with mortality among patients receiving venovenous extracorporeal membrane oxygenation for COVID-19: a systematic review and meta-analysis. Lancet Respir Med 2023;11(3):235–44.
[106] Oh TK, Song IA. Extracorporeal Membrane Oxygenation Support and Critically Ill COVID-19 Patient Outcomes: A Population-Based Cohort Study. Am Soc Artif Intern Organs J 2023.
[107] Kurihara C, Manerikar A, Querrey M, et al. Clinical characteristics and outcomes of patients with COVID-19-associated acute respiratory distress syndrome who underwent lung transplant. JAMA 2022;327(7):652–61.
[108] Kehara H, Mangukia C, Sunagawa G, et al. Lung transplantation for COVID-19 pulmonary sequelae. Transplantation 2023;107(2):449–56.
[109] Mohanka MR, Joerns J, Lawrence A, et al. ECMO long haulers: a distinct phenotype of COVID-19-associated ARDS with implications for lung transplant candidacy. Transplantation 2022;106(4):e202–11.
[110] Florissi IS, Etchill EW, Barbur I, et al. Lung transplantation in patients with COVID-19-the early national experience. Semin Thorac Cardiovasc Surg 2023;35(4):822–30.
[111] Ruck JM, Zhou AL, Florissi I, et al. Uptake and 1-year outcomes of lung transplantation for COVID-19. J Thorac Cardiovasc Surg 2023;167(2):549–55.e1.
[112] Shi S, Qin M, Shen B, et al. Association of cardiac injury with mortality in hospitalized patients with COVID-19 in Wuhan, China. JAMA cardiology 2020;5(7):802–10.
[113] Madjid M, Safavi-Naeini P, Solomon SD, et al. Potential effects of coronaviruses on the cardiovascular system: a review. JAMA cardiology 2020;5(7):831–40.

[114] Guzik TJ, Mohiddin SA, Dimarco A, et al. COVID-19 and the cardiovascular system: implications for risk assessment, diagnosis, and treatment options. Cardiovasc Res 2020;116(10):1666–87.
[115] Bleakley C, Singh S, Garfield B, et al. Right ventricular dysfunction in critically ill COVID-19 ARDS. Int J Cardiol 2021;327:251–8.
[116] Cain MT, Smith NJ, Barash M, et al. Extracorporeal membrane oxygenation with right ventricular assist device for COVID-19 ARDS. J Surg Res 2021;264:81–9.
[117] Mariani S, De Piero ME, Ravaux JM, et al. Temporary mechanical circulatory support for COVID-19 patients: A systematic review of literature. Artif Organs 2022;46(7):1249–67.
[118] Sai Santhosha Mrudula A, Agarwal P, Vempati R, et al. Clinical outcome of established diagnostic and treatment modalities of COVID-19-associated myocarditis: a systematic review. Annals of medicine and surgery (2012) 2023;85(7):3583–94.
[119] Gorder K, Young W, Kapur NK, et al. Mechanical Circulatory Support in COVID-19. Heart Fail Clin 2023;19(2):205–11.
[120] Vasquez DN, Estenssoro E, Canales HS, et al. Clinical characteristics and outcomes of obstetric patients requiring ICU admission. Chest 2007;131(3):718–24.
[121] Pollock W, Rose L, Dennis CL. Pregnant and postpartum admissions to the intensive care unit: a systematic review. Intensive Care Med 2010;36(9):1465–74.
[122] Hegewald MJ, Crapo RO. Respiratory physiology in pregnancy. Clin Chest Med 2011;32(1):1–13.
[123] Ramanathan K, Tan CS, Rycus P, et al. Extracorporeal membrane oxygenation in pregnancy: an analysis of the extracorporeal life support organization registry. Crit Care Med 2020;48(5):696–703.
[124] O'Neil ER, Lin H, Shamshirsaz AA, et al. Pregnant and peripartum women with COVID-19 have high survival with extracorporeal membrane oxygenation: an extracorporeal life support organization registry analysis. Am J Respir Crit Care Med 2022;205(2):248–50.
[125] Kalyanaraman M, Anderson MR. COVID-19 in children. Pediatr Clin 2022;69(3): 547–71.
[126] Palella S, Muscarà L, La Via L, et al. Veno-venous extracorporeal membrane oxygenation for rescue support in pregnant patients with COVID-19: a systematic review. Br J Anaesth 2023;131(4):e130–2.
[127] Byrne JJ, Shamshirsaz AA, Cahill AG, et al. Outcomes Following Extracorporeal Membrane Oxygenation for Severe COVID-19 in Pregnancy or Post Partum. JAMA Netw Open 2023;6(5):e2314678.
[128] Richley M, Rao R. Extracorporeal membrane oxygenation in pregnancy during the SARS-CoV-2 pandemic. Semin Fetal Neonatal Med 2023;28(1):101435.
[129] Favilli A, Mattei Gentili M, De Paola F, et al. COVID-19 and pregnancy: an updated review about evidence-based therapeutic strategies. J Personalized Med 2023;13(7).
[130] Gonzalez-Dambrauskas S, Vasquez-Hoyos P, Camporesi A, et al. Paediatric critical COVID-19 and mortality in a multinational prospective cohort. Lancet regional health Americas 2022;12:100272.
[131] Gerall C, Cheung EW, Klein-Cloud R, et al. Allocation of resources and development of guidelines for extracorporeal membrane oxygenation (ECMO): Experience from a pediatric center in the epicenter of the COVID-19 pandemic. J Pediatr Surg 2020;55(12): 2548–54.
[132] Di Nardo M, Hoskote A, Thiruchelvam T, et al. Extracorporeal membrane oxygenation in children with coronavirus disease 2019: Preliminary Report from the Collaborative European Chapter of the Extracorporeal Life Support Organization Prospective Survey. Am Soc Artif Intern Organs J 2021;67(2):121–4.
[133] Rimensberger PC, Cheifetz IM. Ventilatory support in children with pediatric acute respiratory distress syndrome: proceedings from the pediatric acute lung injury consensus conference. Pediatr Crit Care Med 2015;16(5 Suppl 1):S51–60.

[134] Watanabe A, Yasuhara J, Karube T, et al. Extracorporeal membrane oxygenation in children with COVID-19: a systematic review and meta-analysis. Pediatr Crit Care Med : a journal of the Society of Critical Care Medicine and the World Federation of Pediatric Intensive and Critical Care Societies 2023;24(5):406–16.

[135] Krishnan P, Malik A, Isath A, et al. Nationwide analysis of the outcomes and mortality of hospitalized infants with concomitant diagnosis of COVID-19. Am J Perinatol 2023; https://doi.org/10.1055/a-2149-8810.

[136] Barbaro RP, Odetola FO, Kidwell KM, et al. Association of hospital-level volume of extracorporeal membrane oxygenation cases and mortality. Analysis of the extracorporeal life support organization registry. Am J Respir Crit Care Med 2015;191(8):894–901.

[137] Emanuel EJ, Persad G, Upshur R, et al. Fair allocation of scarce medical resources in the time of covid-19. N Engl J Med 2020;382(21):2049–55.

[138] Sayed AN, Noorizadeh M, Alhomsi Y, et al. Ambulatory extracorporeal membrane oxygenation simulator: The next frontier in clinical training. Perfusion 2023 2676591231201527.

[139] Supady A, Badulak J, Evans L, et al. Should we ration extracorporeal membrane oxygenation during the COVID-19 pandemic? Lancet Respir Med 2021;9(4):326–8.

[140] Supady A, Brodie D, Curtis JR. Ten things to consider when implementing rationing guidelines during a pandemic. Intensive Care Med 2021;47(5):605–8.

[141] Supady A, Curtis JR, Abrams D, et al. Allocating scarce intensive care resources during the COVID-19 pandemic: practical challenges to theoretical frameworks. Lancet Respir Med 2021;9(4):430–4.

[142] Levy D, Lebreton G, Pineton de Chambrun M, et al. Outcomes of patients denied extracorporeal membrane oxygenation during the COVID-19 Pandemic in Greater Paris, France. Am J Respir Crit Care Med 2021;204(8):994–7.

[143] ELSO. ECMO availability map. Available at: https://www.elso.org/membership/ecmoavailabilitymap.aspx. [Accessed 10 December 2023].

Advances in Surgery 58 (2024) 275–291

ADVANCES IN SURGERY

Young-Onset Rectal Cancer

Is It for Real?

Reena S. Suresh, MBChB, Leonardo E. Garcia, MD, Susan L. Gearhart, MD, MEd*

Department of Surgery, Division of Colorectal Surgery, Johns Hopkins School of Medicine, 600 N. Wolfe Street / Blalock 618, Baltimore, MD 21287, USA

Keywords

• Colorectal cancer • Rectal cancer • Hereditary colorectal cancer • Early-onset colorectal cancer • Young adults

Key points

- There has been a significant rise in the incidence of early-onset colorectal cancer (EOCRC) in the last 2 decades.
- Diagnosis is delayed in EOCRC as symptoms are often overlooked and patients present at a worse stage.
- There are currently no different national or international guidelines for cancer treatment recommendations in patients with early- versus late-onset disease; however, a more aggressive management approach is often taken in younger patients.
- There are unique challenges to be addressed in patients with EOCRC such as financial concerns, fertility, sexual health, and psychosocial well-being.
- The American Cancer Society has lowered the guidelines for the age of screening to begin at 45 years in average-risk patients.

INTRODUCTION

The incidence of colorectal cancer (CRC) has been on a downward trend in patients above the age of 50 years in countries of a higher socioeconomic status. Most epidemiologists theorize that this is likely secondary to effective screening programs. What is alarming is that this has been paralleled by a significant rise since the early 1990s in the incidence of patients diagnosed with CRC under

*Corresponding author. Department of Surgery, Division of Colorectal Surgery, 600 N. Wolfe Street / Blalock 618, Baltimore, MD 21287. *E-mail address:* sdemees1@jhmi.edu

https://doi.org/10.1016/j.yasu.2024.04.015

the age of 50 years. Patients less than 50 years of age diagnosed with CRC are referred to has having young- or early-onset colorectal cancer (EOCRC) and the chosen age limit of 50 years is based on historical recommendations to initiate average-risk screening at this age [1]. As the rate of EOCRC continues to increase, it is predicted to become a significant public health threat. Of most concern, younger patients tend to be diagnosed at more advanced stages (III and IV) with poor histologic features. The origin of this trend is still largely unknown. There have been many proposed risk factors due to shifts in dietary, lifestyle, and social trends in younger populations; however, investigations into these factors have shown controversial and inconsistent findings. Although hereditary syndromes occur in up to 35% of EOCRC [2], there has not been a substantial increase in incidence of these syndromes and studies examining genetic or molecular factors have suggested that perhaps EOCRC represents a new distinct variant. Finally, the mortality rates for CRC have been declining overall; however, this has not been seen in patients with EOCRC (Fig. 1). The purpose of this article is to share with the reader current evidence on risk factors and management options for EOCRC with a focus on rectal cancer and the quality-of-life concerns which accompany this diagnosis at a young age.

EPIDEMIOLOGY

The first evidence of an increase in EOCRC in the United States was reported in the literature in 2003 by O'Connell and colleagues [3]. In this study, Surveillance, Epidemiology and End Result registries (SEER) database was examined between the years of 1973 and 1999. It was noted that there was a 17% rise in the incidence rate in colon cancer in individuals less than 50 years of age and a 75% rise in the incidence rate of rectal cancer in the same age group. Overall, however, the reported incidence of EOCRC was low. In 2009, SEER cancer registries were utilized to examine data from 1992 to 2005 for individuals aged 20 to 49 years and noted an increase in the incidence of EOCRC by 1.5% per year in male individuals and 1.6% per year in female individuals [4]. The largest annual percent increase in CRC incidence was in the youngest age group (20–29 years); 5.2% per year in men and 5.6% per year in women. Further analysis by anatomic site demonstrated a predilection for the distal colon and rectum in both sexes. Siegel and colleagues [5] reported again from an analysis of SEER data that US adults born after 1990 have a 2x fold higher risk of developing colon cancer and a 4x higher risk of developing rectal cancer. The investigator went on to predict that by 2030, 11% of all colon cancers and 23% of all rectal cancers will be diagnosed in individuals less than 50 years of age.

In parallel to these findings, large European population-based studies reported a similar increase in EOCRC. Vuik and colleagues examined national and regional cancer registries in Europe from 2004 to 2016 [6]; the study demonstrated a dramatic rise in CRC rates among individuals aged 20 to 49 years over the past 25 years. In particular, the incidence of rectal cancer rose among adults aged 20–29 years by 3.5%. In a recent review examining international trends in CRC, it was noted that several other countries had reported increasing

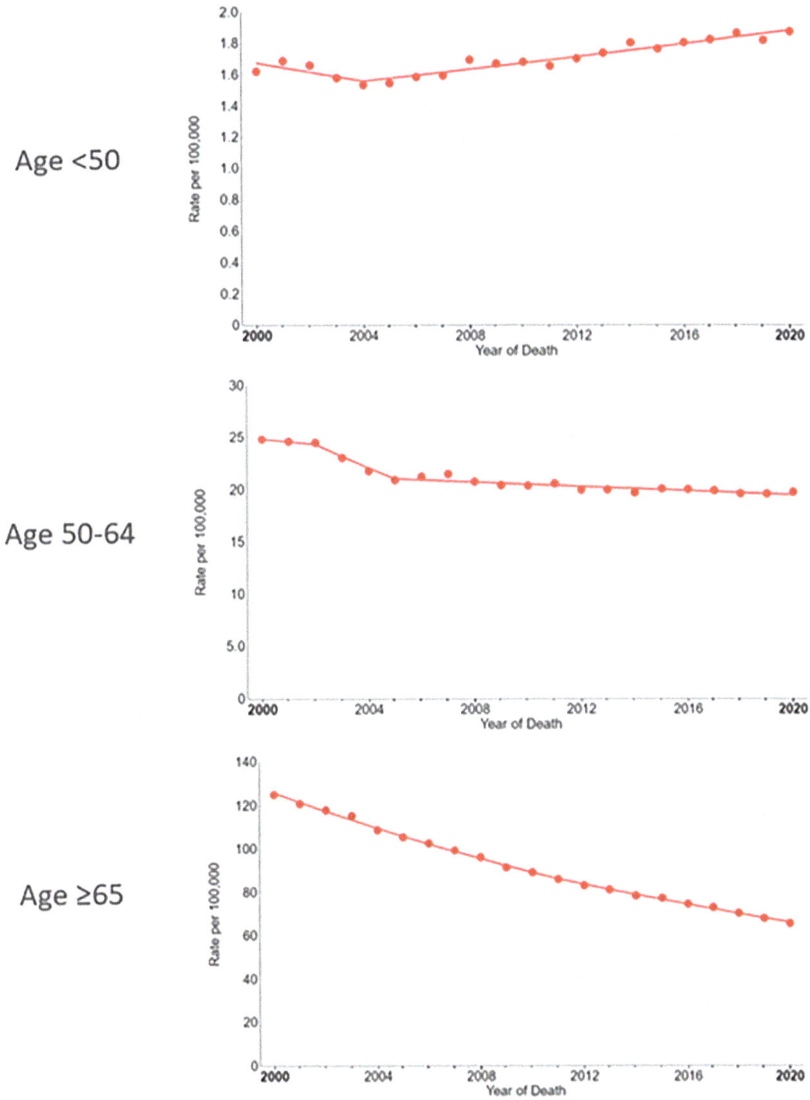

Fig. 1. Age-adjusted Surveillance, Epidemiology and End Results (SEER) mortality rates of colon and rectal cancer in the United States from 2000 to 2020 by age. (Data plotted by accessing SEER*Explorer [https://seer.cancer.gov/explorer/index.html].)

trends in the incidence of EOCRC. On examination of the Annual Average Percentage Change (AAPC) in several countries over the past 2 decades, the United Kingdom had the highest AAPC of 3.3%, followed by Canada with an AAPC of 2.8%, the United States 2.2%, and Germany 1.3% [7].

Of most concern is the changes seen in the incidence of rectal cancer. SEER data comparing colon and rectal cancer incidence rates by age can be seen from Fig. 2,

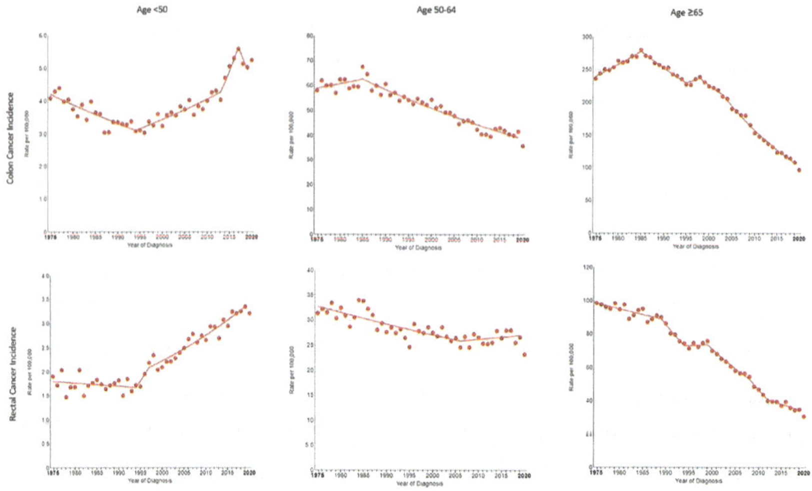

Fig. 2. Age-adjusted SEER incidence rates of colon and rectal cancer from 1975 to 2020 by age.Data plotted by accessing SEER*Explorer.

where the largest rise can be seen in rectal cancer incidence. Examining trends between 1973 and 2005 in SEER data demonstrated a significant increase in early-onset rectal cancer rates, with an annual percentage increase of 2.6%, and this was independent of sex or race [8]. This rise in the incidence of rectal cancer has been noted outside the United States. Wong and colleagues [9] examined registries from 36 countries and noted a rising rate of rectal cancer in Europe and Asia (Fig. 3). As a result of this notable trend, in May 2021, the US Preventative Services Task Force updated the guidance for CRC screening, decreasing the recommended age for average-risk patients from 50 to 45 years [10].

WHAT ARE THE EXPLANATIONS FOR THE INCREASE IN EARLY-ONSET RECTAL CANCER?

When evaluating risk factors for the development of rectal cancer, it is important to note that most etiologic studies examining risks for EOCRC group colon and rectal cancers together as a single disease. However, there is a need to separate the data as the findings for colon cancer may not necessarily apply to rectal cancer, given their inherent differences in incidence, clinicopathological features, and microbiome data [11]. Nevertheless, the rise in incidence of EOCRC remains a challenging area to study; most young adults diagnosed with EOCRC have no obvious risk factors (such as family history or inflammatory bowel disease) and would be classified as average risk by current screening guidelines. Evolving lifestyle factors alongside genetic/molecular features (Fig. 4) have been implicated, and differences in pathologic and clinical presentation raise the possibility of early-onset rectal cancer being a unique disease with different mechanisms of pathogenesis.

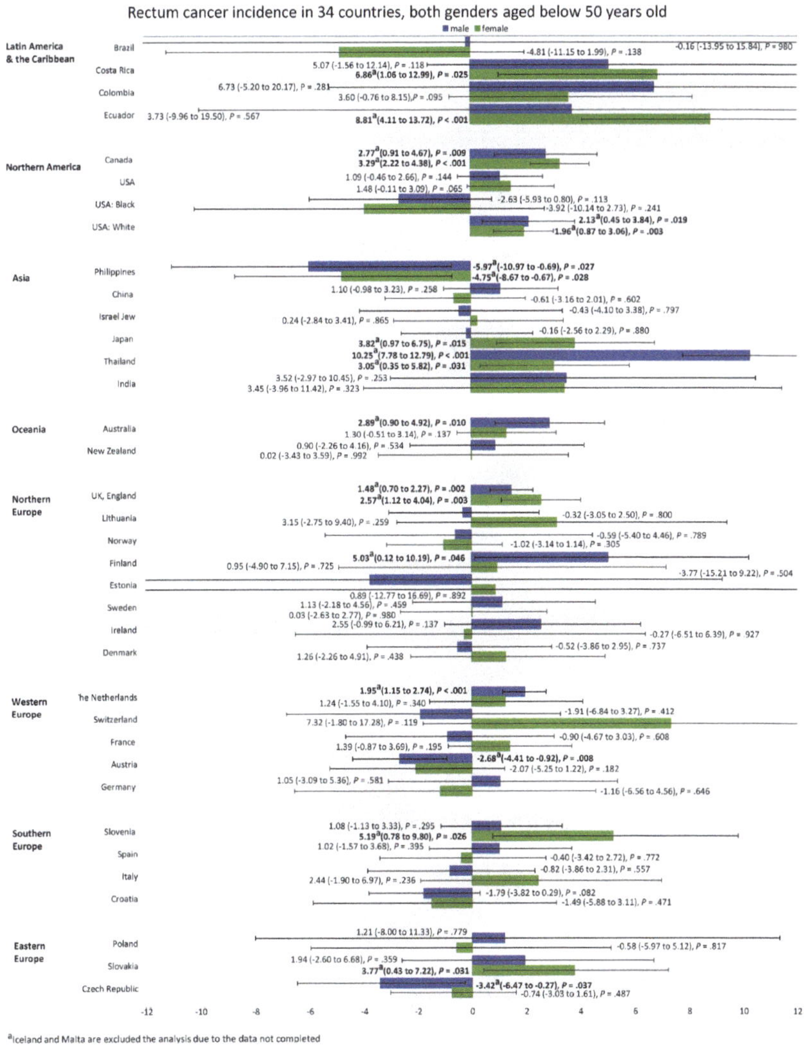

Fig. 3. Rectal cancer incidence in 34 countries for both sexes, age younger than 50 years. (*From* Wong MCS, Huang J, Lok V, Wang J, Fung F, Ding H, Zheng ZJ. Differences in Incidence and Mortality Trends of Colorectal Cancer Worldwide Based on Sex, Age, and Anatomic Location. Clin Gastroenterol Hepatol. 2021 May;19(5):955-966.e61.)

A mechanism to understand the impact of lifestyle risk factors on the development of CRC is to examine potentially modifiable risk factors. Islami and colleagues [12] examined several prevalent cancers to understand this impact using several different cancer registries and population survey data. This study reported that 54.6% of all CRC cases in the United States in 2014 were attributable to the evaluated modified risk factors. These risk factors are listed in

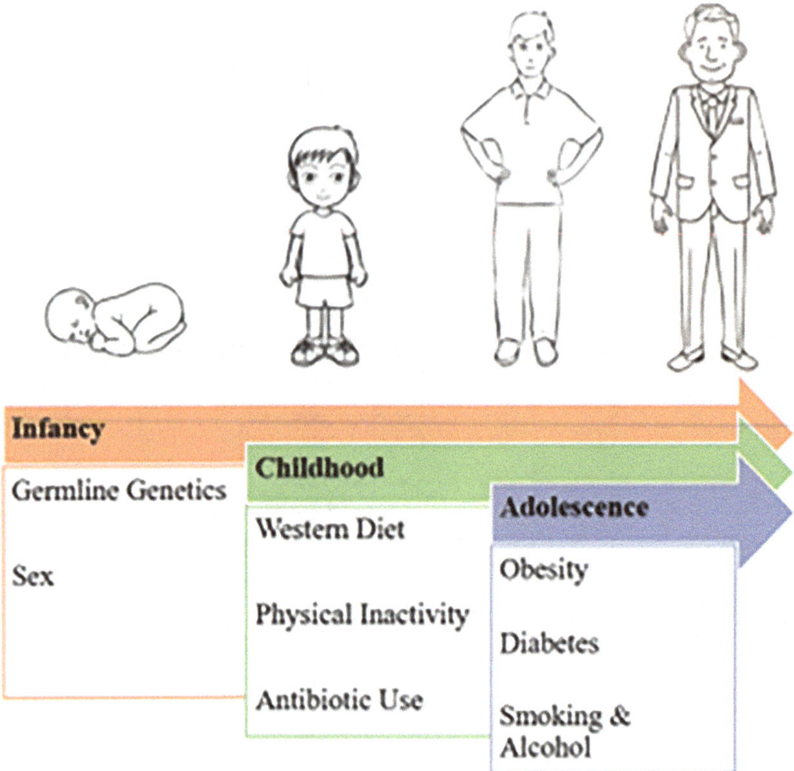

Fig. 4. Factors influencing the risk of colorectal cancer. Germline genetics, sex, diet, lifestyle exposures, and health conditions interact with the gut microbiome over a patient's lifetime and influence the risk of colorectal cancer.

Table 1. Additional evidence for behavioral and lifestyle factors is again seen in population studies such as period cohort analysis performed using data from Siegel's retrospective cohort study of patients 20 years and older diagnosed with CRC in the United States and identified in the SEER database from 1974 to 2013 [13]. This study demonstrated increasing incidences of EOCRC cases in sequential birth cohorts. The rise starts in those born between 1946 and 1964 and is at present, highest for those born in 1965 to 1980. This strong birth cohort effect suggests that population-level changes could have influenced the EOCRC risk. According to the National Program of Cancer Registry data from 2001 to 2015, there is also a geographic variation in incidence of EOCRC where the highest incidence is found in the Mississippi delta region (14 per 100,000) and lowest in the western states (9.5 per 100,000) suggesting environmental and occupational exposures may also contribute [14].

Major established modifiable risk factors for CRC are obesity, smoking, heavy alcohol consumption, and high intake of red or processed meat. An association

Table 1
Potential modifiable risk factors determined by the population attributable fraction for the development of colon and rectal cancer

Risk factor	Site: colon	Site: rectum
Smoking	x	x
Excess body weight	x	x
Excess red meat	x	x
Excess processed meat	x	x
Low dietary fiber	x	x
Low dietary calcium	x	x
Physical inactivity	x	0

Data from Islami F, Sauer A, Miller K et al. Proportion and Number of Cancer Cases and Deaths Attributable to Potentially Modifiable Risk Factors in the United States. Ca Cancer J Clin 2018;68:31-54.

between these factors and the gut microbiome has also been established. However, these associations are based almost entirely on older cohorts. At present, there is insufficient evidence and inconsistent findings regarding risk factors for EOCRC. In this segment, a few known risk factors for CRC that have been implicated for EOCRC will be discussed.

Obesity

Obesity has long been positively associated with risk of CRC. Several studies have implicated obesity to be a strong risk factor for EOCRC. A meta-analysis demonstrated a higher risk for EOCRC for overweight and obese individuals (BMI $\geq$ 25 kg/m^2) compared with normal weights (OR 1.42, 95% CI 1.19–1.68) [15]. The Nurses' Health Study II, a prospective cohort study of 85,256 women (of which 114 cases of EOCRC were identified) demonstrated women who were obese (BMI of $\geq$ 30 kg/m^2) had a nearly doubled risk of EOCRC compared with women of a body mass index (BMI) of 18.5 to 22.9 (multivariable relative risk [RR] 1.93 [95% CI 1.15–3.25]) [16]. Nguyen and colleagues [17] also reported that women who remained sedentary for more than 14 hours a week had a higher risk (RR 1.68, 95% CI 1.09–2.63) of colon cancer. The rates of childhood obesity have increased from 13.9% to 18.5% between 1999 and 2015; the rates of EOCRC may continue to rise as this population ages [18].

Diet

Red meat is described as beef, veal, pork, mutton, and lamb. Processed meats are defined as ham, bacon, sausages, and cured or preserved meats. A meta-analysis of relevant prospective studies demonstrated that the consumption of red or processed meats was associated with an increased risk for CRC [19]. The relative risk of developing CRC after consuming 100 g/day of red or processed meat was 1.14 (95% CI: 1.04–1.24) and higher amounts consumed was associated with a higher relative risk. The mechanism behind this finding is believed to be that diets high in red, processed meats, and low in fiber affect the gut microbiome and promote inflammation. Preparation techniques such as deep-frying, grilling, and roasting generate more advanced glycation end-products which can promote oxidative stress and create a microenvironment encouraging carcinogenesis [20]. While these changes in diet do provide a possible explanation, the rising incidence of EOCRC in countries with low consumption of red meat (eg, India) can question this hypothesis.

Microbiome

There is increasing evidence that changes to the intestinal tract microbiome which is made up of bacteria, viruses, and fungi can allow environmental risk factors to promote the development of CRC. Experts in the microbiome believe that alterations in the microbiome lead to changes in metabolism and immune function which ultimately lead to breakdown of the intestinal membrane and tumorigenesis [21]. Likely suspects include *Bacteroides fragilis* and *Clostridium difficile* as their increased presence/activity in the intestines of patients with EOCRC has been identified [22,23]. Efforts to sustain the health of the intestinal membrane and microbiome may be one mechanism to reduce EOCRC.

Molecular/genetic risk factors

Pathologic germline variants associated with CRC are present in an increased number of patients with EOCRC. Two multigene panel testing studies examined the incidence of germline mutations with EOCRC (450 patients in an Ohio study and 403 patients in a Michigan study); these studies found that 16% (Ohio) and 25% (Michigan) of the patients with EOCRC had germline mutations in cancer susceptibility genes [24,25]. Further findings of interest include a relatively high rate of kirsten rat sarcoma viral oncogene homolog (KRAS) mutations, tumor protein 53 (TP53) mutations, long interspersed nuclear element (LINE-1) hypomethylation, and generally low incidences of BRAF^{V600E} and adenomatous polyposis coli (APC) mutations among EOCRC [26]. These findings suggest that EOCRC may be a distinct entity with a unique set of genetic features.

CLINICAL AND PATHOLOGIC FEATURES

There are multiple differences in the presentation of early- versus late-onset CRC regarding symptoms, anatomic site, histopathology, and stage at diagnosis (Table 2). Studies have reported up to 86% of patients with EOCRC to be symptomatic at the time of diagnosis with the most common symptoms and signs being hematochezia, iron-deficiency anemia, and weight loss [27,28]. EOCRC has a predilection for the left colon and rectum and more frequently demonstrates adverse histopathological features [29]. Data from the National Cancer Database and SEER demonstrated EOCRC to more likely to have a mucinous or signet-ring histology (12.6% vs 10.8%, $P<.01$) and poor or no differentiation (20.4% vs 18%, $P<.01$) compared to the older onset [30]. In addition, EOCRC is more likely to present with more stage III and IV diseases compared to the older onset CRC [31]. Combined incidence data from SEER and the National Program of Cancer Registries data are shown to demonstrate CRC stage distribution by age (Fig. 5) [32].

Table 2
Differences in patterns of presentation, tumor factors, and treatment methods described among patients with EOCRC versus late-onset CRC

Characteristics	Young-onset colorectal cancer	Late-onset colorectal cancer
Presentation	• Delay from symptom onset to presentation • More likely to present with signs and symptoms (hematochezia, iron-deficiency anemia, weight loss)	• Earlier detection (screening) • Asymptomatic disease at presentation is more common
Location	• Distal colon and rectum	• Right colon
Disease Stage at Diagnosis	• More advanced stage at presentation (stages III/IV)	• Reduced likelihood of metastases • Stage I/II more common
Pathologic Features	• Poor differentiation • Mucinous tumors • Signet-ring morphology • Perineural/venous invasion	• The ratio of well-differentiated carcinoma is higher
Molecular Profile	• Microsatellite instability • More likely to exhibit LINE-1 hypomethylation and TP53 sequence variations • Less frequently harbor KRAS, BRAF V600E, and APC sequences	• More frequent APC and BRAF mutations
Treatment	• More likely to have postoperative systemic chemotherapy • Multiagent chemotherapy regimens • More likely to undergo radiation therapy	• The ratio of patients undergoing less aggressive therapy is higher

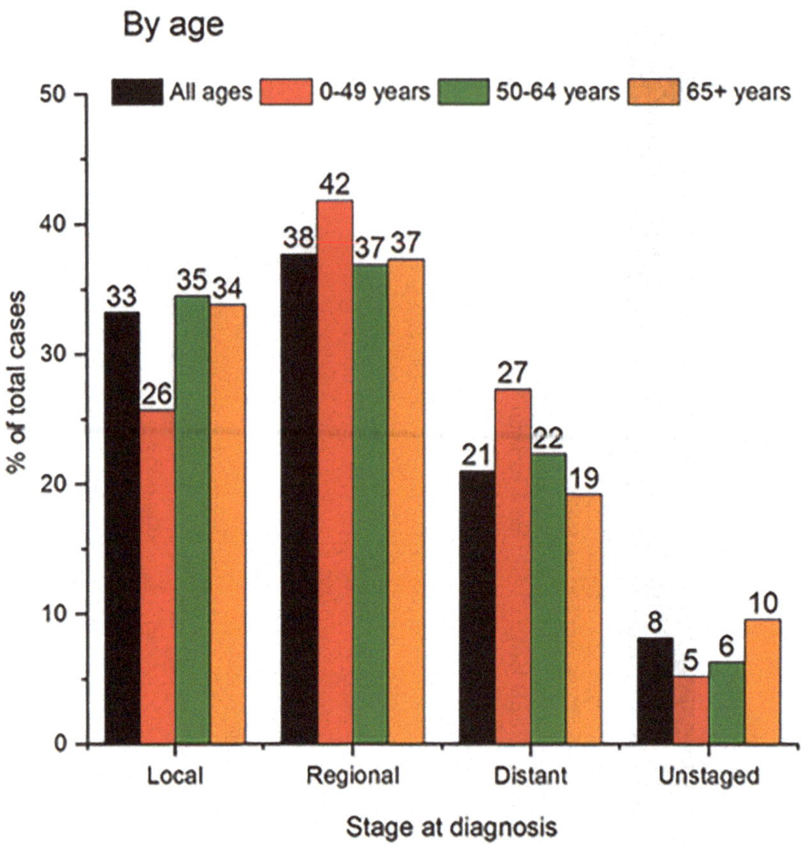

Fig. 5. Colorectal cancer stage distribution (%) by age (Colorectal Cancer Statistics 2023). (*From* Siegel RL, Wagle NS, Cercek A, Smith RA, Jemal A. Colorectal cancer statistics, 2023. *CA: A Cancer Journal for Clinicians.* 2023;73(3). doi:https://doi.org/10.3322/caac.21772.)

TREATMENT

At present, the guidelines in the United States are not age-specific with regard to treatment of EOCRC, and most strategies are based on studies which included older patients with CRC. As younger patients are often more robust and have improved performance status, they are more likely to receive more aggressive multimodal therapies; however, this has not translated into a significant survival benefit [33]. Recent guidelines have been established for the management of EOCRC and endorsed by the Associazone Italiana Familarita Ereditarieta Tumori, the Collaborative Group of the Americas on Inherited Gastrointestinal Cancers, the European Hereditary Tumor Group, and the International Society for Gastrointestinal Hereditary Tumours [34]. These guidelines mandate the following:

1. EOCRC must undergo germline multigene panel testing and complete a family history. Germline multigene panel testing can provide guidance on surgical planning and the use of chemotherapy or immunotherapy. A discussion of prophylactic colectomy for patients with polyposis syndrome and the risk of metachronous CRC and uterine cancer in patients with Lynch syndrome should be conducted. Patients with EOCRC who are mismatch repair deficient may benefit from immunotherapy and should avoid 5-fluorouracil (5-FU)-based treatment.
2. EOCRC should receive information on fertility preservation options. Current options for fertility preservation include ovarian transposition prior to the initiation of radiotherapy. In addition, there is the option of cryopreservation of oocytes, embryos, ovarian tissue, and sperm banking. One must also consider the risk of uterine damage as a result of radiation and recent small studies have explored the benefits of uterine transposition for preservation of fertility [35].
3. Consider enhanced antiemetic prophylaxis during treatment of EOCRC. Symptom control is imperative to treatment adherence. There is an increased risk of nausea and vomiting among women with EOCRC [36].
4. Patients with EOCRC should not be discharged from follow-up. The risk of metachronous CRC is increased among EOCRC [37]; however, there is insufficient evidence to support increased intensity of current follow-up recommendations or to support discharge from follow-up after a certain observation period.

There are many areas of controversy in the management of EOCRC. At present, there is limited evidence on any added benefit of neoadjuvant and adjuvant chemotherapy beyond standard treatment regimens in the management of EOCRC. A more aggressive approach in the management of EOCRC has been described, and as a result, it has been reported that younger patients were more likely to receive systemic chemotherapy at all stages, with only minimal gain in survival compared to their older counterparts who received less treatment. Moreover, young adults have been reported to be more likely to receive multiagent regimens at all stages [38]. Patient demands and the perception of young adults to tolerate more treatment may have influenced these practices; however, the potential for treatment-related toxicity cannot be overlooked. Long-term data from international studies have demonstrated a 10% to 15% rate of persistent peripheral sensory neuropathy and a 3% rate of persistent toxicities that interfere with daily activity after multiagent chemotherapy [39,40]. In addition to chemotherapy, there is also concern about overtreatment with radiotherapy. Analyzing the National Cancer Database, younger patients were more likely to receive radiotherapy for all stages—including stage I disease (41.9% in the young onset vs 31.7% in the late onset, $P<.01$) [41].

It has also been demonstrated that patients with EOCRC with distant metastases were more likely to undergo surgery for their primary tumor compared to their older counterparts (72% vs 63%, $P<.001$) [42]. This may be secondary to more emergent or symptomatic presentations, or an increased willingness to pursue more aggressive therapy by patients with EOCRC and their surgeons. Furthermore, it is not recommended to perform more extensive surgical resection for patients with EOCRC who do not have a high-risk predisposition (such as a hereditary syndrome or ulcerative colitis) [43]. Gynecologic cancers also need to be considered as patients with Lynch syndrome have a higher risk of endometrial/ovarian cancer before the age of 50 years. Simultaneous hysterectomy with or without oophorectomy may be required for patients with Lynch syndrome [44]. These decisions should be individualized, and patients should be appropriately counseled.

ADDITIONAL CARE CONSIDERATIONS IN EARLY-ONSET COLORECTAL CANCER

With the rising incidence of EOCRC, unique challenges need to be addressed including financial and psychological impacts (Fig. 6).

Financial impact

Patients with EOCRC are particularly susceptible to the financial hardships posed by cancer treatments [45]. These patients are more likely to lack savings and employment security; patients can also face indirect costs through lost wages and lower earning potential [46]. Many patients will often feel the need to continue to work soon after treatment which presents an additional stressor to patients. Some may have families with young children who are

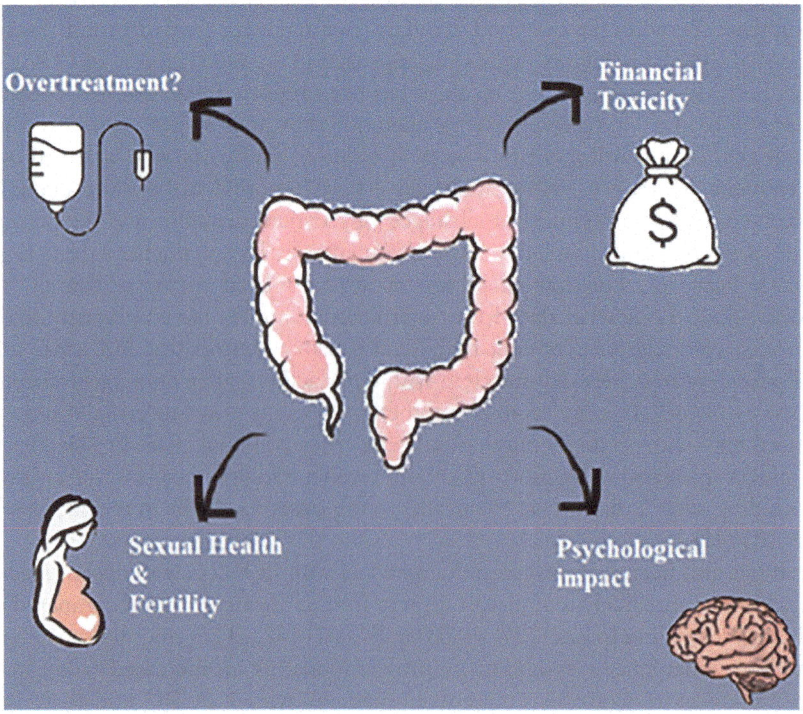

Fig. 6. Graphic abstract of additional care considerations in EOCRC.

dependent on them for support [47]. It is imperative to seek opportunities and openly discuss and address financial hardships for patients and their families; this requires engagement of the multidisciplinary team to provide resources for support.

Psychological impact

There is a paucity of research focusing on survivorship issues, including the mental and social implications of survivorship and the impact on dependents. As mentioned earlier, the incidence of rectal cancer is rising faster than colon cancer in young adults. Unfortunately, many long-term survivors of rectal cancer can experience late effects on their quality of life including sexual dysfunction, fecal incontinence, urinary incontinence, neuropathy, and psychosocial impacts of having an ostomy. Cancer treatment survivors have reported significant rates of sexual dysfunction; erectile dysfunction was more often present in those following rectal cancer treatment compared to colon cancer [48]. Studies have also reported patients with a present or past ostomy to have worse sexual function and to struggle more with body image-related issues [49]. Patients with EOCRC will undergo a vastly different psychosocial experience compared to elderly patients. International studies have demonstrated younger patients with cancer to have a worse quality of life, increased depression and anxiety, increased disruptions to social and sexual health, and greater emotional distress than older patients with CRC [50,51]. There is a clear need to empower patients and medical caregivers to proactively discuss sexual health and long-term impacts of therapies, especially with the rising number of EOCRC.

Future research

The incidence of EOCRC is rising at an alarming rate and there is an urgent need for research to address this important public health concern. There should be a focus on addressing important gaps in research including screening and diagnostic delays in young populations, assessing outcomes after oncologic and surgical therapies, and addressing financial concerns, psychosocial well-being, and fertility. There are many factors that could lead to overall poorer outcomes among EOCRC; most significant would be a lack of awareness by patients and providers as rectal cancer is commonly associated with older age. A 2019 survey demonstrated that patients with EOCRC were unaware that CRC can arise in individuals under 50 years and symptomatic patients often waited over 6 months to seek medical attention [52]. There are also significant delays by primary care physicians referring to specialists for diagnostic evaluation [53]. The advanced stage at presentation has led to aggressive therapies and a significant decrease in quality of life. Patients with EOCRC have suffered from neuropathy, anxiety, depression, and sexual dysfunction [54]. No survival benefit in younger patients or occasionally even lower survival in young patients has been reported when compared with their older counterparts. There is a significant need for a multifactorial approach to address this rising number of younger onset cases. This should include patient and provider education, research exploring trends and potential etiologic factors, and addressing knowledge gaps in management such as whether patients with EOCRC should receive different surgical, adjuvant, neoadjuvant, and supportive treatments.

CLINICS CARE POINTS

Diagnosis	• The most common symptoms and signs found for EOCRC were hematochezia (46%), iron-deficiency anemia (13.0%), and weight loss (10%). • These should prompt early evaluation and an expedited diagnostic colonoscopy. • The US screening guidelines now recommend average risk screening begins at age 45 years.
Risk factors	• A thorough family history should be taken to inform risk assessment for CRC. • There is insufficient evidence at present to implicate factors such as sex, ethnicity, obesity, diet, and hyperlipidemia as risk factors to recommend earlier screening.
Genetics	• All newly diagnosed patients with EOCRC should receive genetic testing, ideally before surgery, to determine the possible hereditary nature of their disease.
Treatment	• There is no evidence to suggest that neoadjuvant, adjuvant therapy, and surgery should differ in EOCRC without a high-risk predisposition.
Fertility and sexual health	• Clinicians should refer patients with EOCRC to a specialist in reproductive medicine before treatment to discuss risks of infertility, preservation options, and pregnancy. • Discussions regarding fertility, sexual health, and psychological counseling should be had early.

Disclosure

The authors have nothing to disclose.

References

[1] Pignone M, Rich M, Teutsch SM, et al. Screening for Colorectal Cancer in Adults at Average Risk: A Summary of the Evidence for the U.S. Preventive Services Task Force. Ann Intern Med 2002;137(2):132.

[2] Mork ME, You YN, Ying J, et al. High Prevalence of Hereditary Cancer Syndromes in Adolescents and Young Adults With Colorectal Cancer. J Clin Oncol 2015;33(31):3544–9.

[3] O'Connell JZB, Maggard MA, Liu JH, et al. Rates of colon and rectal cancers are increasing in young adults. Am Surg 2003;69:866–72.

[4] Siegel R, Jemal A, Ward E. Increase in Incidence of Colorectal Cancer Among Young Men and Women in the United States. Cancer Epidemiol Biomarkers Prev 2009;18:1695–8.

[5] Siegel R, Fedewa S, Anderson W, et al. Colorectal Cancer Incidence Patterns in the United States, 1974-2013. JNCI Natl Cancer Inst 2017;109:1–6.
[6] Vuik F, Nieuwenburg S, Bardou M, et al. Increasing incidence of colorectal cancer in young adults in Europe over the last 25 years. Gut 2019;68:1820–6.
[7] Li N, Lu B, Luo C, et al. Incidence, mortality, survival, risk factor, and screening of colorectal cancer: A comparison among China, Europe, and Northern America. Cancer Lett 2021;522:255–68.
[8] Meyer JE, Narang T, Schnoll-Sussman FH, et al. Increasing incidence of rectal cancer in patients aged younger than 40 years. Cancer 2010;116(18):4354–9.
[9] Wong MCS, Huang J, Lok V, et al. Differences in Incidence and Mortality Trends of Colorectal Cancer Worldwide Based on Sex, Age, and Anatomic Location. Clin Gastroenterol Hepatol 2021 May;19(5):955–66.e61.
[10] Wolf AMD, Fontham ETH, Church TR, et al. Colorectal cancer screening for average-risk adults: 2018 guideline update from the American Cancer Society. CA A Cancer J Clin 2018;68(4):250–81.
[11] Xi Y, Yuefen P, Wei W, et al. Analysis of prognosis, genome, microbiome, and microbial metabolome in different sites of colorectal cancer. J Tansl Med 2019;17:353.
[12] Islami F, Sauer A, Miller K, et al. Proportion and Number of Cancer Cases and Deaths Attributable to Potentially Modifiable Risk Factors in the United States. Ca Cancer J Clin 2018;68: 31–54.
[13] Siegel RL, Fedewa SA, Anderson WF, et al. Colorectal Cancer Incidence Patterns in the United States, 1974-2013. J Natl Cancer Inst 2017;109(8):djw322.
[14] Stoffel EM, Murphy CC. Epidemiology and Mechanisms of the Increasing Incidence of Colon and Rectal Cancers in Young Adults. Gastroenterology 2020;158(2):341–53.
[15] Li H, Boakye D, Chen X, et al. Association of Body Mass Index With Risk of Early-Onset Colorectal Cancer: Systematic Review and Meta-Analysis. Am J Gastroenterol 2021;116(11): 2173–83.
[16] Liu PH, Wu K, Ng K, et al. Association of Obesity With Risk of Early-Onset Colorectal Cancer Among Women. JAMA Oncol 2019;5(1):37–44.
[17] Nguyen LH, Liu PH, Zheng X, et al. Sedentary Behaviors, TV Viewing Time, and Risk of Young-Onset Colorectal Cancer. JNCI Cancer Spectr 2019;2(4).
[18] Sanyaolu A, Okorie C, Qi X, et al. Childhood and Adolescent Obesity in the United States: a Public Health Concern. Global Pediatric Health 2019;6(6).
[19] Chan DS, Lau R, Aune D, et al. Red and processed meat and colorectal cancer incidence: meta-analysis of prospective studies. PLoS One 2011;6(6):e20456.
[20] Azizian-Farsani F, Abedpoor N, Hasan Sheikhha M, et al. Receptor for Advanced Glycation End Products Acts as a Fuel to Colorectal Cancer Development. Front Oncol 2020;10.
[21] Ahmad Kendong SM, Raja Ali RA, Nawawi KNM, et al. Gut Dysbiosis and Intestinal Barrier Dysfunction: Potential Explanation for Early-Onset Colorectal Cancer. Front Cell Infect Microbiol 2021;11:744606.
[22] Song M, Chan AT, Sun J. Influence of the Gut Microbiome, Diet, and Environment on Risk of Colorectal Cancer. Gastroenterology 2020;158(2):322–40.
[23] Drewes J, Chen J, Markham N, et al. Human Colon Cancer-Derived *Clostridiole difficile* Strains Drive Colonic Tumorigenesis. Cancer Discov 2022;12:1873–85.
[24] Pearlman R, Frankel WL, Swanson B, et al. Prevalence and Spectrum of Germline Cancer Susceptibility Gene Mutations Among Patients With Early-Onset Colorectal Cancer. JAMA Oncol 2017;3(4):464.
[25] Stoffel EM, Koeppe E, Everett J, et al. Germline Genetic Features of Young Individuals With Colorectal Cancer. Gastroenterology 2018;154(4):897–905.
[26] REACTT Collaborative, Zaborowski AM, Abdile A, et al. Characteristics of Early-Onset vs. Late-Onset Colorectal Cancer: A Review. JAMA Surgery 2021;156:865–74.

[27] Siegel RL, Jakubowski CD, Fedewa SA, et al. Colorectal cancer in the young: Epidemiology, prevention, management. American Society of Clinical Oncology Educational Book 2020;40(40):e75–88.
[28] Dozois EJ, Boardman LA, Suwanthanma W, et al. Young-Onset Colorectal Cancer in Patients With No Known Genetic Predisposition. Medicine 2008;87(5):259–63.
[29] Patel SG, Ahnen DJ. Colorectal Cancer in the Young. Curr Gastroenterol Rep 2018;20(4).
[30] You YN, Xing Y, Feig BW, et al. Young-Onset Colorectal Cancer: Is It Time to Pay Attention? Arch Intern Med 2012;172(3):287.
[31] Chen FW, Sundaram V, Chew TA, et al. Advanced Stage Colorectal Cancer in Persons Younger Than 50 Years not Associated With Longer Duration of Symptoms or Time to Diagnosis. Clinical gastroenterology and 2017;15(5):728–37.
[32] Siegel RL, Wagle NS, Cercek A, et al. Colorectal cancer statistics, 2023. CA A Cancer J Clin 2023;73(3); https://doi.org/10.3322/caac.21772.
[33] Siegel RL, Miller KD, Jemal A. Colorectal Cancer Mortality Rates in Adults Aged 20 to 54 Years in the United States, 1970-2014. JAMA 2017;318(6):572.
[34] Cavestro Giulia Martina, Mannucci Alessandro, Balaguer F, et al. Delphi Initiative for Early-Onset Colorectal Cancer (DIRECt) International Management Guidelines. Clin Gastroenterol Hepatol 2023;21(3):581–603.e33.
[35] Ribeiro R, Baiocchi G, Moretti-Marques R, et al. Uterine transposition for fertility and ovarian function preservation after radiotherapy. Int J Gynecol Cancer 2023;33(12):1837–42.
[36] Fontana E, Meyers JP, Sobrero AF, et al. Early-onset colorectal adenocarcinoma in the IDEA database: treatment adherence, toxicities, and outcomes with 3 and 6 months of adjuvant fluoropyrimidine and oxaliplatin. J Clin Oncol 2021;39:4009–19.
[37] Liang J, Huang K, Cheng AL, et al. Clinicopathological and molecular biological features of colorectal cancer in patients less than 40 years of age. Br J Surg 2003;90(2):205–14.
[38] Kneuertz PJ, Chang GJ, Hu CY, et al. Overtreatment of Young Adults With Colon Cancer. JAMA Surgery 2015;150(5):402.
[39] Braun MS, Seymour MT. Balancing the efficacy and toxicity of chemotherapy in colorectal cancer. Therapeutic Advances in Medical Oncology 2011;3(1):43–52.
[40] Kidwell KM, Yothers G, Ganz PA, et al. Long-term neurotoxicity effects of oxaliplatin added to fluorouracil and leucovorin as adjuvant therapy for colon cancer: Results from National Surgical Adjuvant Breast and Bowel Project trials C-07 and LTS-01. Cancer 2012;118(22): 5614–22.
[41] Kolarich A, George TJ Jr, Hughes SJ, et al. Rectal cancer patients younger than 50 years lack a survival benefit from NCCN guideline-directed treatment for stage II and III disease. Cancer 2018;124(17):3510–9.
[42] Abdelsattar ZM, Wong SL, Regenbogen SE, et al. Colorectal cancer outcomes and treatment patterns in patients too young for average-risk screening. Cancer 2016;122(6): 929–34.
[43] Klos CL, Montenegro G, Jamal N, et al. Segmental versus extended resection for sporadic colorectal cancer in young patients. J Surg Oncol 2014;110(3):328–32.
[44] Schmeler KM, Lynch HT, Chen L, et al. Prophylactic Surgery to Reduce the Risk of Gynecologic Cancers in the Lynch Syndrome. N Engl J Med 2006;354(3):261–9.
[45] Zheng Z, Jemal A, Han X, et al. Medical financial hardship among cancer survivors in the United States. Cancer 2019;125(10):1737–47.
[46] Mehnert A. Employment and work-related issues in cancer survivors. Crit Rev Oncol Hematol 2011;77(2):109–30.
[47] Blum-Barnett E, Madrid S, Burnett-Hartman A, et al. Financial burden and quality of life among early-onset colorectal cancer survivors: A qualitative analysis. Health Expect 2019;22(5):1050–7.
[48] Den Oudsten BL, Traa MJ, Thong MSY, et al. Higher prevalence of sexual dysfunction in colon and rectal cancer survivors compared with the normative population: A population-based study. Eur J Cancer 2012;48(17):3161–70.

[49] Reese JB, Finan PH, Haythornthwaite JA, et al. Gastrointestinal ostomies and sexual outcomes: a comparison of colorectal cancer patients by ostomy status. Support Care Cancer: Official Journal of the Multinational Association of Supportive Care in Cancer 2014;22(2): 461–8.
[50] Waddell O, Mclauchlan J, McCombie A, et al. Quality of life in early-onset colorectal cancer patients: systematic review. BJS Open 2023;7(3).
[51] Howren A, Sayre EC, Cheng V, et al. Risk of Anxiety and Depression after Diagnosis of Young-Onset Colorectal Cancer: A Population-Based Cohort Study. Curr Oncol 2022;29(5): 3072–81.
[52] Scott RB, Rangel LE, Osler TM, et al. Rectal cancer in patients under the age of 50 years: the delayed diagnosis. Am J Surg 2016;211(6):1014–8.
[53] Yarden RI, Newcomer KL, Board NTYA. Young onset colorectal cancer patients are diagnosed with advanced disease after multiple misdiagnoses. Cancer Res 2019;79(13_Supplement): 3347.
[54] Buccafusca G, Proserpio I, Tralongo AC, et al. Early colorectal cancer: diagnosis, treatment and survivorship care. Crit Rev Oncol-Hematol 2019;136:20–30.

Advances in Surgery 58 (2024) 293–309

ADVANCES IN SURGERY

The Role of Surgery for Stage IV Breast Cancer

Baraah M.A. Mohamed, MD[a,1], Lisa Jacobs, MD, MSPH[b,*]

[a]York WellSpan Health, 1001 South George Street, PO Box 15198, York, PA 17405-7198, USA; [b]Johns Hopkins University, 600 N. Wolfe Street, Blalock 688, Baltimore, MD 21287, USA

Keywords

• Metastatic breast cancer • Surgery • Palliative surgery
• Surgery with curative intent • Liver metastases • Lung metastases
• Brain metastases • Breast cancer subtypes

Key points

- The role of surgery for palliation of metastatic breast cancer is well established. Palliation may be needed for an intact primary tumor or systemic metastases.
- Surgery of an intact primary breast cancer has been investigated in 4 randomized trials. The results of those trials are reviewed.
- Surgery of systemic secondary metastases is supported for palliative purposes. The therapeutic benefit is controversial and depends on the site and the goal of surgery.

BACKGROUND

Breast cancer is the most common cancer in the United States with an estimated 297,790 people diagnosed in 2023 accounting for 15.2% of all cancer cases with an overall survival (OS) 90.8%. There will be an estimated 43,170 deaths from breast cancer accounting for 7.1% of all cancer deaths making it the fourth leading cause of cancer death. Based on the Surveillance, Epidemiology and End Results (SEER) database 6% of the newly diagnosed patients will be stage IV at the time of diagnosis (de novo metastatic disease; Fig. 1). Metastatic breast cancer can also occur at a time remote to the initial diagnosis most commonly presenting with bone, liver, lung, or brain metastases (secondary metastases). The incidence and death rate of breast cancer has been

[1]Present address: 3204 Rowen Court, York, PA 17403.

*Corresponding author. 600 N. Wolfe Street, Blalock 688, Baltimore, MD 21287. *E-mail address:* Ljacob14@jh.edu

https://doi.org/10.1016/j.yasu.2024.04.016

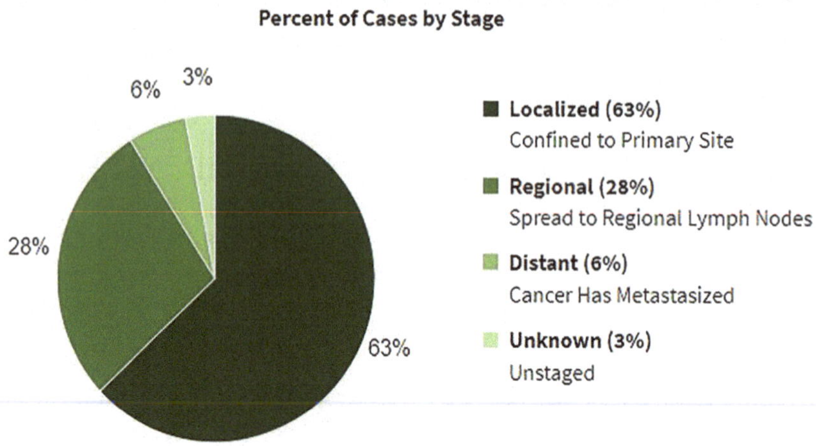

Fig. 1. Breast cancer stage at presentation as reported by the National Cancer Institute using data from the Surveillance, Epidemiology, and End Results (SEER) Program.

decreasing over the last 20 years. The observed 5 year survival in 1995 was 87.3%, and in 2015, it was 92.8%. From 1999 to 2019, the observed rate of new breast cancers per 100,000 people decreased from 142.3 to 136.3. During the same time frame, the observed death rate per 100,000 people decreased from 26.6 to 19.4. The reductions in death rate and improvement in 5 year survival rate are likely due to improvements in systemic therapies. With those improvements, the number of patients living with metastatic disease is increasing with a 31% 5 year survival of those diagnosed with stage IV disease (Fig. 2) [1]. This leads to the question of whether surgical management of metastatic disease should be pursued.

Traditionally, metastatic breast cancer has been considered incurable with surgery done only for palliative purposes. In the early 2000s, a number of retrospective reviews were completed using national and single-institution databases evaluating the role of surgical management of the primary tumor in de novo metastatic breast cancer. While these studies were flawed by selection bias due to the retrospective nature of the data, many showed an improvement in survival with surgical management. These results prompted the initiation of randomized trials to address the value of surgery in the face of metastatic disease. This article first discusses the management of de novo disease and then addresses secondary metastatic disease.

IMPACT OF TUMOR SUBTYPES ON METASTATIC DISEASE

Breast cancer subtypes have been developed for both the prognostic and predictive value. The tumor features used to determine the subtypes are the presence/absence of hormone receptors (HRs), the presence of human epidermal

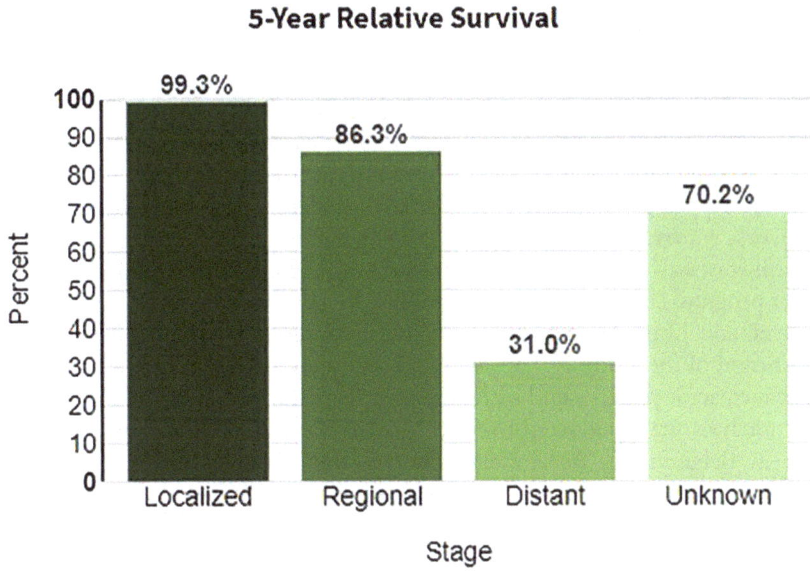

Fig. 2. The 5 year breast cancer survival rates based on stage at diagnosis as reported by the National Cancer Institute using data from the Surveillance, Epidemiology, and End Results (SEER) Program.

growth factor receptor 2 (HER2) over expression, and the Ki-67 level of greater or less than 20%. The 4 subtypes are (1) Luminal A which is HR+/HER2−/Ki-67 low, (2) Luminal B which is HR+/HER2−/Ki-67 high, (3) HER2 which is HR ± HER2+, and (4) triple negative (TN) which is HR−/HER2−. The subtypes are prognostic providing estimates of risk of recurrence and survival and correlates with location and frequency of metastatic disease. The subtypes are also predictive providing insight into the likelihood of successful treatment with targeted therapies such as hormone therapy and HER2 targeting therapies. Luminal A tumors have the lowest risk of recurrence with metastatic disease most commonly occurring in bone with fewer visceral and central nervous system (CNS) metastases. Survival with metastatic disease is longer with Luminal A tumors. Luminal B tumors have a worse prognosis as compared to Luminal A due to the higher proliferation rate. These tumors also develop bone metastases but have a higher rate of visceral metastases compared to Luminal A tumors. HER2 tumors are more aggressive than the luminal tumors and have a lower survival. However, the development of HER2-targeted therapies has increased the survival of HER2+ tumors. These tumors also develop bone metastases but have a higher rate of visceral metastases when compared to the luminal tumors. TN is the most aggressive breast cancer subtype and is the subtype most likely to present with de novo metastatic disease and to develop secondary metastases [2].

To further evaluate the role of subtypes on the pattern and frequency of metastases, Xiao analyzed the SEER database including 295,213 patients from the years 2010 to 2014 [3]. Of the patients with de novo metastatic breast cancer, 3.28% had bone metastases, 1.52% had lung metastases, 1.20% had liver metastases, and 0.35% had brain metastases. The median survival is best with bone metastases (30 months) and worst with brain metastases (11 months). The survival of all types of metastases is best for HR+/HER2+ tumors. TN tumors have the worst survival with all types of metastatic disease. Of those patients with bone metastases or lung metastases, those with HR+/HER2− tumors have a better prognosis than those with HR−/HER2+ tumors. The same did not apply to liver and brain metastases where the prognosis was similar. The overall conclusion of the study is that the tumor subtypes are associated with both de novo metastatic patterns and with prognosis from the metastases. A similar database analysis was conducted by Van Mechelen using a single-institution database in Belgium [4]. As a cross-sectional study, it included both de novo metastatic disease and secondary metastases. Of the 5972 patients included in the study from the years of 2000 to 2010, 308 presented with de novo breast cancer. After a median follow-up of 103.6 months, 817 of the 5664 (14.4%) patients developed secondary metastases. The tumor subtype was predictive of both risk of development of metastases and the risk of death from disease. The rate of metastases was 11.8% for Luminal A, 24.9% for Luminal B, 26.3% for HER2, and 29.2% for TN. Bone metastases were most common in Luminal A and B tumors and least common in TN. Liver metastases were most common in HER2 and least common in TN. Lung metastases were most common in TN and least common in Luminal A. Brain metastases were most common in TN and least common in Luminal A. Tumor subtype was also prognostic with the highest breast cancer-specific survival in Luminal A tumors and in tumors that are HR+/HER2+ treated with trastuzumab. The survival was lower in TN. The site of the metastasis was also predictive of survival when it was a single site. Median survival of brain metastases was 13.9 months, and for bone metastases, it was 48.4 months. Using a Cox regression analysis, the investigators identified age, subtype, de novo versus secondary metastasis, and number of metastases as predictors of breast cancer-specific survival. The findings of these 2 studies are consistent and show that tumor subtype is predictive of site of metastases and overall prognosis.

Over the last 20 years, there have been a number of research studies both retrospective reviews and more recently randomized trials addressing the topic of surgical management of the primary tumor in cases of de novo metastatic disease. In addition, surgical management of distant metastatic disease has also been investigated. Both are addressed in this article.

MANAGEMENT OF DE NOVO METASTATIC BREAST CANCER

Retrospective data

Over the last 20 years, a number of retrospective reviews of prospective databases have been completed to evaluate the benefit of surgery for de novo breast cancer. Large national and single-institution databases have been used attempting to determine the benefit of surgical management of the primary in de novo metastatic breast cancer. All of these studies identify selection bias as having a potential impact on the results. Varied approaches were used in these studies to attempt to identify populations of patients that may benefit from treatment of the primary tumor. These studies as a group generally found an improvement in survival with treatment of the primary tumor. A meta-analysis of 15 retrospective case series completed by Petrelli [5] identified a consistent improvement in survival associated with surgery of the primary tumor with a hazard ratio of 0.69 ($P < .00001$). The survival benefit is independent of age, tumor burden, type of surgery, margin status, site of metastases, HR status, and HER2 status. In addition to the surgery, the use of systemic therapy (ST) and radiation therapy was associated with improvements in survival.

Cochrane review of randomized trials

A Cochrane review was completed to evaluate the role of surgery in de novo metastatic breast cancer [6]. The inclusion criteria were randomized controlled trials of women with metastatic breast cancer at initial diagnosis comparing breast surgery plus ST versus ST alone. The primary outcomes were OS and quality of life. Secondary outcomes were progression-free survival (local and distant control), breast cancer-specific survival, and toxicity from local therapy. Two trials enrolling 624 women were included in the review [7,8]. The review is unable to make conclusions about the ability of breast surgery to improve OS because the quality of the evidence has been assessed as very low (hazard ratio [HR] 0.83, 95% CI 0.53–1.31; 2 studies; 624 women). The 2 studies included did not report quality-of-life assessments. The conclusion from the review is that "breast surgery may improve local progression-free survival (HR 0.22, 95% CI 0.08–0.57; 2 studies; 607 women; low-quality evidence), while it probably worsened distant progression-free survival (HR 1.42, 95% CI 1.08–1.86; 1 study; 350 women; moderate-quality evidence)." The 2 included studies did not measure breast cancer-specific survival. Toxicity from local therapy was reported by 30 day mortality and did not appear to differ between the 2 groups (RR 0.99, 95% CI 0.14–6.90; 1 study; 274 women; low-quality evidence). The Cochrane review was completed before the POSYTIVE [9] and Khan [10] trials were reported.

Randomized controlled trials

Dr Khan initiated the conversation about surgery for the intact primary in patients with metastatic breast cancer with her retrospective review of the National Cancer Data Base (NCDB) database in 2002 where she found that surgery may have a beneficial effect on survival [11]. Her publication and several others retrospective reviews over 15 years highlighted the need for controlled randomized trials to definitively answer the question. Four randomized controlled trials have been reported (Table 1). The accrual in the reported trials varies from 90 to 350. The timing of surgery and the use of ST have varied among the trials.

Table 1
Randomized trials evaluating surgical treatment of the primary tumor in de novo metastatic breast cancer

Trial	N	OS (Months)		Local Disease-free Progression		Timing of Randomization	Biopsy of Metastatic Site Required	Sequencing of Treatment	Systemic therapy	Radiation Therapy	Axillary Surgery
		Surgery	No Surgery	Surgery	No Surgery						
Tata Badwe et al,[7] 2015	350	19.2	20.5	Median not attained	18.2 mo	After chemotherapy	No	Chemotherapy prior to surgery	Chemotherapy in 336 and hormone therapy in 14; did not include HER2-targeted therapies	Nonmetastatic standard	Complete axillary dissection
MF07–01 Soran et al,[8] 2018	278	60% at 36 mo 45% at 40 mo 42% at 60 mo 19% at 120 mo	51% at 36 mo 26% at 40 mo 24% at 60 mo 5% at 120 mo	1%	11%	Prior to any treatment	No	Chemotherapy prior to surgery	Chemotherapy	Nonmetastatic standard	SLND and ALND for positive nodes
ABCSG-28 POSYTIVE Fitzal et al,[9] 2019	90 closed early due to poor accrual	Median survival 34.6 mo	Median survival 54.8 mo	8.9%	17.8%	Prior to any treatment	No	Chemotherapy alone vs surgery followed by chemotherapy	Nonmetastatic standard	Investigator's discretion 20% in surgery group and 4% in systemic therapy group	Required SLNB vs ALND at discretion of investigator ALND for positive nodes
E2108 Khan et al,[10] 2021	256	68.4% at 36 mo	67.9% at 36 mo	16.3% at 36 mo	39.8% at 36 mo	After assessment of response to systemic therapy	Yes	Surgery vs continued chemotherapy	Nonmetastatic standard	Nonmetastatic standard	Nonmetastatic standard

The first trial randomizing patients after neoadjuvant chemotherapy was published in 2015 by Badwe and colleagues [7]. Patients were enrolled at the Tata Medical Center in Mumbai, India. Of the 716 patients presenting with metastatic breast cancer, 350 were randomized with 173 in the local regional treatment (LRT) arm and 177 in the no LRT arm. All of the patients received ST prior to surgery except patients with HR+ resectable tumors who were randomized at enrollment. The HR+ group accounted for only 25 of the 716 total patients. All of the other patients had ST prior to randomization. Patients with unresectable disease in the breast received 6 to 8 cycles of chemotherapy. If an objective response was achieved, the patient was randomized. Of the 691 patients eligible for ST, 276 were ineligible for the study due to inadequate tumor response, progression, or life expectancy less than 6 months. The remaining 415 patients were enrolled in the study. Of the 440 patients (25 HR+ patients and 415 HR− patients) enrolled 350 were randomized with 14 receiving endocrine therapy and 336 receiving chemotherapy. Of the 177 assigned to no LRT, 18 had a palliative mastectomy and 1 had a mastectomy off protocol. Analysis was done on an intention to treat basis. Median follow-up was 23 months with an OS of 19.2 months in the LRT group and 20.5 months in the no LRT group. The 2 year survival was 41.9% in the LRT group and 43% in the no LRT group. This study has been criticized by the lack of HER2-targeted therapies in the patients who were HER2-positive. The conclusion from the study is that there is no benefit to surgical management of the intact primary. Subgroup analysis using menopausal status, metastatic burden, HR status, and HER2 status did not identify a group that benefited from surgery. In addition, the investigators concluded that surgery to prevent local disease progression is not routinely justified because only 10% of those patients in the no LRT arm required mastectomy.

Soran published the initial results of the MF07-01 study in 2018 [8]. This is a multicenter trial completed in Turkey that enrolled 274 patients with treatment-naive stage IV breast cancer to LRT followed by ST (LRT + ST) or ST alone. In the LRT + ST group, the surgery was performed as standard surgical management with either breast preservation or mastectomy with negative margins and standard axillary staging with sentinel lymph node biopsy for clinically node-negative disease and axillary node dissection for clinically node-positive disease. Axillary dissection was also performed on those with positive sentinel lymph nodes. Survival at 40 months was 45% in the LRT + ST group and 26% in the ST group with a hazard ratio of 0.66; 95% CI 0.49 to 0.88; $P=$ .005. The investigators note that at 3 years, the survival between the 2 groups was similar but by the 5th year of follow-up the survival was improved in patients in the LRT + ST group (41.6%) as compared to the ST group (24.4%). An unplanned subgroup analysis demonstrated improved survival in the LRT + ST group for patients with the following characteristics: HR+, HER2−, age younger than 55 years, and bone only metastases. In those patients with multiple pulmonary or liver metastases, the survival at 3 years was greatest in the ST group (67%) as compared to the LRT + ST group

(31%). The rate of local regional progression/relapse was lower in the LRT + ST group (1%) as compared to the ST group (11%). Of those patients in the ST group 18% went on to have palliative surgery. Radiation therapy was not found to affect survival. Patients with TN tumors had no difference in survival between the study arms. The investigators conclude that local regional therapy may play a role in improving the local regional progression/relapse and survival rates but age, performance status, comorbidities, tumor type, and metastatic burden must be considered when making recommendations. One concern for this study is that the groups were not well matched with the LRT + ST group having a higher rate of HR-positive tumors (86% vs 73%, P =.01) and lower rates of TN tumors (7% vs 18%, P= .01) as compared to the ST group.

The Soran study was updated with 10 year follow-up in 2021 [12]. At 10 years of follow-up, the LRT + ST group had an OS of 19% with a median survival of 46 months as compared to OS of 5% and median survival of 35 months in the ST group. The hazard ratio was 0.71; 95% CI 0.59 to 0.86; P= .0003 for death in the LRT + ST group compared to the ST group. Subgroup analysis again showed that the features of HR-positive, HER2-negative, age less than 55 years, and solitary bony metastases had an improved survival when treated with LRT + ST versus ST alone. The subgroup analysis also showed that HER2-positive tumors had an improved survival in the LRT + ST arm as compared to the ST arm (Hazard Ratio of 0.69; 95% CI 0.85–0.98; P= .04). Those patients with TNBC continued to have a poor prognosis that was not changed by local regional therapy. The study also showed that the greater the metastatic burden is, the lower the survival. However, those patients with solitary liver/lung metastases did see a possible benefit to local regional therapy of the primary tumor with OS of 38% (n = 5) in the LRT + ST group and 7% (n = 1) in the ST group; however, the number of patients in each category was very small making conclusions impossible. Quality-of-life assessments completed as a part of the study demonstrated no effect of local regional therapy on quality of life as compared to ST alone.

The ABCSG-28 POSYTIVE trial is a multicenter randomized trial completed in Austria and published by Fitzal [9]. The trial was stopped early due to poor accrual after enrollment of 90 patients. The study randomized patients prior to any systemic treatment and patients were randomized to surgery followed by ST (LRT + ST) versus ST alone. This trial did not have the power to assess the primary outcome. However, the results while underpowered did not detect a difference between the arms. There was a trend for improvement in local disease control in the LRT + ST group. Another weakness of the study is that 20% of the patients in the LRT + ST group were resected with positive margins. The quality-of-life assessments show similar overall quality of life between the 2 groups. Both groups had declines in quality of life during and shortly after treatment which later improved.

The final study is a multicenter randomized trial E2108 which was coordinated by the ECOG-ACRIN (Eastern Cooperative Oncology Group-) Cancer Research Group, completed in the United States, and published by Khan [10].

The hypothesis of the study is that treatment of the primary tumor prolongs survival if the metastatic disease is not resistant to ST. In this study, all patients were treated with ST for 4 to 8 months. The systemic therapies included endocrine therapy in 117 patients, chemotherapy in 113 patients, combined chemotherapy and endocrine therapy in 39 patients, and chemotherapy with HER2-targeting agents in 105 patients. Those patients who had a response to ST or stable disease were randomized to local regional treatment (LRT) of the primary site or continued ST. The LRT included surgery and radiation therapy using the nonmetastatic standard of care. Biopsy of the metastatic disease was required, which was unique to this study. The ST given was per standard of care for nonmetastatic disease. The study enrolled 389 patients with 256 showing nonprogressive disease after the ST making them eligible for randomization. The remaining enrolled but not randomized patients were followed.

Of those patients randomized to LRT, 86% had surgery with 70% having a mastectomy and 30% having breast preservation. The margins were negative in 92% and radiation therapy after breast preservation was performed in 84%. Of those patients who were randomized to ST, 17% subsequently had surgery. The OS at 3 years was 68.4% in the LRT group and 67.9% in the ST group. Of those patients not eligible for randomization, the 3 year OS was 44.8% and 5 year OS was 29.7%. Local progression was evaluated in the study. Local progression occurred in 40% of the ST group and 16% of the LRT group. The recurrences in the LRT group were associated with positive margins. The use of radiation therapy was not associated with the recurrence risk. Health-related quality-of-life evaluations showed no significant differences in quality-of-life scores, symptoms, worry, or functionality between the groups. The investigators conclude that there is no support for the use of surgery to the intact primary tumor in de novo breast cancer treated with ST prior to surgery to improve survival but there is evidence of an improved local progression-free survival and that if no surgery is performed there is approximately a 20% chance that local palliation may be needed.

Two additional controlled randomized trials have been initiated but not reported. The Dutch Breast Cancer Trialists' Group initiated the SUBMIT: ST with or without upfront surgery of the primary tumor in patients with breast cancer with distant metastases at initial presentation and the Japan Clinical Oncology Group initiated a randomized controlled trial comparing primary tumor resection plus ST with ST alone in metastatic breast cancer (PRIM-BC): Study JCOG1017. Both were initiated in 2012. The Submit trial was closed with no publication [13]. The JCOG1017 was presented at ASCO 2023 [14]. The design of the study is similar to the study completed by Khan in the United States. Patients were enrolled and received ST based on tumor subtype. Those who showed a response were randomized to further ST versus primary tumor resection plus ST. A total of 570 patients were enrolled with 407 eligible for randomization. There was no difference in OS. However, the local relapse-free survival was better in the resection arm and the percentage of patients with progression at the metastatic sites was lower in the resection arm. Subset analysis showed improved survival with the following features: HR+ tumors, premenopausal status, or single-organ metastasis. The investigators conclude that primary tumor excision should not be recommended for all patients with de novo metastatic breast cancer but is acceptable in some patients for local disease control.

With the results of these studies, the NCCN guidelines state that for M1 disease, "Routine surgical resection of the primary breast tumor is generally not indicated in the management of patients presenting with de novo stage IV (M1) disease. Although there is no survival benefit, it may be considered for local control of the primary tumor. Discussion regarding management of the primary tumor in this setting must be individualized" [15].

Breast reconstruction with de novo metastatic breast cancer

Two retrospective reviews of breast reconstruction in de novo metastatic breast cancer have been completed using the NCDB [16] and the SEER databases [17]. The NCDB study evaluated patients who received ST and mastectomy with or without reconstruction from 2004 to 2013. To control for bias, propensity score-matched analysis was used. The SEER study included patients treated with mastectomy with or without reconstruction from 1998 to 2015. Both studies found an increasing trend for reconstruction over the time of the study and no difference in survival between those with and without reconstruction. Predictors of breast reconstruction in the NCDB study are age 49 to 58 years, HR+, low grade, fewer metastasis, and receipt of ST. Predictors of breast reconstruction in the SEER study included recent year of diagnosis, age less than 60 years, married status, higher socioeconomic status, ductal histology, tumor stage 1-3 (T1-3), receipt of chemotherapy, and lack of lung metastasis. The NCDB study also evaluated 30 day mortality and readmissions to assess complications of the procedures. There were no differences between the groups indicating no significant increased risk of complications with reconstruction. The conclusions from the studies are that more women with metastatic disease are undergoing breast reconstruction and that there is no change in survival or complications associated with the reconstruction. Because the studies are from retrospective databases, quality-of-life assessments are not possible.

MANAGEMENT OF SECONDARY METASTASIS

Introduction

The controversies over the value of treating secondary metastatic sites are similar to those regarding treatment of the primary tumor in de novo metastatic breast cancer. A number of retrospective studies have been completed with many reporting some improvement in survival. However, the retrospective nature of the studies makes them prone to bias. In addition, the heterogeneity of breast cancer makes it difficult to complete a study with an adequate sample size. A systematic review of ablative therapies for metastatic breast cancer was performed by Kucharczyk and colleagues [18] who found that of the 41 studies identified as a part of the systematic review, all were observational cohort studies with a level of evidence of 2B to 4. The investigators were not able to identify predictors of improved outcome and concluded that a clinical trial is needed to address this topic. NRG oncology (a multicenter cooperative research group in the United States) conducted a phase II randomized trial in patients with oligometastatic breast cancer defined as fewer than 4 extracranial metastases [19]. The study randomized patients to ST versus metastasis-directed therapy (MDT) with either stereotactic body radiation therapy (SBRT) or surgical resection (SR). In the MDT arm, all sites of metastases were treated. Of the 129 patients randomized, 125 were eligible with 79% HR+, 13% HER2+, and 8% TN. The majority (60%) had a single metastasis and 20% had de novo disease. In the MDT arm, 93% of the patients received SBRT and 2% received SR. With a median follow-up of 30 months, there were no differences in progression-free survival, OS, or adverse events. Because there was no improvement in progression-free survival, the study did not proceed on to the phase III stage. Similar to the treatment of the primary disease in de novo breast cancer, this study does not support local therapies for metastatic sites.

The NCCN guidelines do not identify a subtype of breast cancer, volume of metastatic disease, or site of metastatic disease where surgical treatment is a part of the algorithm [15].

Metastasis to the liver

Of the 5% to 8% of patients with de novo metastatic breast cancer, 50% to 70% of these patients will have liver metastasis. Of those, only 5% to 18% have isolated liver metastases [20]. The prognosis for these patients is poor, approximately 4 to 8 months without intervention and 2 to 3 years with treatment. The 5 year survival is 8% to 12% [21].

According to the National Cancer Institute's SEER database, liver metastases were present more frequently with breast cancer subtypes that are HER2+. HER2+/ER−/PR− is the most common subtype found in 32.7% to 46.5% of patients with liver metastases. HER2+/ER+/PR+ subtype is present in 20.3% of stage IV disease with hepatic metastases. TN breast cancer has a lower rate of liver metastasis when compared to enriched HER2+ tumors; however, TN tumors continue to have a worse OS compared to HER2+ breast cancer with liver metastasis [3]. Unfortunately, the majority of patients with liver metastases have disseminated deposits throughout the liver and are therefore not good candidates for local therapy. For those who are candidates, local therapies for breast cancer liver metastasis include surgical resection, stereotactic body radiation therapy (SBRT), and radiofrequency ablation (RFA).

Liver resection

Surgical resection is the most common local treatment of liver metastases. Millen used the NCDB to evaluate the use of liver resection (LR) in patients with metastatic breast cancer [22]. Query of the NCDB for the years of 2010 to 2014 identified 9244 patients with breast cancer liver metastases. Isolated liver metastases were found in 28.5%. Treatments included chemotherapy in 78.2%, LR in 3.6%, and chemotherapy and LR in 3.2%. OS for the whole group was 18.3 months and was 29 months for those with isolated liver metastases. Chemotherapy with LR had a survival of 69.7 months and chemotherapy alone had a survival of 49.2 months. Predictors of survival in this study included receipt of chemotherapy, LR, HR+, and HER+. Patients with isolated liver metastases were more likely to receive treatment of the intact primary tumor, receive chemotherapy, and to have an LR. In those patients with multiorgan metastases, there was an improvement in survival with chemotherapy but no improvement in survival with LR. Those patients with HR+ tumors had an improvement in survival with chemotherapy and LR as compared to chemotherapy alone. TN tumors also had an improved survival with chemotherapy and LR as compared to chemotherapy alone.

In 2017, there were 2 systematic reviews evaluating the role of LR in metastatic breast cancer with similar conclusions [21,23]. Both reviews included studies with isolated liver metastases and studies with extrahepatic metastases. In both reviews, the survival is similar with 3 year rates of 54% to 83% and 5 year survival rates of 25% to 78%. The survival rates in patients with extrahepatic disease are similar to those without extrahepatic disease. The morbidity and mortality of LR are considered low in both studies with morbidity rates of 17% to 36% and mortality rates of 0.7% to 2.5%. Because the morbidity and mortality were considered low and there was a prolongation of survival over that achieved with chemotherapy alone, both studies conclude that LR is an effective treatment that can be considered as an option for patients with breast cancer liver metastases. Both studies call for randomized trials to further evaluate the treatment. These were published before the randomized phase II trial showing no benefit to treatment of metastatic disease.

RFA, a minimally invasive technique, uses targeted electrical and thermal energy to kill cancer cells. Compared to resection, this technique has fewer complications, decreased length of stay, and a median OS of 29.9 months. Age and increasing comorbidities reduce the survival. RFA is often pursued in patients with who are not candidates for LR either due to the site of disease, number of metastatic lesions, or comorbidities [20].

SBRT uses targeted radiation therapy to ablate the metastatic sites. This is an alternative to a surgical procedure for local therapy of metastatic lesions [24]. A phase II nonrandomized trial was conducted to evaluate SBRT in the management of oligometastatic liver and lung breast cancer metastases [25]. In this study, oligometastases was defined as up to 5 lesions. The size of the largest lesion had to be less than 5 cm and disease had to be confined to the liver and lung. The study allowed stable or responding extrahepatic or extrapulmonary disease. All breast cancer subtypes were included in the study. Morbidity occurred in 31% and included acute radiation toxicity in 23% and late radiation toxicity in 14%. They reviewed their results with 24 months of follow-up. Responses were seen in 87% of patients with 60.8% having a complete response and 26.1% having a partial response. The remaining 13.1% had a local progression of the treated lesion. Progression in a different site was seen in 86.9%. A small number of patients, 13.1% remained disease free at last follow-up visit. In this study, good local control was achieved at the treated metastatic sites but the inability to control disease at other sites resulted in a very low disease-free survival.

Each of the methods of treating metastatic disease to the liver shows success of controlling the disease at the treated site. In retrospective reviews and non-randomized phase II studies, there have been some improvements in survival; however, these studies have biases. For patients with symptomatic disease, it is reasonable to pursue local therapies but counseling of patients should not state survival benefits for these patients.

Metastases to lung

Management of a solid pulmonary nodule in a patient with breast cancer will often involve attempts to obtain diagnostic material to confirm whether the nodule represents metastatic disease. As interventional pulmonology improves, many of these lesions are biopsied through percutaneous or endoscopic methods. However, some may require more invasive surgical techniques for diagnosis. The least invasive surgical method is video-assisted thoracic surgery which is a minimally invasive technique allowing removal of the pulmonary nodule for histologic examination. In a series of 79 patients evaluated for solitary pulmonary nodule and a history of breast cancer, 38 had primary lung cancer, 27 had metastatic breast cancer, and 14 had other histology [26]. For those with metastatic breast cancer, this represented oligometastatic disease. The average disease-free interval for those who were found to have metastatic breast cancer was 50 months, which was shorter than the interval between breast cancer diagnosis and lung cancer diagnosis which was 179 months. Survival from metastatic breast cancer to the lung was 38% at 5 years and 18% at 10 years. In cases of known pulmonary metastases from breast cancer, the ability to improve survival with surgical management or other ablative techniques has not been demonstrated with a high level of evidence and therefore remains controversial.

Metastases to bone

Bone metastases are commonly associated with HR+ tumors and therefore are often responsive to hormone therapy and patients with bone only metastases have longer survival than patients with metastases in other sites. Surgical management of bone metastases is primarily used to ensure stability of the bony elements to prevent impending fractures or to stabilize existing fractures and to control pain. For symptomatic bone disease that is refractory to ST, patients may receive radiation therapy to bony metastases [27].

Metastases to the central nervous system

Brain metastases from breast cancer have been investigated but many of the studies are retrospective and include a variety of tumor types. The only randomized trials are old and also included a variety of tumor types. A retrospective review of patients treated by radiation oncology at Allegheny General Hospital

[28] showed that at presentation, 68% had multiple lesions, 17% had a solitary metastasis, and 15% had leptomeningeal disease. The median survival after diagnosis of metastases was 9.7 months. The presence of leptomeningeal disease and TN or HER2 subtypes predicted for lower median survival of only 3.1 months for any of those factors. CNS involvement is most commonly associated with the TN subtype (25%–27%) and the HER2 subtype (11%–20%). In the TN setting, the brain metastases are commonly associated with extracranial metastases. The brain metastases that occur in HER2+ patients are isolated to the brain in 50% of patients when the remaining systemic disease is controlled by HER2-targeted therapies. Survival rates with brain metastases are best in Luminal B tumors (19–21 months) and worst with TN tumors (3–4 months) [29]. The European Association of Neuro-Oncology and the European Society for Medical Oncology issued guidelines for management of brain metastases in 2021 [30]. The goal of treatment of brain metastases is to prevent or delay neurologic decline and, in some cases, to improve survival while maintaining quality of life. The recommendations for surgery in the presence of brain metastases include (1) diagnostic uncertainty or need for pathologic data, (2) presence of a solitary metastasis, (3) multiple resectable brain metastases may be considered for resection, (4) patients requiring steroids and are eligible for treatment with immune checkpoint inhibitors, and (5) presence of acute symptoms of increased intracranial pressure. The resection should be followed by a brain MRI 48 hours after surgery to determine the adequacy of resection. In some patients, stereotactic radio surgery (SRS) is an alternative or adjunct to surgery. It is recommended with 1 to 10 brain metastases or in combination with surgical resection. The use of ST in the presence of brain metastases remaining an important component of the patient's care.

SUMMARY

The value of surgery in the presence of metastatic disease, either de novo or secondary, has been the subject of recent randomized trials. The most extensive investigations have been in the evaluation of management of the primary tumor in de novo metastatic breast cancer. These trials have generally not provided adequate support to recommend resection of the primary for a survival benefit. However, the studies show a benefit in local control and remains recommended for palliation. The value of surgery for secondary metastases and systemic disease has primarily been investigated with retrospective reviews or nonrandomized prospective studies. These indicate a possible benefit to metastasis-targeted therapies. However, the most recent phase II randomized trial done for systemic metastases did not show a benefit to surgery; therefore, the planned phase III study was not completed. This study excluded brain metastases. While the phase II study did not show a survival benefit, it showed good local control of the disease sites treated. As with treatment of the intact primary in de novo disease, surgical resection can be considered in symptomatic disease or situations where local control is more important due to the location. In some cases where surgical resection was previously used, minimally invasive techniques such as RFA in the liver or lung, SBRT, SRS, and radiation therapy are now used with similar rates of disease control with lower morbidity.

Management of metastatic disease is most successful when there are systemic therapies available that are effective against the individual patient's tumor. Treatment with ST first to determine the effectiveness of the therapy was a common plan in the randomized studies that were conducted for de novo breast cancer. This approach is also often used for secondary metastases. Treatment with a standard regimen and then proceeding on to surgery at the conclusion of that regimen or treating to maximal effect with ST and then proceeding to surgery for residual disease that may become symptomatic are both options for management. Proceeding to surgery prior to ST is most commonly used in cases that have an urgent palliative need.

CLINICS CARE POINTS

- Control of symptomatic metastatic disease both de novo and secondary can be reliably controlled with local therapies either surgery or radiation therapy, however, randomized trials show no survival benefit.
- Current randomized trials evaluating treatment of de novo or secondary metastatic disease do not show a survival benefit to local therapies.
- Survival with metastatic breast cancer is improving, likely due to more effective systemic therapies.

Disclosure

The authors have nothing to disclose.

References

[1] Cancer stat facts: female breast cancer. 2023. Available at: https://seer.cancer.gov/statfacts/html/breast.html. [Accessed 16 December 2023].

[2] Orrantia-Borunda E, Anchondo-Nuñez P, Acuña-Aguilar LE, et al. Subtypes of breast cancer. In: Mayrovitz HN, editor. Breast cancer. Brisbane (AU): Exon Publications; 2022. p. 31–42.

[3] Xiao W, Zheng S, Yang A, et al. Breast cancer subtypes and the risk of distant metastasis at initial diagnosis: a population-based study. Cancer Manag Res 2018;10:5329–38.

[4] Van Mechelen M, Van Herck A, Punie K, et al. Behavior of metastatic breast cancer according to subtype. Breast Cancer Res Treat 2020 May;181(1):115–25, Epub 2020 Mar 19. Erratum in: Breast Cancer Res Treat. 2021 Apr;186(2):587-589.

[5] Petrelli F, Barni S. Surgery of primary tumors in stage IV breast cancer: an updated meta-analysis of published studies with meta-regression. Med Oncol 2012 Dec;29(5):3282–90.

[6] TosellоG TorloniMR, MotaBS NeemanT, Mota BS, et al. RieraR. Breast surgery for metastatic breast cancer. Cochrane Database Syst Rev 2018;(3):CD011276; https://doi.org/10.1002/14651858.CD011276.pub2.

[7] Badwe R, Hawaldar R, Nair N, et al. Locoregional treatment versus no treatment of the primary tumour in metastatic breast cancer: an open-label randomised controlled trial. Lancet Oncol 2015;16:1380–8.

[8] Soran A, Ozmen V, Ozbas S, et al. Randomized trial comparing resection of primary tumor with no surgery in stage iv breast cancer at presentation: protocol MF07-01. Ann Surg Oncol 2018;25:3141–9.
[9] Fitzal F, Bjelic-Radisic V, Knauer M, et al, on behalf of the ABCSG. Impact of breast surgery in primary metastasized breast cancer outcomes of the prospective randomized phase III ABCSG-28 POSYTIVE Trial. Ann Surg 2019;269:1163–9.
[10] Khan S, Zhao F, Goldstein L, et al. Early local therapy for the primary site in de novo stage iv breast cancer: results of a randomized clinical trial (EA2108). J Clin Oncol 2022;40: 978–87.
[11] Khan SA, Stewart AK, Morrow M. Does aggressive local therapy improve survival in metastatic breast cancer? Surgery 2002 Oct;132(4):620–6, discussion 626-7.
[12] Soran A, Ozmen V, Ozbas S, et al, MF07-01 Study Group. Primary surgery with systemic therapy in patients with de novo stage iv breast cancer: 10-year follow-up; protocol MF07-01 randomized clinical trial. J Am Coll Surg 2021;233:742e752.
[13] Available at Clinical.trials.gov. Accessed December 16, 2023.
[14] Shien T, Hara F, Aogi K, et al. A randomized controlled trial comparing primary tumor resection plus systemic therapy with systemic therapy alone in metastatic breast cancer (PRIM-BC): Japan Clinical Oncology Group study JCOG1017. J Clin Oncol 2023;41(16_suppl):523.
[15] Gradishar W.J., Moran M.S., Abraham J., et al., NCCN guidelines version 5.2023 breast cancer, Available at: https://www.nccn.org/professionals/physician_gls/pdf/breast.pdf (Accessed 26 December 2023).
[16] Weiss A, Chu CK, Lin H, et al. Reconstruction in the metastatic breast cancer patient: results from the national cancer database. Ann Surg Oncol 2018;25(11):3125–33.
[17] Chen H, Zhang M, Wang M, et al. Immediate breast reconstruction in de novo metastatic breast cancer: an analysis of 563 cases based on the SEER database. Clin Breast Cancer 2019;19(1):e135–41.
[18] Kucharczyk MJ, Parpia S, Walker-Dilks C, et al. Ablative therapies in metastatic breast cancer: a systematic review. Breast Cancer Res Treat 2017;164(1):13–25.
[19] Chmura S, Winter K, Woodward W, et al. NRG-BR002: A phase IIR/III trial of standard of care systemic therapy with or without stereotactic body radiotherapy (SBRT) and/or surgical resection (SR) for newly oligometastatic breast cancer (NCT02364557). J Clin Oncol 2022;40(suppl 16):abstr 1007.
[20] Kümler I, Parner VK, Tuxen MK, et al. Clinical outcome of percutaneous RF-ablation of non-operable patients with liver metastasis from breast cancer. Radiol Med 2015;120(6): 536–41.
[21] Yoo T, Cranshaw I, Broom R, et al. Systematic review of early and long-term outcome of liver resection for metastatic breast cancer: is there a survival benefit? Breast 2017;32:162–72.
[22] Millen J, Hofmann A, Mesquita-Neto J, et al. Evolving role of liver resection in selected patients with metastatic breas. Cancer JSR 2021;259:363–71.
[23] Tasleem S, Bolger J, Kelly M, et al. The role of liver resection in patients with metastatic breast cancer: a systematic review examining the survival impact. J Med Sci 2018;187:1009–20.
[24] Scorsetti M, Franceschini D, De Rose F, et al. Stereotactic body radiation therapy: a promising chance for oligometastatic breast cancer. Breast 2016;26:11–7.
[25] Franceschini D, Comito T, Gallo A, et al. Stereotactic body radiation therapy for lung and liver oligometastases from breast cancer: toxicity data of a prospective non-randomized phase ii trial. Curr Oncol 2022;29:7858–67.
[26] Rena O, Papalia E, Ruffini E, et al. The role of surgery in the management of solitary pulmonary nodule in breast cancer patients. EJSO 2007;33:546–50.
[27] Shehadi J, Sciubba D, Suk I, et al. Surgical treatment strategies and outcome in patients with breast cancer metastatic to the spine: a review of 87 patients. Eur Spine J 2007;16: 1179–92.
[28] Quigley MR, Fukui O, Chew B, et al. The shifting landscape of metastatic breast cancer to the CNS. Neurosurg Rev 2013 Jul;36(3):377–82.

[29] Soffietti R, Pellerino A, Ruda R. Neuro-oncology perspective of treatment options in metastatic breast cancer. Future Oncol 2018;14(17):1765–74.

[30] Le Rhun E, Guckenberger M, Smits M, et al, EANO Executive Board and ESMO Guidelines Committee. EANO-ESMO Clinical Practice Guidelines for diagnosis, treatment and follow-up of patients with brain metastasis from solid tumours. Ann Oncol 2021;32(11):1332–47.

Advances in Surgery 58 (2024) 311–327

ADVANCES IN SURGERY

Current Status of Laparoscopic Liver Resection

Hala Muaddi, MD, MSc, PhD[a], Hallbera Gudmundsdottir, MD[a], Sean Cleary, MD, MSc, MPH[b,*]

[a]Division of Hepatobiliary and Pancreas Surgery, Mayo Clinic, Rochester, MN, USA; [b]Division of Hepatobiliary and Pancreas Surgery, University of Toronto, Toronto, Ontario, Canada

Keywords

• Laparoscopic • Minimally invasive • Liver resection

Key points

- Various scoring systems like Iwate, IMM, Southampton, and Hasegawa aid in assessing laparoscopic liver resection complexity, guiding surgeons in case selection and predicting outcomes.
- Laparoscopic liver resection is preferred for small, solitary tumors in accessible segments, with considerations for patient comorbidities, anatomy, and technical expertise influencing decision-making.
- Positioning, pneumoperitoneum, intraoperative visualization, and vascular-parenchymal transection techniques are crucial for successful laparoscopic liver resection, with evolving methods like ICG staining and stapling improving outcomes.
- From benign tumors to complex malignancies like colorectal liver metastasis and hepatocellular carcinoma, laparoscopic resections offer comparable oncological outcomes, reduced morbidity, and shorter hospital stays.

INTRODUCTION

The evolution of laparoscopic liver resection over the past decades, from initial skepticism to widespread acceptance, reflects a journey marked by innovation and continuous refinement of minimally invasive solutions to complex hepatobiliary challenges. In this study, we provide a comprehensive overview of

*Corresponding author. Division of Hepatobiliary and Pancreas Surgery, University of Toronto, Toronto General Hospital, 10 E N 216 200, Elizabeth Street, Toronto, ON M5G 2C4, Canada. *E-mail address:* Sean.Cleary@uhn.ca

https://doi.org/10.1016/j.yasu.2024.05.002
0065-3411/24/

laparoscopic liver resection, including its historical development, indications, technical nuances, and clinical outcomes. From its early beginnings to its contemporary applications, this study highlights the impact of laparoscopic liver resection that continues to shape the landscape of liver surgery, profoundly enhancing patient care worldwide.

The development of safe laparoscopic liver surgery was facilitated by cross-institutional and international collaboration and communication through consensus and guidelines meetings including gatherings in Louisville, United States [1]; Morioka, Japan [2]; and Southampton, United Kingdom [3]. To facilitate research on safety, patient outcomes, and selection criteria, consensus guidelines established 3 distinct categories [1]. These categories include (1) biopsies and small wedge resections; (2) resections of the left lateral section or anterior hepatic segments (4b, 5, 6); and (3) hemihepatectomies, trisectionectomies, and resections of the difficult posterior segments (4a, 7, 8). These classifications serve as a common ground to describe laparoscopic liver resections and associated implications.

HISTORY

Laparoscopic surgery made its debut in the 1960s, initially finding application primarily in gynecologic and urologic procedures. Several decades later, in 1987, the evolution of laparoscopy in general surgery began with Phillipe Mouret, based in Lyon, France, who reported the first laparoscopic cholecystectomy using the modern technique [4]. Over the subsequent decades, the horizon of laparoscopic surgery expanded steadily across a spectrum of surgical disciplines. In the early 1990s, the pioneering study of Reich and colleagues marked a pivotal moment with the reporting of the first laparoscopic liver resection [5]. As surgical technology evolved, enabling more intricate procedures, the boundaries of laparoscopic liver surgery continued to expand [5,6]. As surgeons gained more comfort and experience, the first reported laparoscopic anatomic hepatectomy was performed by Azagra and Kaneko in 1996 [7–9]. In 1997, Huscher and colleagues achieved another milestone by successfully performing the first laparoscopic major hepatectomy [10].

Several hurdles had to be surmounted before laparoscopic liver resection could soar to its current prominence [11]. First, it was imperative to develop laparoscopic techniques capable of matching the precision of open procedures, facilitating the mobilization, dissection, Pringle maneuver, and transection of critical structures safely. Second, strategies had to be devised to mitigate anticipated intraoperative complications. Third, widespread acceptance within the surgical and oncological community was indispensable for establishing laparoscopic liver resection as a noninferior alternative to open surgery.

DIFFICULTY SCORING SYSTEMS AND LEARNING CURVES

To facilitate the assessment of laparoscopic liver resection complexity, several difficulty scoring systems have been developed and validated. These scoring systems aid in evaluating the suitability of a laparoscopic approach for specific cases. Among the most employed are the Iwate score [12], Institute Mutualiste Montsouris (IMM) score [13], Southampton score [14], and Hasegawa score [15]. The Iwate criteria include tumor location, tumor size, proximity of the tumor to major vessels, liver function, and technical consideration. Based on these factors, patients are stratified into 1 of 4 groups, which range in difficulty [12]. The IMM score focuses on intraoperative variables including operative time, blood loss, and conversation to an open procedure. Laparoscopic liver resections were then stratified based on difficulty into 3 groups [13]. The Southampton score includes lesion type, lesion size, neoadjuvant chemotherapy, previous open liver resections, and the classification of resection to divide patients into 4 groups of complexity [14]. Lastly, the Hasegawa score includes extent of resection, location of tumor, obesity, and platelet count to derive 3 different classifications of complexity [15]. These scores have been validated and proven effective in predicting the difficulty of laparoscopic liver resection procedure [16,17]. Comparisons on the utility of these scores in clinical practice have not been published, but the scores demonstrate significant commonalities that contribute to assessing technical difficulty and surgical risks and have been derived on different patient populations. All these factors do not serve as contraindications but rather as a guide for surgeons to assess the feasibility and potential challenges in performing laparoscopic liver resection within the context of the experience of the surgeon and institution. When combined with each individual surgeon's learning curve, these scores help delineate the technical limitations of laparoscopic liver resection, guide surgeons in taking the necessary precautions to ensure patient safety to optimize surgical outcomes, and provide a context for comparisons across institutions and publications.

The development in competence in laparoscopic liver surgery includes a stepwise progression in the development of minimally invasive surgical skills, progressive comfort in managing intraoperative adverse events, progressive increase in case difficulty, and thoughtful assessment of outcomes and progress. The importance of case selection cannot be understated, and the use of difficulty/complexity scores, described earlier, can be a useful guide. Based on this, early cases should focus on resection of small solitary tumors located in the left lateral section or anterolateral segments. A key component of the learning curve and safeguarding patient safety is familiarity and comfort of the surgical team in dealing with bleeding from the liver parenchyma and intrahepatic vascular structures [18]. Achieving this surgical competence and overcoming the learning curve for laparoscopic liver resection varies among surgeons and may depend on their prior expertise and the specific center where they practice. Several studies have evaluated the learning curve of laparoscopic liver surgery, using operative time, blood loss, conversion rate, and complication rate as the outcomes of interest [19–21]. Evidence suggests that approximately 25 to 40 cases are needed to achieve proficiency in minor liver resections, while proficiency in major liver resections may require 50 to 70 cases [19–21]. Studies on learning curves must be interpreted with caution, as there are many opportunities for biased results. For each individual surgeon, the learning curve will depend on multiple factors, including prior experience with open liver resection and nonliver laparoscopic surgery, as well as case complexity.

INDICATIONS AND PATIENT SELECTION

The primary determinant of performing a laparoscopic liver resection remains technical feasibility. Laparoscopic liver resections of small solitary tumors located in the left lateral sections (segments 2 and 3) and the anterior segments (segments 4b, 5, and 6) are generally well accepted and within the capabilities of many medium-volume and high-volume centers [1–3,22]. Surgeons typically favor laparoscopic liver resection for tumors smaller than 5 cm located away from major blood vessels and hilar structures. While those are guidelines, it is important to acknowledge that multifocal lesions, lesions in other segments, and larger tumors do not preclude the use of laparoscopy [1–3,23,24]. However, due to the challenges associated with caudal visualization of the liver during laparoscopy, laparoscopic liver resection for posterior and superior segments may be avoided by surgeons and centers with early experience in laparoscopic liver resections, as these locations have been linked to a higher risk of bleeding and a greater likelihood of conversion to open surgery [2,25]. In other words, the decision to perform laparoscopic liver resection is contingent on the surgeon's and the center's expertise [24]. For instance, major liver resections such as right hepatectomies, though technically demanding, can be executed successfully with the appropriate surgical proficiency [26,27]. Similarly, resection of large, bilateral or central tumors located close to the hilum or inferior vena cava (IVC) can be achieved laparoscopically with the appropriate expertise in selected patient populations [26–29].

Laparoscopic liver resection can be an appropriate approach for both benign and malignant liver lesions, including primary and secondary neoplastic conditions [18]. Additionally, recent evidence supports laparoscopic living donor liver harvest, further emphasizing its versatility [30]. The decision to opt for a laparoscopic approach may be reconsidered when comorbidities and anatomic constraints of the liver lesion make it less amenable to this technique [1–3,18].

A patient population worth special mention is patients with cirrhosis. These patients have a higher risk of intraoperative and postoperative complications related to any liver resection, laparoscopic or open, and thus, the presence of cirrhosis is accounted for in many difficulty scores. The increased fibrosis in the hepatic parenchyma and higher portal pressures can contribute significantly to the increased difficulties of transection and management of intraoperative bleeding. However, several studies have shown improved outcomes in this population when a laparoscopic approach is utilized, including decreased intraoperative blood loss, reduced postoperative ascites, maintenance of important porto-venous collaterals in the abdominal wall and lower rate of posthepatectomy liver failure, while achieving similar overall and recurrence-free survival [31–33].

Aside from technical considerations, there are few contraindications to a laparoscopic approach to liver resection. Most importantly, patients must be fit enough from a cardiopulmonary standpoint to tolerate pneumoperitoneum. Patients with impaired right heart function, valvular heart disease as well as diastolic and systolic dysfunction may not tolerate the decreased venous return associated with increased intra-abdominal pressures associated with laparoscopy. Additionally, patients with extensive upper abdominal surgical history may require extensive lysis of adhesions and are at higher risk of conversion if the anatomy is significantly distorted or the surgeon is unable to gain enough working space to safely perform the procedure laparoscopically.

TECHNICAL ASPECTS

Positioning

Positioning the patient is a crucial initial step in laparoscopic liver resection. The most widely employed position is the reverse Trendelenburg, with or without split legs, which optimizes visualization of the surgical field [2]. Having the patient in split legs/stirrups, also known as the "French position," has favorable ergonomics for the operating surgeon between the legs and accessing the upper abdomen. This positioning serves multiple purposes: it facilitates the establishment of a low central venous pressure (CVP) and displaces the omentum, colon, and intestines inferiorly, thereby enhancing the surgeon's view of the liver. In standard laparoscopic liver resections, a supraumbilical or infraumbilical port is used in addition to 4 to 6 trocar ports. The subcostal ports serve as the main working ports, and additional ports can be strategically placed for assistance and retraction. However, it is worth noting that the supine position can be challenging for accessing superior and posterior lesions due to poor visibility and unfavorable working angles, promoting some surgeons to perform laparoscopic liver resection in the left lateral position for those locations [34,35].

Pneumoperitoneum

Pneumoperitoneum is established using carbon dioxide (CO_2), with pressure generally set between 10 and 15 mm Hg. Initial concerns regarding clinically significant CO_2 embolisms were dispelled using animal models that demonstrated this as a rare occurrence [36,37]. CO_2 is rapidly reabsorbed and, therefore, only large influxes of CO_2 through large defects in the hepatic veins or IVC are likely to be of hemodynamic significance [36,37]. The hemodynamic effects of pneumoperitoneum may be particularly impactful in patients with impaired cardiac function, as described earlier, or hypovolemia, which can be either intentional as part of maintaining low CVP for hepatic transection or blood loss. Careful management of intra-abdominal pressures, volume status, and pulmonary end expiratory pressures may be useful in managing these situations. Other preliminary concerns include port seeding or peritoneal implants were quickly dissipated through subsequent studies [38,39].

Intraoperative visualization

Technological advancements, such as laparoscopic intraoperative ultrasonography (IOUS) and adaptation of electrosurgical tools to minimally invasive surgery (MIS), have facilitated important improvements in surgical technique and adoption [18]. While laparoscopic IOUS has yet to be integrated into several consensus guidelines [1–3], its value lies in the ability to visualize tumor extent, dimensions, and their relationship to vascular structures, thereby precisely delineating the dissection plane [40]. This is especially critical in laparoscopic procedures, due to the limited tactile feedback and constrained 3 dimensional visualization. Furthermore, IOUS can reveal small tumors or liver lesions that were not evident on preoperative imaging [41].

Intraoperative visualization techniques using indocyanine green (ICG) have gained prominence as an adjunct in laparoscopic liver resection to improve quality and precision of anatomic resection and transection. Multiple approaches to ICG administration exist, most frequent of which are the positive staining and negative staining techniques [42–45]. Positive staining including injection of ICG into the portal branch of the targeted resection segment under percutaneous-guided laparoscopic ultrasound to allow for the visualization of clear demarcation planes. A small amount of ICG is injected into the portal branch slowly to prevent retrograde flow into adjacent portal segments. Negative staining includes the injection of ICG after clamping of the segmental portal pedicle of the target resection segment. Failure of positive staining could occur due to retrograde flow or puncturing wrong branches, while failure of negative staining could be due to collateral circulation or aberrant circulation. However, both methods have been described to assist in anatomic liver resection by rendering the segment hypofluorescent or hyperfluorescent, thereby facilitating the identification of transection lines [42–45].

Vascular and parenchymal transection

Several devices have been described and developed to facilitate laparoscopic parenchymal transection, yet consensus on the optimal modality remains elusive [46]. Frequently described devices for parenchymal transection include ultrasonic scalpel, bipolar electrocautery, stapler, cavitron ultrasonic surgical aspirator, and water jet. For the management of surface bleeding, monopolar and bipolar cautery, argon beam coagulator, and microwave coagulator are commonly employed.

In terms of the overarching concepts of resection, laparoscopic liver resection aligns closely with open procedures. In anatomic liver resections, inflow vessels are isolated and occluded to minimize bleeding before liver parenchymal transection. Laparoscopic staplers are frequently used to divide large major hepatic vessels. During parenchymal transection, vessels with diameters ranging from 3 to 7 mm are typically managed with clips or vessel-sealing devices, while those less than 2 mm can be divided using a bipolar sealing device. Techniques using microwave ablation and radiofrequency ablation as a precoagulation technique have been described with low risk of bleeding but possible increases in bile leak [47–49].

Retrospective studies demonstrated that stapling across the parenchyma can reduce bleeding, operative time, and transfusion requirements [50]. Despite stapling raising concerns related to defining precise oncological margins, this did not translate into an increased recurrence rate [50]. Another retrospective study explored the use of bipolar compression and ultrasonic devices for parenchymal transection during laparoscopic liver resection, revealing that bipolar compression led to decreased transection and total operative times [51]. There were no differences observed in blood loss or postoperative complication [51]. It is worth noting that while argon beam coagulators excel at maintaining hemostasis, several centers have reported an increased risk of gas embolism, limiting their widespread adoption [2].

OUTCOMES

In a pivotal article published in 2009, Nguyen and colleagues demonstrated the safety of laparoscopic liver resection, with morbidity and mortality rates comparable to open surgery for both minor and major liver resections in a carefully selected group of patients [52]. The primary advantages of laparoscopic liver resection are related to improved short-term perioperative outcomes. Multiple studies have shown that laparoscopic approaches are associated with decreased intraoperative blood loss, lower complication rates, and shorter hospital lengths of stay [53,54]. When conversion to an open procedure is required, perioperative outcomes are similar to those observed after upfront open surgery [55]. It is noteworthy that much of the evidence supporting laparoscopic liver resection comes from observational studies rather than randomized controlled trials. Despite the absence of level one evidence, the existing literature consistently highlights the safety, feasibility, and benefit of laparoscopic liver resection when compared to open surgery. Over time, laparoscopic liver resection has progressively extended its purview to encompass increasingly complex anatomic and nonanatomical resections of both benign and malignant lesions.

Benign liver tumors

The early experience of laparoscopic liver resection focused on resection of benign liver tumors such as hemangiomas or hepatocellular adenomas. Several studies published in the early 2000s demonstrated both feasibility and safety of laparoscopic liver resection for carefully selected patients with small tumors located in the left lateral or anterior segments [56–59]. Multiple studies consistently demonstrated that within this selected group of patients, laparoscopic liver resection offered several advantages, including shorter hospital length of stay, quicker resumption of oral intake, and reduced overall morbidity [59]. Early studies did indicate relatively high conversion rates to open surgery, primarily to manage bleeding–a reflection of the challenges faced during the early stages of the learning curve [59]. The high rate of resection of benign liver lesions with no malignant potential in early series of laparoscopic liver resection prompted significant debate. This led to the convening of consensus conferences and guidelines recommending laparoscopic resection be considered only in cases with an appropriate and identical indication for open surgery. In essence, the emphasis is not only on the technical capability of performing laparoscopic resections but also on the judicious and evidence-based selection of patients that truly warrant consideration of resection.

The first randomized controlled trial comparing laparoscopic and open liver resections was conducted by Ding and colleagues in 2015 [60]. This trial included 98 patients undergoing treatment of hepatolithiasis within the left lateral lobes, revealing that laparoscopic liver resection exhibited similar safety and feasibility for this condition, with no significant differences in the overall complication rate. Furthermore, the laparoscopic approach offered advantages in terms of shorter operating time, reduced blood loss, and shorter length of stay in hospital [60].

Colorectal liver metastasis

As evidence accumulated for the safety and feasibility of laparoscopic liver resection for benign liver lesions, several surgical groups expanded their practice to include malignant liver lesions. Among the first groups to report their technical experience and patient outcomes in laparoscopic resection of colorectal liver metastases (CRLM) were Vibert and colleagues [61]. Their series was the first to include a combination of both minor and major liver resections for malignant lesions. While the follow-up was relatively short, their data demonstrated feasibility and, importantly, acceptable oncological outcomes.

A subsequent systematic review and meta-analysis summarized all available evidence comparing laparoscopic and open liver resection for CRLM [62,63]. In this study, laparoscopic liver resection was associated with several advantages, including significantly less overall morbidity, reduced blood loss, decreased transfusion requirement, shorter length of hospital stay, but longer operative time. For oncological outcomes, no significant differences were observed in negative surgical margins (R0 resection), tumor recurrence, 3 year disease-free survival, 5 year disease-free survival, or 5 year overall survival between the 2 surgical approaches. It is prudent to mention that all included studies were retrospective in design.

Shortly thereafter, in 2018, the Oslo laparoscopic versus open liver resection for colorectal metastases (OSLO-COMET) randomized controlled trial compared laparoscopic and open liver resections for CRLM [64]. The trial included 280 patients randomized to open and laparoscopic resections. The results showed significant differences favoring the laparoscopic approach, including lower postoperative pain medication requirement, lower complication rate (Dindo–Clavien > II), shorter intensive care unit and hospital stay, and improved quality of life [64].

Further studies delving into more complex cases, such as repeat liver resections and large malignant tumors, have demonstrated that laparoscopic resections are feasible in selected groups of patients with the appropriate surgical expertise. Repeat resections are often characterized by abdominal adhesions and altered liver anatomy. A propensity score matched study showed that laparoscopic liver resection was associated with reduced blood loss and shorter duration of operation and length of stay in hospital when compared to open surgery, with equal postoperative morbidity and mortality [65]. A prospective study examined large tumors (>5 cm) and demonstrated that despite their technical challenges in terms of mobilization and the risk of tumor rupture, they can be safely and feasibly resected laparoscopically [66]. However, tumors exceeding 10 cm in size demonstrated higher blood loss and longer operating time [66]. Complex resections, including those involving multiple bilobar CRLM, can be performed through a 2 stage laparoscopic approach at experienced centers, with less blood loss, fewer perioperative complications, shorter hospital length of stay, and earlier administration of chemotherapy when compared to a propensity-score matched open cohort [67]. Importantly, there were no differences in oncological outcomes in terms of recurrence and survival [67].

Hepatocellular carcinoma

The first experience with laparoscopic resection of hepatocellular carcinoma (HCC) was reported in 2000, and it yielded promising results [56]. A single randomized controlled study compared laparoscopic to open liver resection, involving the randomization of 50 patients into the 2 surgical approaches. All patients had early-stage HCC (tumor size <5 cm) with compensated cirrhosis (Child-Pugh Class A) [68]. The results of the trial demonstrated comparable outcomes of laparoscopic and open liver resections. Most supportive evidence for laparoscopic resections is primarily derived from observational studies [69–73]. A systematic review and meta-analysis that included 51 articles encompassing 6812 patients indicated that the evidence available to date from these studies is in support of laparoscopic liver resection [74]. In this group, laparoscopic liver resection results in fewer blood transfusions, shorter length of stay in hospital, and lower 30 day mortality and morbidity rate [74]. Additionally, there were no differences observed in achieving R0 resection or margin size [74].

Several research groups ventured into examining the outcomes of patients with Child-Pugh B cirrhosis or those with HCC in more challenging locations. The results have been encouraging, demonstrating that the intraoperative and postoperative outcomes were similar among patients who underwent laparoscopic liver resection with HCC in favorable and unfavorable locations [75]. Furthermore, in a highly selected group of patients, the laparoscopic approach was found to be equally safe with Child-Pugh A and Child-Pugh B patients with cirrhosis [76].

Intrahepatic cholangiocarcinoma

Intrahepatic cholangiocarcinoma (iCCA) poses unique challenges in comparison to other liver lesions. These challenges primarily stem from the location and nature of the disease, often necessitating extended liver resection, hilar lymphadenectomy, and possible biliary reconstruction. Consequently, fewer surgical groups have ventured into performing these complex procedures laparoscopically.

With these technical challenges in mind, a systematic review encompassing 4 retrospective studies including 204 patients with iCCA was published in 2020 [77]. The existing evidence suggests that, in a carefully selected group of patients, laparoscopy can be associated with several advantages, including reduced blood loss, fewer blood transfusions, shorter Pringle time, shorter length of stay, and decreased morbidity [77]. However, laparoscopic liver resection was associated with lower rates of lymphadenectomy, although this did not impact disease recurrence or R0 resection margin [77,78]. This was further corroborated by a study, which utilized a large administrative database to examine quality of nodal resections for open and laparoscopic resections of CCA [79]. Examination of 2309 patients with CCA showed worse nodal evaluation for patients undergoing laparoscopic liver resection. However, due to database limitations, recurrence could not be examined [79].

An additional technical challenge encountered with hilar cholangiocarcinoma (hCCA) is the need for biliary reconstruction. Early case series demonstrated its feasibility, with no notable differences in estimated blood loss, blood transfusions requirements, pathologic outcomes, bile leaks, length of hospital stay, or severe postoperative complications [80]. However, the laparoscopic group did experience longer operative time than the open group. Nonetheless, this provided support of the safety and feasibility of laparoscopic resection of hCCA in experienced hands.

Living donor liver transplantation

To minimize the impact on living donors, laparoscopic left lateral sectionectomy emerged as an alternative to the open approach [81]. The left lobe, with its minimal vascular and biliary anatomic variations, offers ideal conditions for laparoscopic liver procurement. The ample length of the extrahepatic vessels allows for straightforward control, and its anterior position permits access with minimal mobilization. Furthermore, modern imaging techniques enable precise and reliable characterization of both vascular and biliary anatomy. These advancements have not only popularized laparoscopy in liver resection but also have extended its utility into the realm of organ procurement.

While living donor liver transplant outcomes have shown success, they remain predominantly within the purview of high-volume centers [82,83]. Several groups demonstrated that laparoscopic donor hepatectomies yield outcomes comparable to open procedures marked by low morbidity and mortality rates [84,85]. However, early evidence suggests an association with higher rate of biliary complications in recipients who received a liver from a laparoscopic donor compared to open donors [86].

CHALLENGES AND TECHNICAL LIMITATIONS

Several strategies have been proposed to overcome the limitations of laparoscopic liver resection. The 2 most commonly accepted are hand-assisted laparoscopic surgery and hybrid approach. Both are accepted as safe and a feasible approach to a pure laparoscopic approach [87,88].

To address the challenges posed by technically demanding tumor locations, some surgeons choose to combine the laparoscopic approach with a hand-assisted or a combined open approach. This hybrid approach expands the spectrum of MIS, particularly for lesions located in technically challenging anatomic locations [87]. Additionally, these approaches are helpful during the learning curve as a bridge to laparoscopic liver resection or more complex liver resections [89].

Other approaches brought forward to overcome the challenges of laparoscopic liver resection for superior and posterior lesions include placing patients in the lateral decubitus position. Other approaches include either transthoracic approaches or placement of intercostal trocars for improved visualization [90–93]. Both are in their early stages with only case-series data reported [91–93]. Other technical approaches described include the diamond technique, which is reported to allow for safe parenchymal sparing liver resections of lesions in posterosuperior segments [94–96]. All these approaches require center and hospital expertise in MIS.

The integration of robotic surgery into liver resections represents a promising advancement in the field of minimally invasive hepatobiliary procedures. Robotic-assisted surgery, although still in its early stages of development for liver resections, holds significant potential for the future. The current body of evidence is largely derived from retrospective studies, which have demonstrated that robotic liver resections can offer equivalent outcomes to laparoscopic procedures. Its role may lay in its ability to offer patients a minimally invasive approach when laparoscopic surgery is not achievable for patients who would otherwise be subject to open surgery. As the field of robotic liver resections continues to evolve, the challenge lies in standardizing techniques and defining safety protocols. Furthermore, the limited availability and development of specific instruments for hepatic transection are limiting factors for many centers. Building on the current evidence, ongoing research and clinical experience will help refine the indications and guidelines for robotic liver resections. This, in turn, will contribute to a broader adoption of robotic-assisted procedures, further expanding the toolkit available to surgeons in their pursuit of safer and more effective liver resections.

SUMMARY

This study provides a comprehensive exploration of the evolution and intricacies of laparoscopic liver resection, a transformative force in the field of surgery. Beginning with its historical development, indications, and technical aspects, the study delves into the outcomes and safety of laparoscopic liver resection, covering both benign and malignant liver lesions. It highlights the transition from initial skepticism to the current acceptance of laparoscopic liver resection as a viable alternative to open surgery, supported by accumulating evidence and observational studies. The study underscores the importance of patient selection and surgical expertise in achieving successful outcomes. Furthermore, it discusses the growing role of laparoscopic liver resection in addressing various liver pathologies, from benign tumors to CRLM and intrahepatic carcinoma. In a constantly evolving field, this study encapsulates the journey of laparoscopic liver resection and its significant impact on the landscape of liver surgery, emphasizing the need for continued research and expertise to maximize its potential in patient care.

The future of laparoscopic liver resection is marked by exciting possibilities. Advances in technology, including improved surgical instruments and imaging techniques, are poised to enhance the precision and safety. Machine learning algorithms, in combination with advanced imaging and data analytics, have the potential to revolutionize the way surgeons plan and execute laparoscopic liver resection. These algorithms can assist in preoperative planning by accurately assessing the anatomic variations and vascular structures of the liver, providing invaluable insights for precise surgical navigation. Furthermore, predictive models driven by machine learning can assess patient-specific risk factors and recommend optimal surgical approaches, personalized to each case, thus optimizing outcomes. These innovations are expected to expand the scope of laparoscopic liver surgery, making it applicable to even more complex and challenging cases, such as large malignant tumors, hCCA, and repeat liver resections. Moreover, ongoing research into minimizing postoperative complications, optimizing patient outcomes, and refining the learning curve for surgeons is likely to solidify the role of laparoscopic liver resection as a standard of care. The increasing recognition of the benefits of minimally invasive approaches in terms of reduced blood loss, shorter hospital stays, and quicker postoperative recovery is expected to encourage its adoption in a broader range of clinical settings. As high-volume centers continue to accumulate experience and publish valuable data, the future of laparoscopic liver resection holds the promise of becoming an essential component of modern liver surgery, continually shaping and advancing the field for the benefit of patients around the world.

CLINICS CARE POINTS

- Utilize scoring systems such as Iwate score, IMM score, Southampton score, or Hasegawa score to evaluate the difficulty of laparoscopic liver lesion resection.
- Consider surgeons' learning curve and their comfort in managing intraoperative adverse events when considering laparoscopic liver resection.
- Benign and malignant lesions may be resected laparoscopically if there are no clinical or technical barriers.
- In appropriately selected patients with the required technical expertise, laparoscopic liver resection may offer benefits such as reduced blood loss, fewer complication rates, and shorter hospital stay.

DISCLOSURE

No disclosures of conflict of interest to declare.

References

[1] Buell JF, Cherqui D, Geller DA, et al. The international position on laparoscopic liver surgery: The Louisville Statement, 2008. Ann Surg 2009;250(5):825–30.
[2] Wakabayashi G, Cherqui D, Geller DA, et al. Recommendations for laparoscopic liver resection: a report from the second international consensus conference held in Morioka. Ann Surg 2015;261(4):619–29.
[3] Abu Hilal M, Aldrighetti L, Dagher I, et al. The southampton consensus guidelines for laparoscopic liver surgery: from indication to implementation. Ann Surg 2018;268(1):11–8.
[4] Litynski GS. Profiles in laparoscopy: mouret, dubois, and perissat: the laparoscopic breakthrough in europe (1987-1988). J Soc Laparoendosc Surg 1999;3(2):163–7.
[5] Reich H, McGlynn F, DeCaprio J, et al. Laparoscopic excision of benign liver lesions. Obstet Gynecol 1991;78(5 Pt 2):956–8.
[6] Katkhouda N, Fabiani P, Benizri E, et al. Laser resection of a liver hydatid cyst under videolaparoscopy. Br J Surg 1992;79(6):560–1.
[7] Azagra JS, Goergen M, Gilbart E, et al. Laparoscopic anatomical (hepatic) left lateral segmentectomy-technical aspects. Surg Endosc 1996;10(7):758–61.
[8] Kaneko H, Takagi S, Shiba T. Laparoscopic partial hepatectomy and left lateral segmentectomy: technique and results of a clinical series. Surgery 1996;120(3):468–75.
[9] Gagner M. Laparoscopic partial hepatectomy for liver tumor. Abstract Surg Endosc 1992;6:99.
[10] Huscher CG, Lirici MM, Chiodini S, et al. Current position of advanced laparoscopic surgery of the liver. J R Coll Surg Edinb 1997;42(4):219–25.
[11] Coelho FF, Kruger JA, Fonseca GM, et al. Laparoscopic liver resection: Experience based guidelines. World J Gastrointest Surg 2016;8(1):5–26.
[12] Ban D, Tanabe M, Ito H, et al. A novel difficulty scoring system for laparoscopic liver resection. J Hepatobiliary Pancreat Sci 2014;21(10):745–53.
[13] Kawaguchi Y, Fuks D, Kokudo N, et al. Difficulty of laparoscopic liver resection: proposal for a new classification. Ann Surg 2018;267(1):13–7.
[14] Halls MC, Berardi G, Cipriani F, et al. Development and validation of a difficulty score to predict intraoperative complications during laparoscopic liver resection. Br J Surg 2018;105(9):1182–91.
[15] Hasegawa Y, Wakabayashi G, Nitta H, et al. A novel model for prediction of pure laparoscopic liver resection surgical difficulty. Surg Endosc 2017;31(12):5356–63.
[16] Tanaka S, Kawaguchi Y, Kubo S, et al. Validation of index-based IWATE criteria as an improved difficulty scoring system for laparoscopic liver resection. Surgery 2019;165(4):731–40.
[17] Kawaguchi Y, Tanaka S, Fuks D, et al. Validation and performance of three-level procedure-based classification for laparoscopic liver resection. Surg Endosc 2020;34(5):2056–66.
[18] Vigano L, Tayar C, Laurent A, et al. Laparoscopic liver resection: a systematic review. J Hepatobiliary Pancreat Surg 2009;16(4):410–21.
[19] Brown KM, Geller DA. What is the learning curve for laparoscopic major hepatectomy? J Gastrointest Surg 2016;20(5):1065–71.
[20] Swaid F, Sucandy I, Tohme S, et al. Changes in performance of more than 1000 minimally invasive liver resections. JAMA Surg 2020;155(10):986–8.
[21] Chua D, Syn N, Koh YX, et al. Learning curves in minimally invasive hepatectomy: systematic review and meta-regression analysis. Br J Surg 2021;108(4):351–8.
[22] Dokmak S, Raut V, Aussilhou B, et al. Laparoscopic left lateral resection is the gold standard for benign liver lesions: a case-control study. HPB (Oxford) 2014;16(2):183–7.
[23] Gobardhan PD, Subar D, Gayet B. Laparoscopic liver surgery: An overview of the literature and experiences of a single centre. Best Pract Res Clin Gastroenterol 2014;28(1):111–21.
[24] Ishizawa T, Gumbs AA, Kokudo N, et al. Laparoscopic segmentectomy of the liver: from segment I to VIII. Ann Surg 2012;256(6):959–64.

[25] Troisi RI, Montalti R, Van Limmen JG, et al. Risk factors and management of conversions to an open approach in laparoscopic liver resection: analysis of 265 consecutive cases. HPB (Oxford) 2014;16(1):75–82.
[26] Abu Hilal M, van der Poel MJ, Samim M, et al. Laparoscopic liver resection for lesions adjacent to major vasculature: feasibility, safety and oncological efficiency. J Gastrointest Surg 2015;19(4):692–8.
[27] Gringeri E, Boetto R, Bassi D, et al. Totally laparoscopic caudate lobe resection: technical aspects and literature review. Surg Laparosc Endosc Percutaneous Tech 2014;24(6):e233–6.
[28] Kwon Y, Han HS, Yoon YS, et al. Are large hepatocellular carcinomas still a contraindication for laparoscopic liver resection? J Laparoendosc Adv Surg Tech 2015;25(2):98–102.
[29] Nomi T, Fuks D, Louvet C, et al. Outcomes of laparoscopic liver resection for patients with large colorectal liver metastases: a case-matched analysis. World J Surg 2016;40(7):1702–8.
[30] Bekheit M, Khafagy PA, Bucur P, et al. Donor safety in live donor laparoscopic liver procurement: systematic review and meta-analysis. Surg Endosc 2015;29(11):3047–64.
[31] Cipriani F, Ratti F, Fornoni G, et al. Conversion of minimally invasive liver resection for hcc in advanced cirrhosis: clinical impact and role of difficulty scoring systems. Cancers 2023;15(5); https://doi.org/10.3390/cancers15051432.
[32] Morise Z, Ciria R, Cherqui D, et al. Can we expand the indications for laparoscopic liver resection? A systematic review and meta-analysis of laparoscopic liver resection for patients with hepatocellular carcinoma and chronic liver disease. J Hepatobiliary Pancreat Sci 2015;22(5):342–52.
[33] Troisi RI, Berardi G, Morise Z, et al. Laparoscopic and open liver resection for hepatocellular carcinoma with Child-Pugh B cirrhosis: multicentre propensity score-matched study. Br J Surg 2021;108(2):196–204.
[34] Ikeda T, Mano Y, Morita K, et al. Pure laparoscopic hepatectomy in semiprone position for right hepatic major resection. J Hepatobiliary Pancreat Sci 2013;20(2):145–50.
[35] Ikeda T, Toshima T, Harimoto N, et al. Laparoscopic liver resection in the semiprone position for tumors in the anterosuperior and posterior segments, using a novel dual-handling technique and bipolar irrigation system. Surg Endosc 2014;28(8):2484–92.
[36] Jayaraman S, Khakhar A, Yang H, et al. The association between central venous pressure, pneumoperitoneum, and venous carbon dioxide embolism in laparoscopic hepatectomy. Surg Endosc 2009;23(10):2369–73.
[37] Schmandra TC, Mierdl S, Hollander D, et al. Risk of gas embolism in hand-assisted versus total laparoscopic hepatic resection. Surg Technol Int 2004;12:137–43.
[38] Gaillard M, Tranchart H, Dagher I. Laparoscopic liver resections for hepatocellular carcinoma: current role and limitations. World J Gastroenterol 2014;20(17):4892–9.
[39] Tranchart H, Dagher I. Laparoscopic liver resection: a review. J Vis Surg 2014;151(2):107–15.
[40] Araki K, Conrad C, Ogiso S, et al. Intraoperative ultrasonography of laparoscopic hepatectomy: key technique for safe liver transection. J Am Coll Surg 2014;218(2):e37–41.
[41] Muaddi H, Silva S, Choi WJ, et al. When is a ghost really gone? a systematic review and meta-analysis of the accuracy of imaging modalities to predict complete pathological response of colorectal cancer liver metastases after chemotherapy. Ann Surg Oncol 2021;28(11):6805–13.
[42] Ishizawa T, Saiura A, Kokudo N. Clinical application of indocyanine green-fluorescence imaging during hepatectomy. Hepatobiliary Surg Nutr 2016;5(4):322–8.
[43] Ishizawa T, Zuker NB, Kokudo N, et al. Positive and negative staining of hepatic segments by use of fluorescent imaging techniques during laparoscopic hepatectomy. Arch Surg 2012;147(4):393–4.

[44] Kudo H, Ishizawa T, Tani K, et al. Visualization of subcapsular hepatic malignancy by indocyanine-green fluorescence imaging during laparoscopic hepatectomy. Surg Endosc 2014;28(8):2504–8.
[45] Sakoda M, Ueno S, Iino S, et al. Anatomical laparoscopic hepatectomy for hepatocellular carcinoma using indocyanine green fluorescence imaging. J Laparoendosc Adv Surg Tech 2014;24(12):878–82.
[46] Otsuka Y, Kaneko H, Cleary SP, et al. What is the best technique in parenchymal transection in laparoscopic liver resection? comprehensive review for the clinical question on the 2nd international consensus conference on laparoscopic liver resection. J Hepatobiliary Pancreat Sci 2015;22(5):363–70.
[47] Rao Z, Ling W, Dai X, et al. Precoagulation with microwave ablation for hepatic parenchymal transection during liver partial resection. Int J Hyperther 2019;36(1):146–50.
[48] Tan K, Du X, Yin J, et al. Microwave tissue coagulation technique in anatomical liver resection. Biomed Rep 2014;2(2):177–82.
[49] Reccia I, Kumar J, Kusano T, et al. A systematic review on radiofrequency assisted laparoscopic liver resection: Challenges and window to excel. Surg Oncol 2017;26(3): 296–304.
[50] Buell JF, Gayet B, Han HS, et al. Evaluation of stapler hepatectomy during a laparoscopic liver resection. HPB (Oxford) 2013;15(11):845–50.
[51] Mbah NA, Brown RE, Bower MR, et al. Differences between bipolar compression and ultrasonic devices for parenchymal transection during laparoscopic liver resection. HPB (Oxford) 2012;14(2):126–31.
[52] Nguyen KT, Gamblin TC, Geller DA. World review of laparoscopic liver resection-2,804 patients. Ann Surg 2009;250(5):831–41.
[53] Ciria R, Cherqui D, Geller DA, et al. Comparative short-term benefits of laparoscopic liver resection: 9000 cases and climbing. Ann Surg 2016;263(4):761–77.
[54] Dagher I, O'Rourke N, Geller DA, et al. Laparoscopic major hepatectomy: an evolution in standard of care. Ann Surg 2009;250(5):856–60.
[55] Gudmundsdottir H, Fiorentini G, Essaji Y, et al. Circumstances and implications of conversion from minimally invasive to open liver resection: a multi-center analysis from the AMILES registry. Surg Endosc 2023; https://doi.org/10.1007/s00464-023-10431-0.
[56] Cherqui D, Husson E, Hammoud R, et al. Laparoscopic liver resections: a feasibility study in 30 patients. Ann Surg 2000;232(6):753–62.
[57] Descottes B, Lachachi F, Sodji M, et al. Early experience with laparoscopic approach for solid liver tumors: initial 16 cases. Ann Surg 2000;232(5):641–5.
[58] Descottes B, Glineur D, Lachachi F, et al. Laparoscopic liver resection of benign liver tumors. Surg Endosc 2003;17(1):23–30.
[59] Troisi R, Montalti R, Smeets P, et al. The value of laparoscopic liver surgery for solid benign hepatic tumors. Surg Endosc 2008;22(1):38–44.
[60] Ding G, Cai W, Qin M. Pure laparoscopic versus open liver resection in treatment of hepatolithiasis within the left lobes: a randomized trial study. Surg Laparosc Endosc Percutaneous Tech 2015;25(5):392–4.
[61] Vibert E, Kouider A, Gayet B. Laparoscopic anatomic liver resection. HPB (Oxford) 2004;6(4):222–9.
[62] Cheng Y, Zhang L, Li H, et al. Laparoscopic versus open liver resection for colorectal liver metastases: a systematic review. J Surg Res 2017;220:234–46.
[63] Zhang XL, Liu RF, Zhang D, et al. Laparoscopic versus open liver resection for colorectal liver metastases: A systematic review and meta-analysis of studies with propensity score-based analysis. Int J Surg 2017;44:191–203.
[64] Fretland AA, Edwin B. Response: the oslo-comet randomized controlled trial of laparoscopic versus open liver resection for colorectal metastases. Ann Surg 2018;268(6):e69–70.

[65] van der Poel MJ, Barkhatov L, Fuks D, et al. Multicentre propensity score-matched study of laparoscopic versus open repeat liver resection for colorectal liver metastases. Br J Surg 2019;106(6):783–9.
[66] Shelat VG, Cipriani F, Basseres T, et al. Pure laparoscopic liver resection for large malignant tumors: does size matter? Ann Surg Oncol 2015;22(4):1288–93.
[67] Okumura S, Goumard C, Gayet B, et al. Laparoscopic versus open two-stage hepatectomy for bilobar colorectal liver metastases: A bi-institutional, propensity score-matched study. Surgery 2019;166(6):959–66.
[68] El-Gendi A, El-Shafei M, El-Gendi S, et al. Laparoscopic versus open hepatic resection for solitary hepatocellular carcinoma less than 5 cm in cirrhotic patients: a randomized controlled study. J Laparoendosc Adv Surg Tech 2018;28(3):302–10.
[69] Andreou A, Struecker B, Raschzok N, et al. Minimal-invasive versus open hepatectomy for hepatocellular carcinoma: Comparison of postoperative outcomes and long-term survivals using propensity score matching analysis. Surg Oncol 2018;27(4):751–8.
[70] Belli G, Fantini C, D'Agostino A, et al. Laparoscopic versus open liver resection for hepatocellular carcinoma in patients with histologically proven cirrhosis: short- and middle-term results. Surg Endosc 2007;21(11):2004–11.
[71] Cheung TT, Dai WC, Tsang SH, et al. Pure laparoscopic hepatectomy versus open hepatectomy for hepatocellular carcinoma in 110 patients with liver cirrhosis: a propensity analysis at a single center. Ann Surg 2016;264(4):612–20.
[72] Xu HW, Liu F, Li HY, et al. Outcomes following laparoscopic versus open major hepatectomy for hepatocellular carcinoma in patients with cirrhosis: a propensity score-matched analysis. Surg Endosc 2018;32(2):712–9.
[73] Yoon YI, Kim KH, Kang SH, et al. Pure laparoscopic versus open right hepatectomy for hepatocellular carcinoma in patients with cirrhosis: a propensity score matched analysis. Ann Surg 2017;265(5):856–63.
[74] Xiangfei M, Yinzhe X, Yingwei P, et al. Open versus laparoscopic hepatic resection for hepatocellular carcinoma: a systematic review and meta-analysis. Surg Endosc 2019;33(8):2396–418.
[75] Levi Sandri GB, Ettorre GM, Aldrighetti L, et al. Laparoscopic liver resection of hepatocellular carcinoma located in unfavorable segments: a propensity score-matched analysis from the I Go MILS (Italian Group of Minimally Invasive Liver Surgery) Registry. Surg Endosc 2019;33(5):1451–8.
[76] Cipriani F, Fantini C, Ratti F, et al. Laparoscopic liver resections for hepatocellular carcinoma. Can we extend the surgical indication in cirrhotic patients? Surg Endosc 2018;32(2):617–26.
[77] Guerrini GP, Esposito G, Tarantino G, et al. Laparoscopic versus open liver resection for intrahepatic cholangiocarcinoma: the first meta-analysis. Langenbeck's Arch Surg 2020;405(3):265–75.
[78] Pery R, Gudmundsdottir H, Nagorney DM, et al. Laparoscopic versus open liver resections for intrahepatic cholangiocarcinoma and gallbladder cancer: the Mayo clinic experience. HPB (Oxford) 2023;25(3):339–46.
[79] Martin SP, Drake J, Wach MM, et al. Laparoscopic approach to intrahepatic cholangiocarcinoma is associated with an exacerbation of inadequate nodal staging. Ann Surg Oncol 2019;26(6):1851–7.
[80] Zhang Y, Dou C, Wu W, et al. Total laparoscopic versus open radical resection for hilar cholangiocarcinoma. Surg Endosc 2020;34(10):4382–7.
[81] Cherqui D, Soubrane O, Husson E, et al. Laparoscopic living donor hepatectomy for liver transplantation in children. Lancet 2002;359(9304):392–6.
[82] Scatton O, Katsanos G, Boillot O, et al. Pure laparoscopic left lateral sectionectomy in living donors: from innovation to development in France. Ann Surg 2015;261(3):506–12.

[83] Soubrane O, Cherqui D, Scatton O, et al. Laparoscopic left lateral sectionectomy in living donors: safety and reproducibility of the technique in a single center. Ann Surg 2006;244(5):815–20.
[84] Jeong JS, Wi W, Chung YJ, et al. Comparison of perioperative outcomes between pure laparoscopic surgery and open right hepatectomy in living donor hepatectomy: Propensity score matching analysis. Sci Rep 2020;10(1):5314.
[85] Soubrane O, Eguchi S, Uemoto S, et al. Minimally invasive donor hepatectomy for adult living donor liver transplantation: an international, multi-institutional evaluation of safety, efficacy and early outcomes. Ann Surg 2022;275(1):166–74.
[86] Hong SK, Tan MY, Worakitti L, et al. Pure laparoscopic versus open right hepatectomy in live liver donors: a propensity score-matched analysis. Ann Surg 2022;275(1):e206–12.
[87] Cardinal JS, Reddy SK, Tsung A, et al. Laparoscopic major hepatectomy: pure laparoscopic approach versus hand-assisted technique. J Hepatobiliary Pancreat Sci 2013;20(2): 114–9.
[88] Nitta H, Sasaki A, Otsuka Y, et al. Impact of hybrid techniques on laparoscopic major hepatectomies. J Hepatobiliary Pancreat Sci 2013;20(2):111–3.
[89] Wabitsch S, Schoning W, Kastner A, et al. A propensity-matched study of full laparoscopic versus hand-assisted minimal-invasive liver surgery. Surg Endosc 2021;35(5):2021–8.
[90] Inoue Y, Suzuki Y, Fujii K, et al. Laparoscopic liver resection using the lateral approach from intercostal ports in segments VI, VII, and VIII. J Gastrointest Surg 2017;21(12):2135–43.
[91] Aikawa M, Miyazawa M, Okamoto K, et al. Thoracoscopic hepatectomy for malignant liver tumor. Surg Endosc 2014;28(1):314.
[92] Lee W, Han HS, Yoon YS, et al. Role of intercostal trocars on laparoscopic liver resection for tumors in segments 7 and 8. J Hepatobiliary Pancreat Sci 2014;21(8):E65–8.
[93] Ogiso S, Conrad C, Araki K, et al. Laparoscopic transabdominal with transdiaphragmatic access improves resection of difficult posterosuperior liver lesions. Ann Surg 2015;262(2): 358–65.
[94] Cipriani F, Shelat VG, Rawashdeh M, et al. Laparoscopic parenchymal-sparing resections for nonperipheral liver lesions, the diamond technique: technical aspects, clinical outcomes, and oncologic efficiency. J Am Coll Surg 2015;221(2):265–72.
[95] Haber PK, Wabitsch S, Krenzien F, et al. Laparoscopic liver surgery in cirrhosis - Addressing lesions in posterosuperior segments. Surg Oncol 2019;28:140–4.
[96] Kim JH. Pure laparoscopic anatomical resection of the segment 8 dorsal area using the transparenchymal Glissonean approach (Video). Surg Oncol 2019;31:99–100.